ENDOCRINE THERAPY OF BREAST CANCER

ENDOCRINE THERAPY OF BREAST CANCER

Edited by

JOHN FR ROBERTSON, MD, FRCS
Professorial Unit of Surgery
Nottingham City Hospital
Nottingham, UK

ROBERT I NICHOLSON, PhD
Tenovus Cancer Research Centre
Welsh School of Pharmacy, Cardiff University
Cardiff, UK

DANIEL F HAYES, MD
Division of Hematology/Oncology
Department of Internal Medicine
Comprehensive Cancer Center
University of Michigan
Ann Arbor, USA

MARTIN DUNITZ

© 2002 Martin Dunitz, a member of the Taylor & Francis Group

First published in the United Kingdom in 2002
by Martin Dunitz, Taylor & Francis Group plc, 11 New Fetter Lane, London EC4P 4EE

Tel.:   +44 (0) 20 7583 9855
Fax.:   +44 (0) 20 7842 2298
E-mail: info@dunitz.co.uk
Website: http://www.dunitz.co.uk

First edition 2002
Reprinted 2002

Although every effort has been made to ensure that all owners of copyright material have been acknowledged in this publication, we would be glad to acknowledge in subsequent reprints or editions any omissions brought to our attention.

Although every effort has been made to ensure that drug doses and other information are presented accurately in this publication, the ultimate responsibility rests with the prescribing physician. Neither the publishers nor the authors can be held responsible for errors or for any consequences arising from the use of information contained herein. For detailed prescribing information or instructions on the use of any product or procedure discussed herein, please consult the prescribing information or instructional material issued by the manufacturer.

A CIP record for this book is available from the British Library.

ISBN 1-901865-72-X

Distributed in the USA by
Fulfilment Center
Taylor & Francis
10650 Tobben Drive
Independence, KY 41051, USA
Toll Free Tel.:   +1 800 634 7064
E-mail: taylorandfrancis@thomsonlearning.com

Distributed in Canada by
Taylor & Francis
74 Rolark Drive
Scarborough, Ontario M1R 4G2, Canada
Toll Free Tel.:   +1 877 226 2237
E-mail: tal_fran@istar.ca

Distributed in the rest of the world by
Thomson Publishing Services
Cheriton House
North Way
Andover, Hampshire SP10 5BE, UK
Tel.:   +44 (0)1264 332424
E-mail: salesorder.tandf@thomsonpublishingservices.co.uk

Distributed in the rest of the world by:
Thomson Publishing Services
Cheriton House
North Way
Andover, Hampshire SP10 5BE, UK

Composition by Wearset Ltd, Boldon, Tyne & Wear, UK

Printed and bound in Spain by Grafos S.A. Arte Sobre Papel

Contents

Part III: Future Strategies

Foreword

The development of combination chemotherapy for breast cancer in the 1960s generated increased optimism and heightened expectations for improved management of metastatic and primary breast cancer. As a result, interest in hormonal therapy waned, and most therapeutic research during the 1970s focused on cytotoxic therapy. However, a distinguished group of laboratory scientists and clinical investigators understood that the endocrine influence in the development and progression of breast cancer was of a fundamental nature. Therefore, additional progress in the management of this disease required an in-depth understanding of the biology of breast cancer. It became apparent that endocrine influences played a central role in this field.

Over the past three decades, our understanding of the importance of steroid hormones on the physiology of the breast has expanded dramatically. In keeping with this understanding, the role of dysregulation of these endocrine influences in malignant transformation became apparent, and led to the realization that becoming familiar with this complex network of cell–cell interactions and signaling pathways would provide increasing opportunities for targeted therapeutic interventions. The past two decades have witnessed a quiet revolution in the endocrine therapy of breast cancer – quiet, because progress in this area was often overshadowed by the development of new cytotoxic agents (anthracyclines, platinum compounds, the taxanes), and more recently by biologically targeted therapy. However, progress in endocrine therapy has been major. Starting with the identification of substantial antitumor activity of the prototype selective estrogen receptor modulator (SERM), tamoxifen, in patients with metastatic breast cancer, a number of highly targeted interventions were taken from the laboratory to the clinic. While trastuzumab is often mentioned as the first 'targeted' therapy for breast cancer, tamoxifen clearly deserves that distinction. The estrogen receptor signaling pathway was also the first to be analyzed and understood in detail, although its complex interactions with other families of non-endocrine growth factor receptors are only starting to be appreciated.

From the establishment of tamoxifen as the endocrine agent of choice for both premenopausal and postmenopausal women with metastatic breast cancer to its integration in combined-modality treatments of receptor-positive primary breast cancer many years elapsed. Furthermore, many misconceptions had to be overcome, by generating evidence on the basis of prospective randomized trials. Studies of structure– function correlations led to the development of other SERMs, and their evaluation in the management of several other health conditions.

Major endocrine ablations were replaced

over these past three decades by two types of interventions: luteinizing hormone-releasing hormone (LHRH) analogs and selective aromatase inhibitors. These agents have made major inroads over a relatively short period of time, and now constitute an integral part of combined-modality therapy of breast cancer. The major effect of endocrine treatment has been in the management of patients with primary breast cancer. Randomized trials have shown that, for appropriately selected patients, the effectiveness of tamoxifen, and more recently anastrozole, appears to exceed that of the most commonly used cytotoxic regimens. Furthermore, the combined use of both chemotherapy and endocrine therapy produces additive effects, thus markedly decreasing the odds of recurrence and death. While therapeutic research in endocrine therapy continues, and many new and exciting agents will be produced in years to come, it is in the area of breast cancer prevention where endocrine interventions show major promise.

The editors of this volume, well-known experts in the field of breast cancer endocrinology and endocrine therapy, have put together an outstanding reference for all those who use these treatments or who need detailed understanding of the endocrine physiology of the breast and the pathophysiology of breast cancer. The first part describes the therapeutic agents and their current utilization in the management of primary and metastatic breast cancer. The second part provides a superb and detailed overview of the science behind this field. Our understanding of this biological process will feed the development of additional, novel therapeutic agents and will lead to increased exploration of endocrine preventive strategies. Those involved in the management of breast cancer owe a debt of gratitude to the tens of thousands of women who participated in clinical trials that defined the role of endocrine therapy in metastatic and primary breast cancer, as well as to the clinical trialists who developed and conducted those trials. We are also grateful to the laboratory scientists on whose work progress in breast cancer endocrinology is based. Finally, we thank the editors for organizing this outstanding and timely volume, which should serve clinicians and scientists alike.

Gabriel N Hortobagyi
Professor of Medicine and Chairman
Department of Breast Medical Oncology
UTMD Anderson Cancer Center
Houston, USA

Contributors

Sian Bryant, BSc, PhD
Tenovus Cancer Research Centre
Welsh School of Pharmacy
Cardiff University
Redwood Building
King Edward VII Avenue
Cardiff CF10 3XF
UK

Jenny Chang, MRCP, MD
Baylor-Methodist Breast Care Center
Smith Tower
6550 Fannin, 7th Floor, Suite 701
Houston, TX 77030
USA

Robert Clarke, PhD, DSc
Departments of Oncology and Physiology and
Biophysics
Vincent T Lombardi Cancer Center
Georgetown University School of Medicine
3970 Reservoir Road NW, W401 NRB
Washington DC 20007-2197
USA

Kristof Chwalisz, MD
TAP Pharmaceutical Products
675 N. Field Drive
Lake Forrest, IL 600452
USA

Robert B Dickson, PhD
Departments of Oncology and Cell Biology
Vincent T Lombardi Cancer Center
Georgetown University School of Medicine
3970 Reservoir Road NW, W401 NRB
Washington DC 20007-2197
USA

Richard M Elledge, MD
The Breast Care Center
6550 Fannin, Suite 701, 7th Floor
Houston, TX 77030
USA

Ulrike Fuhrmann, PhD
Research Laboratories
Schering AG
Müllerstrasse 176-176
13342 Berlin
Germany

Julia MW Gee, BSc, PhD
Tenovus Cancer Research Centre
Welsh School of Pharmacy
Cardiff University
Redwood Building
King Edward VII Avenue
Cardiff CF10 3XF
UK

Marius Giurescu
Research Laboratories
Schering AG
Experimental Oncology
Müllerstrasse 176-176
13342 Berlin
Germany

Harold A Harvey, MD
Medical Oncology
Penn State Milton Hershey Medical Center
500 University Drive
Hershey, PA 17033
USA

Daniel F Hayes, MD
Division of Hematology/Oncology
Department of Internal Medicine
Comprehensive Cancer Center
University of Michigan
6-312 Cancer Center
1500 East Medical Center Drive
Ann Arbor, MI 48109-0942
USA

Jens Hoffmann, PhD
Research Laboratories
Schering AG
Müllerstrasse 176-176
13342 Berlin
Germany

Anthony Howell, MBBS, MSc, FRCP
CRC Department of Medical Oncology
Christie CRC Research Centre
Christie Hospital NHS Trust
University of Manchester
Wilmslow Road
Manchester M20 4BX
UK

Stephen RD Johnston, MA, PhD, FRCP
Department of Medicine
Royal Marsden Hospital and
Fulham Road
London SW3 6JJ
UK

Walter Jonat, MD, PhD
Klinikum der Clinstian-Albrechts
University zu Kiel
Frauenklinik und Machaelis-Hebammenschule
Michaelistrasse 16
24105 Kiel
Germany

Frances Kenny, MB, ChB, FRCS
Professorial Unit of Surgery
Nottingham City Hospital
Hucknall Road
Nottingham NG5 1PB
UK

Rosemarie B Lichtner, PhD
Metagen Pharmaceuticals GmbH
Oudenarder Str. 16
13347 Berlin
Germany

Tracie-Ann Madden, BSc
Tenovus Cancer Research Centre
Welsh School of Pharmacy
Cardiff University
Redwood Building
King Edward VII Avenue
Cardiff CF10 3XF
UK

Horst Michna, PhD, MD
Deutsche Sporthochschule
Carl-Diem-Weg 6
50927 Köln
Germany

William R Miller BSc, PhD, DSc
University of Edinburgh
Edinburgh Breast Unit Research Group
Western General Hospital
Edinburgh EH4 2XU
UK

Gil Mor, MD
Department of Obstetrics and Gynecology
Yale University School of Medicine
333 Cedar Street
New Haven, CT 06510
USA

Hyman B Muss, MD
College of Medicine
University of Vermont
MCHV Campus, Patrick 534
Fletcher Allen Health Care
111 Colchester Avenue
Burlington, VT 05401
USA

Fred Naftolin, PhD, MD
Department of Obstetrics and Gynecology
Yale University School of Medicine
333 Cedar Street
New Haven, CT 06510
USA

Günter Neef, PhD
Research Laboratories
Schering AG
Müllerstrasse 176-176
13342 Berlin
Germany

Robert I Nicholson, BSc, PhD
Tenovus Cancer Research Centre
Welsh School of Pharmacy
Cardiff University
Redwood Building
King Edward VII Avenue
Cardiff CF10 3XF
UK

Julie J Olin, MD
College of Medicine
University of Vermont
MCHV Campus, Patrick 534
111 Colchester Ave
Burlington, VT 05401
USA

Karsten Parczyk, PhD
Research Laboratories
Schering AG
Müllerstrasse 176-176
13342 Berlin
Germany

Robert Pauley, PhD
Breast Cancer Program
Cell Line Resources Core
Karmanos Cancer Center
Wayne State University
Detroit, MI 48201
USA

Kathleen I Pritchard, MD, FRCPC
Trials and Epidemiology
Toronto-Sunnybrook Regional Cancer Center
2075 Bayview Avenue
Toronto, Ontario M4N 3M5
Canada

John FR Robertson, MD, FRCS
Professorial Unit of Surgery
Nottingham City Hospital
Hucknall Road
Nottingham NG5 1PB
UK

Richard J Santen, MD
Department of Internal Medicine
Division of Endocrinology and Metabolism
University of Virginia Health Sciences Center
Charlottesville, VA 22908-0746
USA

Martin R Schneider, PhD
Research Laboratories
Schering AG
Müllerstrasse 176-176
13342 Berlin
Germany

Woo-Shin Shim, PhD
Department of Medicine
University of Virginia Health Sciences Center
Charlottesville, VA 22908-0746
USA

Peter C Willsher, MBBS, DM, FRACS
Department of General Surgery
Royal Perth Hospital
Box X2212 GPO
Perth, WA 6001
Australia

Wei Yue, MD
Department of Medicine
University of Virginia Health Sciences Center
Charlottesville, VA 22908-0746
USA

Part I

Use of Endocrine Therapies in Clinical Practice

1

Overview and concepts of endocrine therapy

Daniel F Hayes, John FR Robertson

Perhaps one of the greatest success stories in the history of cancer treatment has been the study and application of endocrine treatment for breast cancer. Endocrine therapy may lack the immediate impact seen with the dramatic cure rates achieved by chemotherapy in patients with lymphoma or germ cell cancers. However, endocrine therapy for breast cancer has arguably benefited far more patients and saved substantially more lives, given the enormous frequency of the disease in Western society. Furthermore, as the latter half of the 20th century unfolded, a series of groundbreaking laboratory investigations, often based on clinical observations, provided nearly unprecedented insight into the mechanism of action and resistance of endocrine therapies. It is fair to say that endocrine therapy can be considered the paradigm for 'molecular medicine' as a whole, with considerable two-way interaction between the laboratory and the clinic. Indeed many of the new 'biologic therapies' such as trastuzumab or epidermal growth factor receptor (EGFR) tyrosine kinase (TK) inhibitors are based on similar principles that have guided the selection of patients for endocrine therapy.

The field was initiated in the late 1890s, when Sir George Thomas Beatson, a surgeon at Glasgow Royal Infirmary, hypothesized that a link might exist between the breast and the ovary. Beatson was aware that in cows that had recently calved, lactation could be prolonged by performing an oopherectomy. He surmised that one organ held sway over another. Beatson also thought there were similarities in the microscopic appearances of the lactating breast and the neoplastic breast. From these observations, he made the conceptual leap that if castration could affect lactation, it might also effect breast cancers.[1] Beatson first reported a single case study of a young woman who had previously had a mastectomy and subsequently returned with inoperable local recurrence.[1] He carried out bilateral oophorectomy and the patient's cancer responded. However, the cancer eventually progressed and the patient eventually died. The following week (18 July 1896), he reported a second case of a young woman who presented with inoperable, locally advanced breast cancer.[1] This patient did not respond to bilateral oophorectomy. Thus, in the very first two reported patients, Beatson identified the major issues that we still struggle to understand fully today. First, why do some tumors respond (i.e. are endocrine-sensitive) but others do not (i.e. are endocrine-resistant, de novo)? Second, even when tumors do respond to endocrine treatment, why do they eventually progress (i.e. develop acquired endocrine resistance)? In the succeeding decade, a series of reports demonstrated that approximately 25% of patients benefited from surgical oophorectomy, and that this type of treatment appeared to be more effective in younger women than in older patients.[2] With the introduction of radiation therapy, it was later reported that ovarian irradiation could also effect ablation of ovarian function.[3]

By mid-century, endocrine therapy, consisting of oophorectomy for young women and pharmacologic doses of estrogenic compounds for postmenopausal women, was the treatment of choice in advanced disease. Some of the earliest prospective randomized clinical trials in all of medicine addressed chest wall radiation therapy after mastectomy in patients with breast cancer. Not long after these radiotherapy studies, prospective randomized clinical trials investigating adjuvant oophorectomy demonstrated reductions in distant recurrence and mortality, and these trials remain positive to this day.[4] Since then, several new approaches – both surgical (e.g. adrenalectomy) and medical (e.g. tamoxifen) – have been introduced that have improved the efficacy and safety of endocrine therapy. Subsequently, endocrine therapy has become one of the main arrows in the quiver for this disease. Although endocrine therapies were initially introduced in the metastatic setting, their importance in the adjuvant setting is widely accepted.[4,5] Remarkably, endocrine therapy (specifically tamoxifen) has recently been identified as a chemopreventive agent for patients at high risk for a new breast cancer – i.e. those with ductal carcinoma in situ (DCIS) – and even in unaffected women whose personal or family histories place them at risk.[6,7] Therefore, a thorough understanding of the role of endocrine therapy is essential for any student or practitioner involved in the evaluation and/or treatment of women who have breast cancer or who are at risk for it.

Fundamentally, endocrine therapy has been divided into two categories: ablative and additive (Table 1.1). Ablative therapies are directed towards removing the sources of estrogen, which are primarily the ovaries in premenopausal women and the adrenal glands in postmenopausal women. Initially, ablative therapies were accomplished by surgical ablation of hormone-producing organs, but more recently the goal of estrogen deprivation can be accomplished by chemical means. Surgical ablative therapies can be direct, such as oophorectomy and adrenalectomy, or indirect, such as hypophysectomy.

Following Beatson's seminal observation, surgical oophorectomy and (soon after) radiation ablation served as the means of blocking ovarian function in premenopausal women. More recently, 'chemical castration' by the administration of agonists and/or antagonists of luteinizing hormone releasing hormone (LHRH) has been shown to prevent ovarian estrogen production. Unlike surgery or radiation, this method is potentially reversible, especially in younger women. However, approximately one-third of circulating estradiol is produced in premenopausal women by peripheral conversion of androstenedione and testosterone by the aromatase enzyme. Although the ovaries are a major source of this enzymatic activity in premenopausal patients, several peripheral organs also serve as sites of peripheral aromatase activity, including fat, liver, and muscle. Indeed, in postmenopausal women, these peripheral sites become the major sources of aromatization into estradiol of male sex steroids (androstenedione and testosterone) secreted by the adrenal glands. Furthermore, approximately two-thirds of breast cancers express the aromatase enzyme. Consequently, the cancer itself may be responsible for 'local' estrogen production.[8,9]

Prospective randomized clinical trials have now demonstrated that aromatase inhibitors (AIs) are as effective, or more so, than previously existing second-line endocrine treatments in the metastatic setting.[10–12] Recently reported studies suggest that selected AIs may even be more effective than tamoxifen as first-line antimetastatic therapy.[13] The first-generation aromatase inhibitors lacked specificity and were associated with substantial toxicity. However, as outlined in Chapter 6, powerful agents that specifically and almost completely inhibit aromatase activity are now in widespread use. Prospective randomized clinical trials are now underway comparing newergeneration AIs with tamoxifen, in combination

Table 1.1 Categories of steroid hormone endocrine therapies for breast cancer	
Additive	**Ablative**
Estrogenic compounds:	*Surgical*
ethinylestradiol	Oophorectomy
diethylstilbestrol	Adrenalectomy
Androgens:	Hypophysectomy
fluoxymestrone	
methyltestosterone	*Medical*
Selective estrogen receptor modulators	Luteinizing hormone-releasing hormone (LHRH)
(SERMs):	agonist/antagonists:
tamoxifen	goserelin
toremifene	leuprolide
droloxifene	Aromatase inhibitors:
idoxifene	aminoglutethimide
raloxifene	formestane
EM 800	fadrozole
Pure antiestrogens:	anastrazole
fulvestrant	letrozole
Progestins:	exemestane
megestrol acetate	vorozole
medroxyprogesterone acetate	
Antiprogestins:	
mifepristone	
onapristone	

with tamoxifen, or in sequence with tamoxifen, in the adjuvant setting.

Additive endocrine therapies, in principle, function by direct action on the hormonally dependent cancer cell. In that regard, estrogen production persists, but its action is blocked at the cellular level by interference with estrogen and its receptor. Enigmatically, the first such agent to be used successfully was an estrogenic compound (diethylstilbestrol, DES) administered at pharmacologic doses. Subsequently, DES was replaced by a triphenylethylamine, tamoxifen, which was originally considered to be an 'antiestrogen'. As described in Chapters 3 and 4 subsequent studies have demonstrated that tamoxifen and other similar agents (e.g. toremifene, raloxifene, idoxifene and droloxifene) have dualistic agonist and antagonist activity, depending on the tissue of interest. Consequently, tamoxifen, and these other similar agents, have been designated selective estrogen receptor (ER) modifiers (SERMs).

As described in Chapter 7, other hormonal therapies, such as progestational agents (megestrol acetate and medroxyprogesterone acetate) and androgens, have been harder to classify. Both of these types of treatment have been proven to be active against breast cancer, although they have been largely replaced or relegated to third- or fourth-line therapy by newer, more active and tolerable agents. In theory, they might exert their effects at the cellular level via the progesterone or androgen receptors respectively. However, it has been speculated that the mechanism of action of progestins and androgens may be a consequence of suppression of the hypothalamic–pituitary axis via a feedback mechanism. In this case, one might consider these strategies as ablative. More recently, studies have been reported of antiprogestins (e.g. mifepristone and onapristone) that have confirmed that these agents are effective endocrine therapies. Since mifepristone causes an elevation in serum estradiol, it has been debated whether antiprogestins act via inhibition of progesterone receptor (PgR) function or by acting indirectly through the ER. In the latter case, one would simply consider these agents to be another form of estrogen or antiestrogen therapy. Chapter 8 focuses on the clinical studies of antiprogestins in human breast cancer and includes data from two previously unreported studies along with biologic data from a phase II study that suggests that at least one of the antiprogestins appears to act via the PgR.

These considerations and several unusual clinical observations have led clinicians to appreciate that not all endocrine therapies are equal with regard to mechanisms of action, efficacy, or toxicity. For example, additive therapies, such as DES and the SERMs, occasionally produce a short-lived syndrome of tumor exacerbation, designated 'clinical flare', that is often followed by clinical response.[14,15] Moreover, some patients who have enjoyed response from these agents and then suffered progression may experience a subsequent clinical benefit from simple removal of the treatment ('withdrawal' or 'rebound' response).[16–18] In contrast, ablative therapies are rarely if ever associated with either tumor flare or withdrawal response. As outlined in Chapters 2–7, it is very common to observe serial therapeutic responses when patients with ER-positive tumors are treated with sequential endocrine therapies. In fact,

recent reports have documented clinical benefit to the aromatase inhibitors even in patients who experienced primary resistance to tamoxifen.[10] If these agents induce response in the same manner, and if resistance is generated via the same mechanism, then these observations are difficult to explain.

Some but not all answers to these contradictory clinical phenomena have been provided by the remarkable molecular biology of endocrine-responsive cancers that has emerged from investigational laboratories over the last 35 years. As described in Chapter 9, it is now well established that steroid hormones, such as estradiol, exert their effect by freely diffusing through the plasma membrane and binding to cytoplasmic peptide receptors. Binding of the steroid ligand with the receptor (in this case, estrogen and ER) induces ER homodimerization, followed by interaction with estrogen response elements (EREs) in the promoter regions of estrogen-dependent genes. Recent work has demonstrated that at least two such ERs exist: ERα and ERβ. Specific genetic function is dictated by carefully orchestrated interaction between the ER/ERE and intranuclear co-activating and co-repressing proteins. The precise cellular/tissue response to estrogen, or to other ligands such as the SERMs, depends on the specific ligand, the balance of ERα and ERβ, and the relative concentrations of multiple co-activators and co-repressors. Perhaps the best example of this exquisite balance is the apparent difference in tissue specificity between tamoxifen and a more recently introduced SERM, raloxifene. Both have antiestrogenic qualities in breast tissue and in the central nervous system, and both appear to be estrogenic in bone and liver. However, while the estrogenic effects of tamoxifen in the uterus account for part, if not all, of the associated increase in endometrial cancer, raloxifene appears, at this stage, to have less agonistic action on the endometrium.[19–25]

Our increasingly sophisticated understanding of the molecular biology of the ER axis may also explain another puzzling clinical observation. During the first 15 years of tamoxifen use, most clinicians assumed that long-term admin-istration should be more effective than shorter courses. Indeed, prospective randomized trials, and a worldwide overview of clinical results, have demonstrated that while 1 year of adju-vant tamoxifen improves disease-free and over-all survival, 2 years and 5 years provide even more benefit.[5] However, in two prospective trials, women who reached 5 years on adjuvant tamoxifen were randomly assigned to ongoing maintenance versus discontinuation of the drug. Results from these individual studies have suggested that not only is there no appar-ent benefit to more than 5 years, there may actually be a higher risk of recurrence and death.[26,27] While larger trials of 5 years versus 10 years are currently ongoing, recent in vitro studies have demonstrated that, as in bone and liver, tamoxifen can become agonistic for the ER in breast cancer tissue, perhaps providing an explanation for this initially confusing clini-cal observation.[28] These considerations con-found the terms 'sensitive' and 'resistant', as classically considered for other antineoplastic agents. For example, does a patient whose tumor initially responded to tamoxifen and subsequently starts to grow in spite of (and per-haps because of) tamoxifen have a 'resistant' tumor? Clinically, the answer is yes, since she has progressive disease in spite of current ther-apy. However, molecularly, the answer is no. Her cancer remains, technically endocrine-'dependent', and tamoxifen is now serving as the agonistic, hormonal ligand. Other mecha-nisms of acquired resistance appear to involve 'crosstalk' with other growth factor pathways such as insulin-like growth factor (IGF) and type 1 (c-ErbB) growth factors (as described in Chapter 10). This discussion is more than semantic, since if a patient's tumor remains hor-mone-dependent, it may still respond to other endocrine manipulations, such a pure ER antagonist and/or an aromatase inhibitor. Thus development of acquired resistance to a particular endocrine agent such as tamoxifen does not, per se, equate to hormone insen-sitivity.

Approximately 30–40% of all breast cancers appear to be endocrine-independent de novo, including 90–100% of ER-negative tumors and 30–40% of ER-positive tumors. This dichotomy is borne out by the recently reported tamoxifen chemoprevention trials, in which tamoxifen only reduced approximately 50% of the cancers that emerged on placebo in high-risk women, and most of the emergent breast cancers on tamoxifen were ER-negative.[7] Large adjuvant trials of women who have never been treated with tamoxifen suggest that the benefits are confined almost exclusively to ER-positive patients. Other breast cancers begin with endocrine dependence, and these cancers are inhibited or even cured by endocrine treatment, especially in the adjuvant setting. In the metastatic setting, many ER-positive cancers are still hormone-dependent, and therefore serial endocrine treatments are effective. Nevertheless most, if not all, metastatic breast cancers become hormone-insensitive by poorly understood mechanisms. Ultimately, these can-cers become truly resistant to further endocrine treatment. Interestingly, in the majority of tumors, these mechanisms do not appear to involve loss of expression of ER. It is in these patients that new therapies are most needed. These new therapies should either be designed to modulate the ER axis to maintain hormone dependence or directed against the non-hormonal (at least non-ER) pathways that now drive the cell to metastasize and proliferate.

What are these pathways? Some evidence suggests other steroidal hormones and their receptors may be functionally important, although less so than the estrogen/ER axis. These pathways include the PgR and various retinoic or retinoic-like receptors (RAR and RXR). Recently, a rapidly growing body of liter-ature has suggested that peptide 'hormones', or growth factors, play important physiologic and pathologic roles in the growth and behavior of epithelial tissues and their associated malignant counterparts. Of these, the ErbB or HER (human epithelial receptor) family has garnered the most excitement. There are four members of the ErbB family (ErbB1, -2, -3, and -4), which variably interact with at least six different extracellular ligands, form homo- or hetero-dimers, and activate one or more of at least four subcellular signal transduction pathways via tyrosine kinase activation. At least two important clinical utilities have emerged from understanding the molecular biology of the ErbB pathway. First, members of this family may be important as prognostic and predictive factors for patients with breast cancer.[29] Several studies have suggested that overexpression of members of the ErbB family, especially ErbB1 (also called the epithelial growth factor receptor, EGFR) and ErbB2 (also called HER2 and c-Neu), are associated with a poorer prognosis in patients with newly diagnosed breast cancer. Amplification and/or overexpression of ErbB1 and ErbB2 may result in decreased hormone dependence for ER-positive cancers, resulting in relative resistance to endocrine therapies.[29] Likewise, other studies have suggested that ErbB2 amplification and/or overexpression may be associated with relative resistance to certain forms of chemotherapy, such as alkylating agents, and relative sensitivity to others, such as anthracyclines.[29] Importantly, agents that are directed towards interruption of the ligand/receptor interaction or of the downstream signalling pathways are now in clinical trials, and one such agent, trastuzumab (Herceptin), is now widely accepted for routine clinical use in patients with HER2-positive metastatic breast cancer.[30–33]

Other peptide growth factor pathways are also under investigation either as de novo axes that breast cancer cells might exploit for hormone independence or as upregulated systems that result in emergence of resistance to endocrine therapy. These include the insulin-like growth factors (IGF-I and IGF-II) and associated receptors[34] and other, less well-studied axes, such as that signalled through Notch receptors. Although none of the studies of non-ErbB pathways has attained clinical utility, it seems likely that future investigations will be fruitful.

In summary, a more thorough understanding of the biology of steroid and peptide hormones has provided explanations for the fascinating and often enigmatic clinical phenomena observed in endocrine treatment of patients with breast cancer. Arguably, endocrine therapy of breast cancer serves as a prime example of molecular medicine and translational science, with substantial bidirectional interaction between clinical observations and laboratory investigations, resulting in increasingly more efficacious and tolerable therapies. The subsequent chapters in this text are meant to provide concise yet sophisticated reviews of both the clinical and laboratory science that has led to endocrine treatment taking its rightful place as the cornerstone of breast cancer therapy.

REFERENCES

1. Beatson GW. On the treatment of inoperable cases of carcinoma of the mamma: Suggestions for a new method of treatment with illustrative cases. *Lancet* 1896; **ii:** 104–7 and 162–5.

2. Lett H. An analysis of ninety-nine cases of inoperable carcinoma of the breast treated by oophorectomy. *Lancet* 1905; **i:** 227–8.

3. Taylor GW. Artificial menopause in carcinoma of the breast. *N Engl J Med* 1934; **211:** 1138–40.

4. Early Breast Cancer Trialists Collaborative Group. Ovarian ablation in early breast cancer: overview of the randomised trials. *Lancet* 1996; **348:** 1189–96.

5. Early Breast Cancer Trialist's Collaborative Group. Tamoxifen for early breast cancer: an overview of the randomised trials. *Lancet* 1998; **351:** 1451–67.

6. Fisher B, Dignam J, Wolmark N et al. Tamoxifen in treatment of intraductal breast cancer: National Surgical Adjuvant Breast and Bowel Project B-24 randomised controlled trial. *Lancet* 1999; **353:** 1993–2000.

7. Fisher B, Costantino JP, Wickerham DL et al. Tamoxifen for prevention of breast cancer: report of the National Surgical Adjuvant Breast and Bowel Project P-1 study. *J Natl Cancer Inst* 1998; **90:** 1371–88.

8. Miller WR, Mullen P, Telford J, Dixon JM. Clinical importance of intratumoral aromatase. *Breast Cancer Res Treat* 1998; **49:** S27–32; discussion S33–7.

9. Miller WR, O'Neil JS. The importance of local synthesis of estrogen within the breast. *Steroids* 1998; **50:** 537–48.

10. Buzdar AU, Jonat W, Howell A et al. Anastrozole versus megestrol acetate in the treatment of postmenopausal women with advanced breast carcinoma: results of a survival update based on a combined analysis of data from two mature phase III trials. Arimidex Study Group. *Cancer* 1998; **83:** 1142–52.

11. Marty M, Gershanovich M, Campos B et al. Letrozole, a new potent, selective aromatase inhibitor (AI) superior to aminoglutethimide in postmenopausal women with advanced breast cancer previously treated with antiestrogens. *Proc Am Soc Clin Oncol* 1997; **16:** Abst 544.

12. Dombernowsky P, Smith I, Falkson G et al. Letrozole, a new oral aromatase inhibitor for advanced breast cancer: double-blind random-ized trial showing a dose effect and improved efficacy and tolerability compared with mege-strol acetate. *J Clin Oncol* 1998; **16:** 453–61.

13. Mouridsen H, Gershanovich M, Sun Y et al. Superior efficacy of letrozole versus tamoxifen as first-line therapy for postmenopausal women with advanced breast cancer: results of a phase III study of the International Letrozole Breast Cancer Group. *J Clin Oncol* 2001; **19:** 2596–606.

14. Clarysse A. Hormone induced tumor flare. *Eur J Cancer Clin Oncol* 1985; **21:** 585.

15. Plotkin D, Lechner JJ, Jung WE, Rosen PJ. Tamoxifen flare in advanced breast cancer. *JAMA* 1978; **240:** 2644–6.

16. Kaufman RJ, Escher GC. Rebound regression in advanced mammary carcinoma. *Surg Gynecol Obstet* 1961; **113:** 635–40.

17. Beex L, Pieters G, Smals A et al. Tamoxifen ver-sus ethinyl estradiol in the treatment of post-menopausal women with advanced breast cancer. *Cancer Treat Rep* 1981; **65:** 179–85.

18. Howell A, Dodwell DJ, Anderson H, Redford J. Response after withdrawal of tamoxifen and progestogens in advanced breast cancer. *Ann Oncol* 1992; **3:** 611–17.

19. Fornander T, Cedermark B, Mattsson A et al. Adjuvant tamoxifen in early breast cancer: occurrence of new primary cancers. *Lancet* 1989; **i:** 117–20.

20. Fornander T, Rutqvist LE, Sjoberg HE et al. Long-term adjuvant tamoxifen in early breast cancer: effect on bone mineral density in post-menopausal women. *J Clin Oncol* 1990; **8:** 1019–24.

21. Fornander T, Rutqvist LE, Wilking N et al. Oestrogenic effects of adjuvant tamoxifen in postmenopausal breast cancer. *Eur J Cancer* 1993; **4:** 497–500.

22. Love RR, Wiebe DA, Newcomb PA et al. Effects of tamoxifen on cardiovascular risk factors in postmenopausal women. *Ann Intern Med* 1991; **115:** 860–4.

23. Love RR, Mazess RB, Barden HS et al. Effects of tamoxifen on bone mineral density in post-menopausal women with breast cancer. *N Engl J Med* 1992; **326:** 852–6.

24. Cauley J, Krueger K, Eckert S et al. Raloxifene reduces breast cancer risk in postmenopausal women with osteoporosis: 40-month data from the ore trial. *Proc Am Soc Clin Oncol* 1999; **18:** 87a (Abst 328).

25. Boss SM, Huster WJ, Neild JA et al. Effects of raloxifene hydrochloride on the endometrium of postmenopausal women. *Am J Obstet Gynecol* 1997; **177:** 1458–64.

26. Fisher B, Dignam J, Bryant J et al. Five versus more than five years of tamoxifen therapy for breast cancer patients with negative lymph nodes and estrogen receptor-positive tumors. *J Natl Cancer Inst* 1996; **88:** 1529–42.

27. Stewart HJ, Prescott RJ, Forrest AP. Scottish Adjuvant Tamoxifen Trial: a randomized study updated to 15 years. *J Natl Cancer Inst* 2001; **93:** 456–62.

28. Osborne CK. Tamoxifen in the treatment of breast cancer. *N Engl J Med* 1998; **339:** 1609–18.

29. Yamauchi H, Stearns V, Hayes DF. When is a tumor marker ready for prime time? A case study of c-erbB-2 as a predictive factor in breast cancer. *J Clin Oncol* 2001; **19:** 2334–56.

30. Baselga J, Tripathy D, Mendelsohn J et al. Phase II study of weekly intravenous recombinant human-ized anti-p185HER2 monoclonal antibody in patients with HER2/neu-overexpressing meta-static breast cancer. *J Clin Oncol* 1996; **14:** 737–44.

31. Cobleigh MA, Vogel CL, Tripathy D et al. Multinational study of the efficacy and safety of humanized anti-HER2 monoclonal antibody in women who have HER2-overexpressing metastatic breast cancer that has progressed after chemotherapy for metastatic disease. *J Clin Oncol* 1999; **17:** 2639.

32. Vogel C, Cobleigh MA, Tripathy D et al. Efficacy and safety of trastuzumab as a single agent in

first-line treatment of HER2-overexpressing metastatic breast cancer. *J Clin Oncol* 2002; **20:** 719–26.

33. Slamon DJ, Leyland-Jones B, Shak S et al. Use of chemotherapy plus a monoclonal antibody against HER2 for metastatic breast cancer that overexpresses HER2. *N Engl J Med* 2001; **344:** 783–92.

34. Ellis MJ. The insulin-like growth factor network and breast cancer. In: *Breast Cancer: Molecular Genetics, Pathogenesis and Therapeutics* (Bowcock AM, ed). Totowa, NJ: Humana Press, 1999: 121–42.

2

Ovarian ablation

Kathleen I Pritchard

CONTENTS • Background • Rationale • Therapy for metastatic disease • Adjuvant therapy • Conclusions and future directions

BACKGROUND

Ovarian ablation was first used by Beatson[1] in the late 19th century, and proved useful in shrinking widespread breast cancer. Around the same time, Schinzinger[2] suggested that oophorectomy be done before or at the time of mastectomy in order to 'involute' the breast, thus 'containing tumour cells'. This was, perhaps, the first call for adjuvant systemic therapy. The subsequent development of methods for radiation ovarian ablation led others to suggest that radiation castration following radical mastectomy might prevent or postpone the development of metastatic disease.[3] A series of small trials of adjuvant ovarian ablation were subsequently carried out, but the small size of the studies, poor study design, lack of sophisticated methodology for analysis, and the apparently minimal effects seen in these trials led to a loss of interest in this modality, which was then overshadowed by the promising early results of adjuvant chemotherapy in the mid 1970s.[4,5]

By the early 1980s, however, it was apparent that combination chemotherapy – at least as given at that time – seemed to provide minimal improvement for postmenopausal women, and even in the premenopausal population was not a panacea. In turn, the more widespread availability of measurements of estrogen receptor (ER) and progesterone receptor (PgR) and the development of several new hormonal agents[6,7] encouraged a re-examination of adjuvant endocrine therapy. It became obvious early in its use that adjuvant tamoxifen, particularly in postmenopausal patients, had an effect that was not dissimilar from that of adjuvant combination chemotherapy in premenopausal women. With this conceptual shift to the use of adjuvant endocrine therapy, there was renewed interest in ovarian ablation in the premenopausal population. The development in 1984 of the Early Breast Cancer Trialists Collaborative Group (EBCTCG) – a consortium of investigators interested in examining adjuvant hormonal and chemotherapy trials with meta-analysis techniques – led to a re-examination of the entire area of adjuvant therapy. It was the results of this first overview analysis that finally made it clear that ovarian ablation in premenopausal women had consistent and significant effects on both relapse-free and overall survival.[8]

RATIONALE

In women with metastatic breast cancer, ablative or additive endocrine therapies produce response rates of 30% in unselected patients, close to 50% in women with ER-positive tumours, and up to 80% in women with ER- and PgR-positive tumours.[9,10] In contrast, fewer than 5–10% of

ER-negative or ER- and PgR-negative tumours will respond to hormonal manipulations.[9,10] Response rates are proportional to the levels of hormone receptor measured.[10,11] Receptor levels measured in primary tumours correspond quite closely to those measured in recurrent disease – at least in the absence of intervening hormonal therapy.[12] Thus, the receptor status of the primary tumour probably represents quite accurately that of any occult metastases left after primary surgery, and so it would seem likely that adjuvant endocrine therapy as well would prove most effective in women with high ER and PgR levels at the time of primary surgery.

THERAPY FOR METASTATIC DISEASE

Ovarian ablation – either medical or surgical – has long been known to be effective therapy in premenopausal women, particularly those who have ER- and/or PgR-positive tumours. Older literature has suggested response rates of about 30% in unselected women, and as high as 60% or more in women with high levels of both ER and PgR.[9–11] In the mid 1980s, two randomized trials comparing tamoxifen with surgical ovarian ablation in premenopausal women with metastatic breast cancer showed that the two approaches are approximately equivalent in effect. A recent large randomized trial showed that response rates to the luteinizing hormone-releasing hormone (LHRH) analogue goserelin are equivalent to those seen with surgical ovarian ablation in premenopausal women with metastatic disease.[13,14]

Several studies have been carried out of an LHRH agonist used as initial hormonal therapy in premenopausal women versus the same LHRH agonist plus tamoxifen.[15,16] A meta-analysis (Table 2.1) of these studies has shown prolonged progression-free survival (Figure 2.1), increased response rate (Figure 2.2), and prolonged survival (Figure 2.3) for the combination as opposed to the LHRH agonist used alone.[16,17] Toxicity was reported to be similar with the combination or with the LHRH agonist used alone. There are some methodological difficulties with these studies, however. First, toxicity data have been collected (or at least published) in a rather sketchy fashion, and it is unclear that toxicities have been measured carefully enough or in enough detail for one to really be certain that there is no toxicity difference between these endocrine approaches. Furthermore, the largest trial, when analysed alone, shows neither a survival benefit nor any difference in time to treatment failure – this trial had a crossover design such that patients who began with the LHRH agonist alone went on to receive subsequent tamoxifen, whereas the other three studies, which contribute most to the survival benefit seen in the meta-analysis, did not have this design feature. The real question is whether an LHRH agonist followed by tamoxifen might produce similar total time without progression, total time without failure, and

---

Table 2.1 European Organization for Research and Treatment of Cancer (EORTC) meta-analysis of LHRH agonist versus LHRH agonist plus tamoxifen in women with metastatic breast cancer

	LHRH agonist	LHRH agonist + tamoxifen	
Overall survival	2.5 years	2.9 years	$p = 0.02^a$
Progression-free survival	5.4 months	8.7 months	$p < 0.001^a$
Response rate	30%	39%	$p = 0.03^b$

[a]Hazard ratio. [b]Odds ratio.

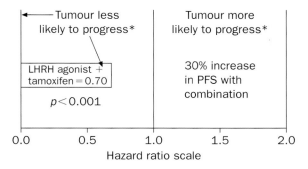

Figure 2.1 EORTC meta-analysis of LHRH agonist versus LHRH agonist plus tamoxifen in women with metastatic breast cancer: progression-free survival (PFS).

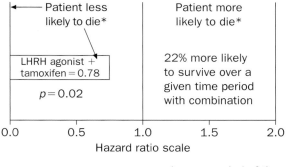

Figure 2.3 EORTC meta-analysis of LHRH agonist versus LHRH agonist plus tamoxifen in women with metastatic breast cancer: overall survival.

similar survival to the two agents used concurrently. Certainly, however, these data provide some suggestion that the use of a concurrent LHRH analogue and tamoxifen may improve overall results. Further data regarding these particular comparisons would be welcome.

A further point in this regard, however, is that currently, most investigators initiate hormonal therapy in premenopausal women with tamoxifen, and only subsequently use ovarian ablation by surgery, irradiation or the use of an LHRH analogue. Thus, it would be of even more interest to know whether adding ovarian ablation, by whatever means, to initial therapy with tamoxifen is a superior approach to tamoxifen alone followed by ovarian ablation. Currently, this comparison is not to our knowledge, being studied.

In summary, ovarian ablation, by either radiation, surgery, or use of an LHRH analogue, remains a useful method of therapy for premenopausal women with metastatic disease that is ER- and/or PgR-positive. Ovarian ablation can be used as either first- or second-line hormonal therapy or can be used concurrently with tamoxifen in this setting.

ADJUVANT THERAPY

Trials of adjuvant ovarian ablation versus no other systemic therapy

Following the proposal of adjuvant oophorectomy by Schinzinger,[2] over 20 trials of ovarian ablation either by surgery or irradiation and

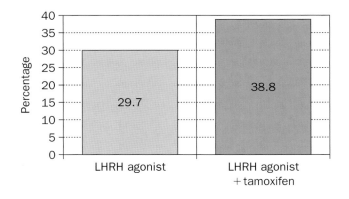

31% increase in objective response with combination

Figure 2.2 EORTC meta-analysis of LHRH agonist versus LHRH agonist plus tamoxifen in women with metastatic breast cancer: objective response rate.

with or without the addition of prednisone were carried out. Many of these trials, however, were done before the era of randomized clinical trials and before the widespread availability of ER and PgR measurements.

The first trials of ovarian ablation consisted mainly of series of patients from single institutions, often with historical non-matched, non-randomized controls. Furthermore, information was seldom present on such now well-

Table 2.2 Randomized trials of ovarian ablation versus no systemic therapy as adjuvant treatment

Trial[a]	Ovarian treatment	Accrual period	Randomized		Data available?	Published?
			<50 years old	≥50 years old		
Paterson (Christie)	450 rad	1948–50	178	11	Yes	Yes[24,68]
Nissen-Meyer (Norwegen)	1000 rad	1957–63	151	195	Yes	Yes[25,69,70]
Nevinny (Boston)	Surgery	1961–[b]	143		No	Yes[30]
Ravdin (NSABP)	Surgery	1961–67	184	0	Yes	Yes[26]
Bryant and Weir (Saskatchewan)	Surgery	1964–74	255	124	Yes	Yes[29]
Meakin and Hayward (Princess Margaret Hospital, Toronto)	2000 rad[c]	1965–72	349	430	Yes	Yes[27,28,31]
Ontario Cancer Research and Treatment Foundation	1500 rad	1968–77	9	323	Yes	Yes[32]
CFRB Cancer Agency	900/1400 rad	1971–76	1	51	Yes	Yes[33]
Bradford Radiotherapy Institute	Surgery	1974–85	42	9	Yes	No
Total (excluding Nevinny)		1948–85	1169	1143	Yes	

[a]NSABP, National Surgical Adjuvant Breast Project; CFRB, Centre Regionale Francois Baclesse.
[b]143 patients were randomized, but no individual patient data are available on accrual period, age distribution, or outcome.
[c]Stratum 1: control versus 2000 rad.

appreciated prognostic factors as nodal status.[18] In spite of the problems with these early studies, however, most suggested some advantage of ovarian ablation. A little later, several studies were carried out with matched but non-randomized control groups.[19–23] Some of these also suggested a degree of benefit for patients who received ovarian ablation,[21,23] although others found neither benefit nor detriment.[19,20,22]

As randomized controlled clinical trials came into more common usage, several prospective randomized trials of ovarian ablation using either surgical or irradiation castration versus control were carried out (Table 2.2).[24–33]

Trials of ovarian ablation plus chemotherapy versus the same chemotherapy used alone

In addition to the randomized studies of ovarian ablation versus no further systemic therapy, there are at least five trials in which women were randomly assigned to receive ovarian ablation by either surgery or irradiation in addition to cytotoxic therapy, versus the same cytotoxic therapy used alone (Table 2.3). These trials in general began somewhat later, and as a result only two of them have been published in individual form,[34,35] although three others have provided updated information to the 1995 Oxford Overview process.

Table 2.3 Randomized trials of ovarian ablation plus chemotherapy versus chemotherapy alone

Trial[a]	Ovarian treatment	Common systemic therapy[b]	Accrual period	Randomized		Data available?	Published?
				<50 years old	≥50 years old		
Bradford Radiotherapy Institute	Surgery	M + TT	1974–85	38	5	Yes	No
Toronto–Edmonton Study Group	1500 rad + prednisone	CMF[c] (some ± TT)	1978–88	241	56	Yes[d]	No
Ragaz (BCCA Vancouver)	1600 rad + prednisone	CMF	1979–85	111	23	Yes[d]	Yes[34]
IBCSG/Ludwig II	Surgery	CMF + P	1978–81	281	75	Yes[d]	Yes[71]
SWOG 7827 B	Surgery	CMFVP	1979–89	262	52	Yes[d]	No
FNCLCC (France)			1989–	244	0	Yes	No
CAMS (China)			1992–	2310	0	Yes	No
Total				3487	211		

[a]BCCA, British Columbia Cancer Agency; IBCSG, International Breast Cancer Study Group; SWOG, Southwest Oncology Group; FNCLCC, Fédération Nationale des Centres de Lutte Contre le Cancer.
[b]M, methotrexate; TT, thiotepa; C, cyclophosphamide; F, 5-fluorouracil; P, prednisone; V, vincristine.
[c]First patients were cross-randomized to receive or not receive immunotherapy with oral BCG (Bacillus Calmette–Guérin).
[d]Estrogen receptors available only in these trials.

Trials of medical ovarian ablation or suppression

At the time of the 1995 Oxford Overview update, four trials in which premenopausal women were randomized to receive medically induced ovarian suppression were registered (Table 2.4). No data were available for the 1995 Overview analysis from any of these trials, but preliminary results from two of these trials as well as from two non-registered trials have now been presented.

The overall results of all of the trials with results available in 1995 were well summarized in the Overview analysis of ovarian ablation published in 1996[36] and summarized below.

EBCTCG or Oxford Overview of ovarian ablation in early breast cancer: the 1995 update

In 1995, the EBCTCG based in Oxford sought information on each patient in any randomized trial of ovarian ablation or suppression versus control that had begun before 1990, for the purpose of an updated overview or meta-analysis. Data were available for 12 of the 13 known studies assessing ovarian ablation by radiation or surgery, but not for any of the four known studies assessing ovarian suppression by drugs, all of which began after 1980. Because menopausal status was not consistently defined across these trials, the 1995 Oxford Overview main analysis has been carried out in women under 50 years of age, as was done in past years.[8,36–39] While the Overview attempted to analyse results according to ER status, these measurements were only available in the later trials – those of ovarian ablation plus chemotherapy versus the same chemotherapy alone.

Effects in women under 50 years of age

The 1995 Overview analysis[36] reports the results from 2102 women aged less than 50 when randomized. At the time of the 1995 analysis, there had been 1130 deaths and an additional 153 recurrences in these women. The analysis showed that the 15-year survival rate was highly significantly improved amongst those allocated to ovarian ablation (52.4% versus 46.1%; difference = 6.3%, ±standard deviation (SD) = 2.3; $p = 0.001$) (Figure 2.4a). The recurrence-free survival rate was even more significantly improved (45% versus 39%; difference = 6.0%, ±SD = 2.3; $p = 0.0007$) (Figure 2.4b).

The numbers of events in the study, although large, are too small for really reliable subgroup analyses. In addition, attempts to analyse the results in node-negative versus node-positive women in the Overview are heavily confounded by the fact that almost all of the node-negative women were entered into trials of ovarian ablation versus no therapy, whereas almost all of the node-positive women were entered into trials of chemotherapy plus ovarian ablation versus the same chemotherapy given alone. Thus, in the overview, the relative effectiveness of ovarian ablation with respect to nodal status could only be assessed in ovarian ablation trials in which chemotherapy was not given. In the trials of ovarian ablation alone versus no other systemic therapy, however, proportional risk reductions for node-positive and for node-negative women appeared to be similar, although the absolute risk reduction was non-significantly greater for node positive women. For both recurrence-free and overall survival, there was a significant improvement within both node-negative ($p = 0.01$ for recurrence; $p = 0.01$ for survival) and node-positive ($p = 0.0002$ for recurrence; $p = 0.0007$ for survival) subgroups of women receiving ovarian ablation (Figure 2.5a,b).

ER measurements on the primary tumour were available for four of the five trials in which women were randomized to receive chemotherapy plus ovarian ablation versus the same chemotherapy used alone. Among the 194 women with ER-poor primary tumours, there was no apparent benefit to the addition of ovarian ablation in terms of recurrence-free or overall survival. Among the 550 women with ER-positive primary tumours, however, the

Table 2.4 Randomized trials of medical ovarian ablation as adjuvant therapy

Trial[a]	Ovarian treatment	Common systemic therapy[b]	Accrual period	Randomized		Data available?	Published?
				<50 years old	≥50 years old		
CRC under 50s (ZIPP)	Goserelin	±Tam ± chemotherapy	1987–99	1191	0	Yes	Yes[41]
FNCLCC France	Triptorelen or goserelin	FAC or FEC	1989–SR[c]	746	120	Yes	No
Southeast Sweden	Goserelin	±Tam	1989–91	40	0	No	No
ECOG EST 5188	Goserelin	FAC ± Tam	1989–94	1382	155	Yes	Yes[42]
University of Pretoria	Goserelin	CMF	1987–94	149	0	No	No
UKCCCR	Goserelin	Tam ± chemotherapy	1993–2000	2095	0	No	No
ICCG	Goserelin	CEF	1991–2000	784	0	No	No
GIVIO	Goserelin	±CMF None vs goserelin vs Tam vs both	1991–96	397	0	No	No
Stockholm Breast Cancer Study Group	Goserelin	±Tam CMF	1990–94	700	0	No	No
Heidelberg + GABG	Goserelin	CMF or CE or CMF	1993–2000	696	0	No	No
IBCSG	Goserelin	CMF vs none vs goserelin vs both	1990–99	1111	0	No	No
Total			1987–2000	9291	275		

[a]CRC, Cancer Research Campaign (UK); ZIPP, Zoladex International; FNCLCC, Fédération Nationale des Centres de Lutte Contre le Cancer; ECOG, Eastern Cooperative Oncology Group; UKCCCR, United Kingdom Co-Ordinating Committee on Cancer Research; ICCG, International Cancer Collaborative Group; GIVIO, Gruppo Interdisciplinare Volutazione Intervention Oncologia; GABG, German Adjuvant Breast Group; IBCSG, International Breast Cancer Study Group.

[b]Tam, tamoxifen; F, 5-fluorouracil; A, doxorubicin; C, cyclophosphamide; E, epirubicin; M, methotrexate.

[c]SR, still randomizing patients.

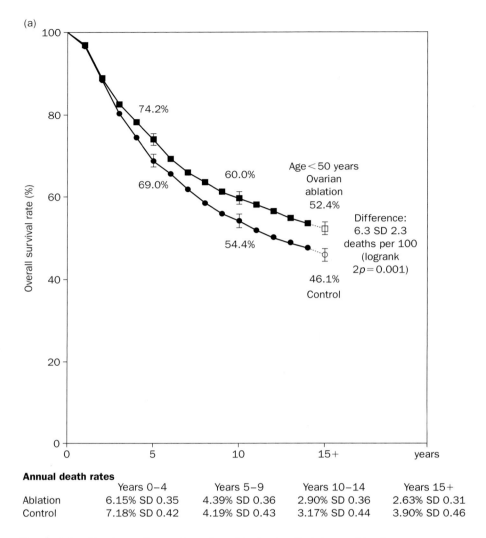

(a)

Annual death rates

	Years 0–4	Years 5–9	Years 10–14	Years 15+
Ablation	6.15% SD 0.35	4.39% SD 0.36	2.90% SD 0.36	2.63% SD 0.31
Control	7.18% SD 0.42	4.19% SD 0.43	3.17% SD 0.44	3.90% SD 0.46

Figure 2.4 Absolute effects of ovarian ablation in all trials combined among women aged under 50 years at entry. Overall survival rate (a) and recurrence-free survival rate (b) for 2102 women aged under 50 when randomized between ovarian ablation (squares) and control (circles). Bars indicate standard deviations (SD).

addition of ovarian ablation appeared to be beneficial both for recurrence-free survival (odds reduction 13%, ±SD = 11; p = non-significant (NS)) and for overall survival (odds reduction 17%, ±SD = 13; p = NS), but these differences were not statistically significant.

Analyses were done to examine the degree of benefit provided by ovarian ablation added to cytotoxic chemotherapy, in comparison with its benefit when given in the absence of cytotoxic chemotherapy. The proportional improvement in annual odds of recurrence in women in the absence of chemotherapy was 25% (±SD = 7; p = 0.0005), while the proportional improvement in annual odds of recurrence in the presence of chemotherapy was only 10% (±SD = 9; p > 0.1, NS) (Figure 2.6a). Similarly, the proportional improvement in annual odds of death

(b)

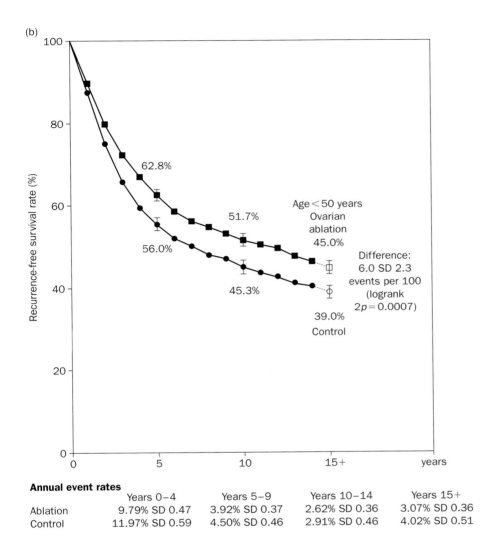

Annual event rates

	Years 0–4	Years 5–9	Years 10–14	Years 15+
Ablation	9.79% SD 0.47	3.92% SD 0.37	2.62% SD 0.36	3.07% SD 0.36
Control	11.97% SD 0.59	4.50% SD 0.46	2.91% SD 0.46	4.02% SD 0.51

was 24% ($\pm$SD = 7; p = 0.0006) in the absence of chemotherapy, but only 8% ($\pm$SD = 10; $p > 0.1$, NS) in the presence of chemotherapy (Figure 2.6b). Because of the small numbers of deaths, however, it is difficult to tell whether these differences are actually reliable. Furthermore, formal statistical testing using tests for heterogeneity, although they are known to lack power, do not confirm a significant difference between the effects of ovarian ablation in the presence and in the absence of chemotherapy.

Effects in women over 50 years of age

In the 1995 Overview analysis, data were available on 1354 women aged 50 or over who were randomly assigned to receive or not receive ovarian ablation. Most of these would have been peri- or postmenopausal. There was only a small and non-significant improvement in survival and in recurrence-free survival in this subset. By year 15 after randomization, there were 3.1 ($\pm$SD = 2.6; p = NS) fewer recurrences or deaths per 100 women allocated to ovarian ablation. There were 32% alive without

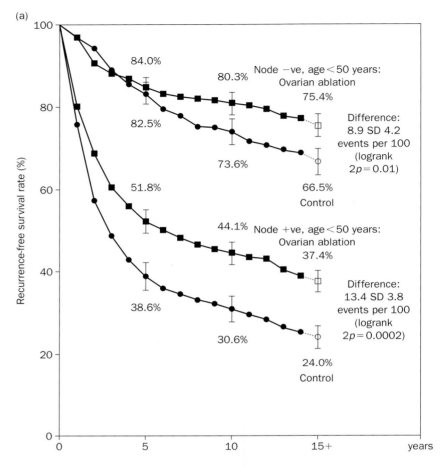

Figure 2.5 Absolute effects of ovarian ablation in the absence of routine chemotherapy in all trials combined among women aged under 50 years at entry: recurrence-free survival rate (a) and overall survival rate (b) for 473 node-negative and 696 node-positive women who were aged under 50 when randomized between ovarian ablation (squares) and control (circles) in the trials, or parts of trials, where cytotoxic therapy was not routinely used. Among node-negative women, in years 0–4 there were 28 deaths out of 1170 person-years in the ablation group versus 25 of 1037 in the controls (annual death rates: 2.4% SD 0.5 versus 2.4% SD 0.5); in years 5–9, there were 15 of 1030 versus 21 of 884 (1.5% SD 0.4 versus 2.4% SD 0.5); in years 10–14, there were 12 of 931 versus 15 of 779 (1.3% SD 0.4 versus 1.9% SD 0.5); and in years 15+ there were 33 of 1580 versus 43 of 1309 (2.1% SD 0.4 versus 3.3% SD 0.5). Among node-positive women, the corresponding values are years 0–4, 166 of 1620 versus 134 of 997 (10.3% SD 0.8 versus 13.4% SD 1.2); years 5–9, 55 of 1077 versus 37 of 577 (5.1% SD 0.7 versus 6.4% SD 1.1); years 10–14, 29 of 870 versus 23 of 426 (3.3% SD 0.6 versus 5.4% SD 1.1); and years 15+, 40 of 1151 versus 28 of 491 (3.5% SD 0.6 versus 5.7% SD 1.1).

(b)

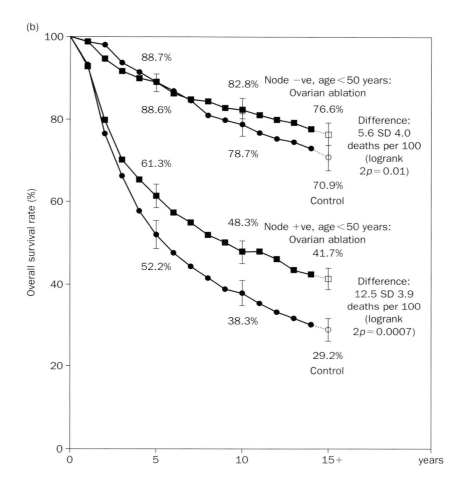

recurrence in the ovarian ablation group versus 28.9% in the controls (*p* = NS) and 36.9% alive overall in the ovarian ablation group versus 34.5% of controls (*p* = NS). It is likely that the lack of benefit of ovarian ablation in this group of women is related to their postmenopausal status rather than to their age per se.

Late effects and effects on non-breast-cancer deaths

The late effects of ovarian ablation can be clearly examined in this Overview analysis. Most of the patients in these trials were randomly assigned before 1970 and for most survivors there is follow-up information going beyond 1990. Thus, there is a large amount of

information available beyond year 15 of follow-up. Even during this later time period, the annual death rates for all women in the Overview remain lower amongst those who were originally allocated to ovarian ablation (2.6%, ±SD = 0.3) than among the controls (3.9%, ±SD = 0.5). Thus, the effects of ovarian ablation appear to persist long after the women underwent this manoeuvre. The Overview also attempted to study cause-specific mortality. Among women under 50 who died without any record of a distant recurrence of their breast cancer, 116 were classified as having died of non-breast-cancer causes. Taking into account the fact that those allocated ovarian ablation survived longer, and were therefore at more

(a)

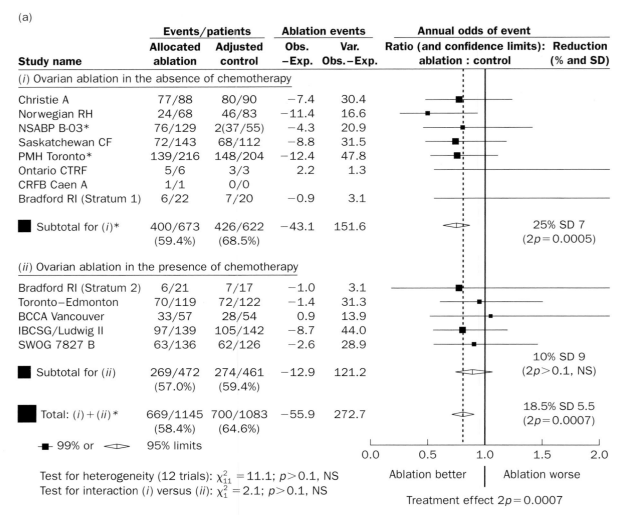

*Adjustment: for balance, control patients in 2:1 randomizations contribute twice.
PMH contributes Stratum 1: 49/68 versus 50/62 plus Stratum 2: 90/148 versus 2(49/71)

Figure 2.6 Proportional effects of ovarian ablation in each trial and overall, with subdivisions by absence or presence of chemotherapy, among women aged under 50 years at entry: recurrence-free survival (a) and overall survival (b) for women aged under 50 when randomized, with subtotals for strata in the absence and in the presence of routine cytotoxic chemotherapy. Each trial, or part of a trial, is described by a single line of information, showing the numbers of events and patients and summary logrank statistics. For each of these strata, the ratio of the annual event rate in the ovarian ablation group to that in the control group (the odds ratio) is plotted as a solid square, with the 99% confidence interval shown. For the subtotals and total, the 95% confidence interval is represented by a diamond. The solid vertical line indicates an odds ratio of 1.0 (i.e. no difference between ovarian ablation and control), whereas the broken vertical line indicates the 'typical odds ratio' in the total of all these trial results. For balance, control patients in the 2 : 1 randomizations (i.e. NSABP and part of PMH) are counted twice in the adjusted control totals but not in the statistical calculations.

(b)

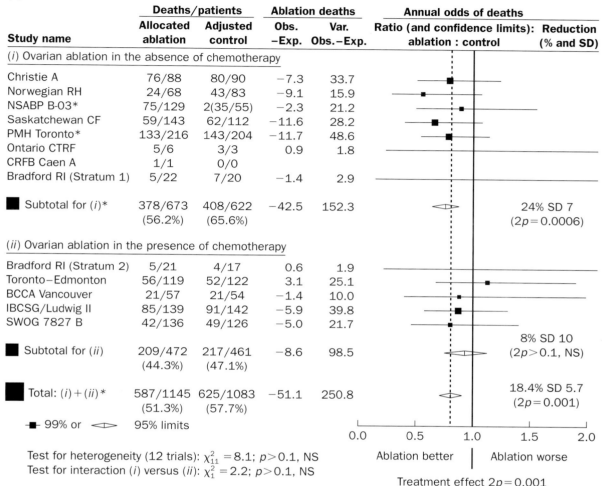

Study name	Deaths/patients		Ablation deaths		Annual odds of deaths	
	Allocated ablation	Adjusted control	Obs. −Exp.	Var. Obs.−Exp.	Ratio (and confidence limits): ablation : control	Reduction (% and SD)
(i) Ovarian ablation in the absence of chemotherapy						
Christie A	76/88	80/90	−7.3	33.7		
Norwegian RH	24/68	43/83	−9.1	15.9		
NSABP B-03*	75/129	2(35/55)	−2.3	21.2		
Saskatchewan CF	59/143	62/112	−11.6	28.2		
PMH Toronto*	133/216	143/204	−11.7	48.6		
Ontario CTRF	5/6	3/3	0.9	1.8		
CRFB Caen A	1/1	0/0				
Bradford RI (Stratum 1)	5/22	7/20	−1.4	2.9		
■ Subtotal for *(i)**	378/673 (56.2%)	408/622 (65.6%)	−42.5	152.3		24% SD 7 (2*p* = 0.0006)
(ii) Ovarian ablation in the presence of chemotherapy						
Bradford RI (Stratum 2)	5/21	4/17	0.6	1.9		
Toronto−Edmonton	56/119	52/122	3.1	25.1		
BCCA Vancouver	21/57	21/54	−1.4	10.0		
IBCSG/Ludwig II	85/139	91/142	−5.9	39.8		
SWOG 7827 B	42/136	49/126	−5.0	21.7		
■ Subtotal for *(ii)*	209/472 (44.3%)	217/461 (47.1%)	−8.6	98.5		8% SD 10 (2*p* > 0.1, NS)
■ Total: *(i)* + *(ii)**	587/1145 (51.3%)	625/1083 (57.7%)	−51.1	250.8		18.4% SD 5.7 (2*p* = 0.001)

■— 99% or <> 95% limits

Ablation better | Ablation worse

Test for heterogeneity (12 trials): $\chi^2_{11} = 8.1$; $p > 0.1$, NS
Test for interaction *(i)* versus *(ii)*: $\chi^2_1 = 2.2$; $p > 0.1$, NS

Treatment effect 2*p* = 0.001

*Adjustment: for balance, control patients in 2:1 randomizations contribute twice.
PMH contributes Stratum 1: 46/68 versus 49/62 plus Stratum 2: 87/148 versus 2(47/71)

prolonged risk of death from other causes, there was then no significant difference between the treatment groups in vascular deaths (22 of 922 in the ovarian ablation group versus 20 of 824 in the controls) in trials for which data were provided. Similarly, there were no differences in non-breast-cancer, non-vascular deaths (44 of 929 versus 30 of 824), or in all non-breast-cancer deaths.

Second breast primaries
An attempt was made to look at the incidence of contralateral breast cancer, but there was not enough information to examine this issue. Thirty contralateral breast cancers were recorded as the first event among 712 women allocated to ovarian ablation, compared with 32 of 679 women in the control arm in trials for which data was provided.

1995 Overview summary

In summary, the Overview confirms suggestions from individual trials that ovarian ablation in premenopausal women provides a statistically significant benefit in terms of recurrence-free and overall survival. This benefit appears to be similar for node-positive and node-negative women. Ovarian ablation provides benefit both in the presence and in the absence of chemotherapy, although the degree of benefit in the presence of chemotherapy is not statistically significant. Furthermore, this appearance is not fully confirmed by formal statistical testing, since tests of heterogeneity suggest no significant difference between the effects of ovarian ablation in the presence and in the absence of chemotherapy. From the few trials for which ER measurements are available, the effect of ovarian ablation appears significant in those women with ER in their tumours and not significant in those without it. The numbers available to examine this issue are very small, however. Similarly, it is difficult to draw firm conclusions regarding non-breast-cancer deaths or regarding the incidence of second primary breast cancers. There is no obvious difference in the incidence of non-cancer deaths in those randomized to ovarian ablation, however.

Summary of subsequent trials using medical ovarian ablation

The development of LHRH analogues has resurrected interest in the use of ovarian ablation in premenopausal women. Various LHRH analogues, in particular goserelin, are currently being tested in the adjuvant setting, in designs that compare goserelin, tamoxifen, or goserelin plus tamoxifen with chemotherapy in the premenopausal setting, or that add goserelin, tamoxifen, or goserelin plus tamoxifen to chemotherapy, in the same group of women. Of particular interest are two trials from which preliminary data have been presented. In one by Jakesz et al[40] 1095 women with stage I and II ER- and/or PgR-positive breast cancer were randomized to receive goserelin plus tamoxifen or

CMF (cyclophosphamide, methotrexate, and 5-fluorouracil (5-FU)) chemotherapy. Women receiving the endocrine therapy had significantly improved disease-free survival ($p < 0.02$). Overall survival, although slightly better than for women receiving goserelin plus tamoxifen, is not significantly improved, at least at this early follow-up. Women who developed amenorrhoea following CMF had significantly better disease-free and overall survival then those who did not ($p = 0.001$ and 0.05). Rutqvist et al[41] also reported results from a large randomized 2×2 factorial study in which premenopausal women with early-stage disease were randomly allocated, after primary surgery to (1) tamoxifen for 2 years, (2) goserelin, 26 monthly subcutaneous injections, (3) tamoxifen plus goserelin, or (4) no endocrine therapy. Some patients electively received tamoxifen or not and were randomly allocated just for goserelin. The study protocol also permitted the use of elective adjuvant chemotherapy in selected patients. A total of 2631 women, of whom 56% were node-negative, were studied. ER status was available in 1577 (60%). At a median follow-up of 4.3 years, fewer recurrences, 261 (20%), were observed among patients allocated to goserelin than among those who did not receive goserelin, 330 (24.9%) (relative hazard (RH) = 0.77; 95% confidence intervals (CI) = 0.66–0.90; $p = 0.001$). This effect was most pronounced amongst those who were known to be ER-positive. The benefit with goserelin appeared to be somewhat less amongst those who received concurrent adjuvant tamoxifen or adjuvant chemotherapy, but the differences compared with patients who did not receive such concurrent treatments were not statistically significant. There were also fewer (but not significantly fewer) deaths in the women allocated to receive goserelin: 140 (10.7%) versus 165 (12.4%) (RH = 0.84; 95% CI = 0.67–1.05; $p = 0.12$). Thus, in this study, medical castration with goserelin for 2 years in premenopausal ER-positive patients produced a statistically significant benefit in terms of disease-free survival and a trend toward improvement in overall survival irrespective of concurrent adjuvant tamoxifen or chemotherapy.

Preliminary results from a study performed by the Eastern Cooperative Oncology Group (ECOG) and US Intergroup were presented at the 1999 ASCO meeting.[42] This study, which compared CAF (cyclophosphamide, doxorubicin, and 5-FU) with CAF plus goserelin or CAF plus goserelin and tamoxifen, in premenopausal node-positive women, showed that the addition of goserelin or goserelin plus tamoxifen gave significantly better results in terms of disease-free survival. It also showed a non-statistically significant trend towards increased overall survival for the addition of goserelin. The addition of tamoxifen to CMF plus goserelin showed only a trend towards improvement for either relapse-free or overall survival. A preliminary subgroup analysis suggested that the addition of goserelin was more effective in younger women and/or women who did not become postmenopausal as a result of chemotherapy, while the addition of tamoxifen seemed more effective in older women and/or in women who became menopausal as a result of chemotherapy. This hypothesis remains to be further explored and substantiated in prospective randomized trials designed to test this question.

In the ZEBRA trial, 1640 women were randomized to receive goserelin for 2 years or CMF for 6 cycles. For ER-positive women, disease-free survival and overall survival were equivalent, while for ER-negative women, CMF was superior.[72,73] The FASG 06 trial randomized 333 premenopausal, 1–3 node-positive women to receive triptorelene and tamoxifen for 3 years or FEC 50 for 6 cycles. At 54 months of follow-up, no significant difference in disease-free or overall survival was seen.[74]

Other studies examining the use of LHRH analogues as adjuvant therapy either in direct comparison with or added to combination chemotherapy or tamoxifen in the premenopausal setting are currently under way (Table 2.4). The results of many of these studies became available for the 2000 Oxford Overview and will shed considerable further light on this situation when they are published in their final form, which is likely to be in 2002 or 2003. These larger and therefore more highly powered studies of medical ovarian ablation will add considerably to what is already known about the role of surgical and irradiation ablation in the adjuvant therapy of premenopausal women.

Relationship between amenorrhoea and response to chemotherapy

The results outlined above suggest that ovarian ablation may not be as effective when it is added to chemotherapy as it is when given alone. An obvious explanation of this observation could involve the degree of ovarian suppression provided by chemotherapy. The incidence of amenorrhoea has been reported from several trials of cytotoxic chemotherapy in premenopausal women, and ranges from 40% to 90%.[43–48] Several investigators have attempted to examine whether chemotherapy acts through ovarian ablation, by attempting to correlate the effectiveness of chemotherapy with amenorrhoea in women within each randomized trial. Three investigations have found that women who develop amenorrhoea have a longer disease-free and/or overall survival,[43–45] but three others have not found this relationship.[46–48] Although conflicting, these data suggest that part of the explanation for the better effects of cytotoxic chemotherapy in younger or premenopausal women arises from the medical castration achieved by many of these women.[43–45] Clearly, however, this effect does not explain the entire action of cytotoxic chemotherapy in this setting.[46–48] Thus, it is probable that the results of the Oxford Overview, in which ovarian ablation does not appear to add as much for women who are also receiving cytotoxic chemotherapy, may relate to the fact that the cytotoxic chemotherapy is already carrying out castration even in the non-ovarian-ablation control groups in these trials. The observation that goserelin may not add as much in older women or in women who have become amenorrhoeic following chemotherapy adds further evidence supporting this theory.[42]

Comparability of ovarian ablation with chemotherapy

There have been very few studies comparing chemotherapy directly with ovarian ablation. The Austrian and ZEBRA studies, described above,[40,72,73] suggest that goserelin or goserelin plus tamoxifen may be equivalent or superior to CMF chemotherapy in women with ER- and/or PgR-positive tumours. One small study by the Scottish Cancer Trials Breast Group[49] compared adjuvant ovarian ablation with combination chemotherapy with CMF in premenopausal women with pathological stage II breast cancer. In this group, ovarian ablation was comparable in its effects to CMF in terms of both disease-free and overall survival for the entire group of women randomized. When one divides the patients by ER positivity and negativity, however, it seems that ovarian ablation produces a substantially better effect in ER-positive women while chemotherapy produces a substantially better effect in ER-negative women. A trial of 732 ER-positive, node-positive or T3 women, presented but never published, suggests that ovarian ablation carried out by irradiation was equivalent to CMF i.v. given for 3 weeks for 9 cycles.[75] The GROCTA trial randomized 244 premenopausal node-positive, ER-positive women to ovarian ablation (by surgery, radiation, or a GNRH agonist for 2 years) plus tamoxifen for 5 years compared to CMF with oral cyclophosphamide. At 75 months of follow-up, disease-free and overall survival were equivalent.[76]

It is worth noting that the CMF given in the Austrian and the Scottish studies was not particularly dose-intensive, and that more aggressive or intensive types of chemotherapy, such as the classic Bonadonna regimen[5] given in full doses, may provide more substantial effects and thus could be superior to ovarian ablation used alone or to goserelin plus tamoxifen. Furthermore, in the last few years, at least two regimens have been reported that are superior to standard adjuvant chemotherapy regimens such as the classic Bonadonna regimen[5] and the AC (doxorubicin and cyclophosphamide) regimen.[50] These include the CEF (cyclophosphamide, epirubicin, and 5-FU) regimen, which has provided superior disease-free and overall survival in comparison with the classic Bonadonna CMF regimen,[51] and the AC–paclitaxel regimen, which has also shown superior disease-free and overall survival in comparison with AC, a regimen that has previously been shown to be equivalent to classic Bonadonna CMF.[50,52] Thus, there are now second-generation chemotherapies such as CEF and AC–taxol that are superior to even the best delivered of the first-generation regimens. As a result, studies that have compared first-generation regimens with endocrine manoeuvres cannot indicate how the latter would compare with second-generation regimens. This sort of indirect conclusion is somewhat unsatisfactory, and it is to be hoped that more direct comparisons of ovarian ablation and chemotherapy will be carried out in the future in order to further delineate their relative roles in premenopausal women.

Comparability of tamoxifen with ovarian ablation and with chemotherapy

There have been no randomized trials comparing tamoxifen with ovarian ablation in the adjuvant setting in premenopausal women. There are, however, three published randomized studies of tamoxifen compared with oophorectomy in premenopausal women with metastatic disease.[53–55] In addition, a meta-analysis of all of the available data on ovarian ablation in comparison to tamoxifen in the metastatic setting has shown equivalence in at least a small group of four trials containing over 300 patients in all.[56] These studies suggest that tamoxifen and ovarian ablation produce similar effects in premenopausal women with metastatic disease. It has also been shown in several of the randomized studies comparing tamoxifen with ovarian ablation that women who have responded to tamoxifen have a 30–60% chance of responding to subsequent oophorectomy, and vice versa. This is in conflict with the data of Hoogstraten and colleagues,[57] which suggested that women responding first to tamoxifen and continued on it had extremely low or no response rates to subsequent ovarian ablation. It would seem that the use of tamoxifen as an adjuvant in the premenopausal setting might be quite comparable to ovarian ablation. This remains to be tested in future adjuvant trials, however.

There have also been very few trials comparing tamoxifen with chemotherapy in the adjuvant setting.[58] The few studies that do exist suggest that tamoxifen may be equivalent or less effective, but this observation may depend completely on the group of patients selected, their levels of ER and/or PgR, and on the type, schedule, and dose intensity of the chemotherapy being tested. Further studies comparing these two approaches are also badly needed.

Equivalence of ovarian medical suppression and surgical or radiation ovarian ablation

Although a number of the newer trials outlined above are now substituting medical ovarian ablation for radiation or surgical ablation, the equivalence of this treatment or indeed the equivalence of ovarian ablation by surgery and by radiation is unclear.

Ovarian irradiation has been assumed to produce an effect similar to that of surgical oophorectomy. There are considerable data, however, to suggest that following ovarian irradiation, depending on the dose and dose schedule, and on the age of the patient, ovarian function may not be totally destroyed. For example, in the study by Nissen-Meyer and colleagues,[25] 13% of the women castrated by irradiation resumed menses at some later date. Similarly, in the study by Meakin et al,[27] 3.3% of women receiving 2000 rad to the ovaries in five fractions resumed menstruation over subsequent years (7% of those over 45 years of age at the time of therapy). Thus, ovarian irradiation may not produce the complete and permanent ablation that is presumably achieved by surgery. Nonetheless, there seems no obvious difference between the results of ovarian abla-

tion and surgical ablation amongst the various individual ovarian ablation trials or in the Oxford Overview analysis.

Similarly, medical ablation with drugs such as goserelin is assumed to be equivalent to surgical oophorectomy. Goserelin has been shown to suppress ovarian function and to produce clinical responses in pre- and perimenopausal women with advanced breast cancer that are similar to those previously reported for other hormonal therapies in phase I and II trials.[59–62] This finding has been confirmed in a small randomized study comparing goserelin with ovarian ablation in premenopausal women with metastatic disease.[13,14] A larger trial would be helpful in increasing the power of this comparison. In ongoing adjuvant trials, however, the LHRH analogues are given for periods of time that range from 2 to 5 years. Depending on the age of the patients involved, 5 years of an LHRH analogue may take them through the time when they would normally reach a physiologic menopause. In younger women, however, the discontinuation of the LHRH analogue would usually lead to resumed ovarian function, since the endocrine effects of these analogues are reversible, with the return of menses usually occurring within 1–2 months after discontinuation of therapy.[63] Presumably the length of the ovarian suppression will affect its efficacy as adjuvant therapy, perhaps in a similar way to the effects demonstrated with varying lengths of tamoxifen.[64,65] The relative importance of length of treatment in this setting has been poorly studied to date, and remains to be clarified in future trials.

Effects of ovarian ablation on other body systems

It is well recognized that premature ovarian ablation can have deleterious effects on the cardiovascular and skeletal systems.[66,67] Whether this assumes a major role in terms of competing risks of death in comparison with the risk of dying from breast cancer has not been clearly established, however. Certainly the most updated information from the Oxford Overview does not suggest any strong trend towards increased cardiac or non-breast-cancer deaths in the women randomized to receive ovarian ablation. The difficulty of establishing cause of death, particularly in a meta-analysis setting in which information is obtained retrospectively from multiple centres, however, may obscure a relatively small or even a moderately large effect on deaths from other causes. Alternatively, the competing risk of death from breast cancer may be so high that it greatly outweighs any effect on deaths from other causes. In particular, deaths related to reduced osteoporosis will not be as frequent as those from breast cancer, nor will they occur until the patients have had 20–30 years of follow-up after ovarian ablation. Cardiac deaths may be of greater concern in that they are both more common and occur at younger ages, but to date increased cardiac deaths have not been demonstrated in any individual study nor in the Overview analysis. Further data concerning these long-term risks of death remain to be accumulated.

CONCLUSIONS AND FUTURE DIRECTIONS

Metastatic disease

In the treatment of metastatic disease, ovarian ablation by surgery, radiation, or the use of an LHRH analogue remains a useful therapeutic modality for ER- and/or PgR-positive women. There is some early suggestion from a small meta-analysis that an LHRH analogue accompanied by tamoxifen may be superior to an LHRH analogue alone, but this meta-analysis is small, has limited toxicity data, and does not address the question of tamoxifen sequenced with an LHRH analogue versus tamoxifen plus a concurrent LHRH analogue. Since tamoxifen is usually used first as therapy for metastatic disease, followed, after response and subsequent relapse, by ovarian ablation by some means, this question would seem of more interest. In any case, it currently seems reasonable to initiate treatment in hormone-responsive premenopausal women with tamoxifen and, if they

respond, then use ovarian ablation as a subsequent endocrine manoeuvre. More data concerning the use of the two agents concurrently is required before this can be recommended as a standard approach.

Adjuvant therapy

In the adjuvant setting, it seems clear from the Oxford Overview that ovarian ablation has a significant effect on disease-free and overall survival in premenopausal women, particularly those with ER-positive tumours. This effect appears to be significant, and fairly similar in both node-positive and node-negative women, although it appears to have a greater absolute effect in the former. The effect appears to be more dramatic when ovarian ablation is used alone than when it is given in the presence of cytotoxic chemotherapy. The indirect comparisons of treatment effects in different circumstances (that is node-negative versus node-positive, or ovarian ablation in the presence versus in the absence of chemotherapy) are, however, to be interpreted with more caution than the results obtained from direct comparisons within each randomized trial and from the summaries of those direct comparisons obtained in the Overview. Much additional follow-up information will be available on each of these individual trials over the next 5–10 years and from the full publication of the 2000 Overview. For example, one Chinese trial of ovarian ablation that began in 1991 has already accrued more than 3000 premenopausal women. In addition, there are over 3000 women in the recent trials of ovarian suppression with LHRH agonists. A large study comparing tamoxifen plus ovarian ablation as adjuvant therapy versus tamoxifen plus ovarian ablation at the time of recurrence has been completed in Vietnam.[77] These trials will add considerable additional information to what is already available.

It would still be useful, however, to undertake further large randomized trials assessing the additional effects of ovarian ablation in the presence of cytotoxic chemotherapy, as well as the additional effects of cytotoxic chemotherapy in the presence of ovarian ablation, and to further assess the effects of both or either of these modalities in the presence of prolonged tamoxifen therapy. Such trials could be designed as three-way comparisons of ovarian ablation versus cytotoxic chemotherapy versus both, which would add data in each of the areas that one might wish to further examine. Until more information becomes available, however, it would seem that there is enough information to conclude that ovarian ablation is useful in premenopausal women with ER-positive tumours, producing effects comparable to those of CMF-type chemotherapy in that setting. Although there is a far larger body of data establishing the role of CMF or comparable types of chemotherapy in the premenopausal setting, certainly enough data exist to suggest that ovarian ablation might be used as an alternative in ER-positive women for whom chemotherapy is either unacceptable or unsuitable for whatever reason. In addition, as increasing data accumulate that being amenorrhoeic following chemotherapy is associated with a better outcome, and that adding ovarian ablation or goserelin to chemotherapy, particularly in younger women or in women who do not become amenorrhoeic,[36,42] may be beneficial, it may be increasingly appropriate to consider adding ovarian ablation by some mechanism to the treatment of young women who do not become amenorrhoeic following adjuvant chemotherapy.

REFERENCES

1. Beatson GT. On the treatment of inoperable cases of carcinoma of the mamma: suggestions for a new method of treatment with illustrative cases. *Lancet* 1896; **ii**: 104–7.
2. Schinzinger A. Ueber carcinoma mammae. *Verh Dtsch Ges Chir* 1889; **18**: 28–29.
3. Taylor GW. Artificial menopause in carcinoma of the breast. *N Engl J Med* 1934; **211**: 1138–40.
4. Fisher B, Carbone P, Economou SG et al. L-phenylalanine mustard (L-PAM) in the manage-ment of primary breast cancer: a report of early findings. *N Engl J Med* 1975; **292**: 117–22.
5. Bonadonna G, Brusamolino E, Valagussa P et al. Combination chemotherapy as an adjuvant treatment in operable breast cancer. *N Engl J Med* 1976; **294**: 405–10.
6. Legha SS, Carter SK. Antiestrogens in the treatment of breast cancer. *Cancer Treat Rev* 1976; **3**: 205–16.
7. Santen RJ, Samojik E, Lipton A et al. Kinetic, hormonal and clinical studies with amino-glutethimide in breast cancer. *Cancer* 1977; **39**: 2948–58.
8. Early Breast Cancer Trialists' Collaborative Group (EBCTCG). Effects of adjuvant tamoxifen and of cytotoxic therapy on mortality in early breast cancer: an overview of 61 randomized trials among 28,896 women. *N Engl J Med* 1988; **319**: 1681–92.
9. Osborne CK, Yochmowitz MG, Knight WA, McGuire WL. The value of estrogen and progesterone receptors in the treatment of breast cancer. *Cancer* 1980; **46**: 2884–8.
10. Bloom ND, Tobin EH, Schreibman B, Degenshein GA. The role of progesterone receptors in the management of advanced breast cancer. *Cancer* 1980; **45**: 2972–7.
11. Leclercq G, Heuson JC. Therapeutic significance of sex-steroid hormone receptors in the treatment of breast cancer. *Eur J Cancer* 1977; **13**: 1205–15.
12. Allegra JC, Barlock A, Huff KK, Lippman ME. Changes in multiple or sequential estrogen receptor determinations in breast cancer. *Cancer* 1980; **45**: 792–4.
13. Taylor CW, Green S, Dalton WS et al. Multicenter randomized clinical trial of goserelin versus surgical ovariectomy in premenopausal patients with receptor-positive metastatic breast cancer: an intergroup study. *J Clin Oncol* 1998; **16**: 994–9.
14. Taylor CW, Green S, Dalton WS et al. A multi-center randomized trial of Zoladex versus surgical ovariectomy in premenopausal patients with receptor positive metastatic breast cancer. *Breast Cancer Res Treat* 1996; **37**: 37.
15. Klijn JG, Seynaeve C, Beex L et al. Combined treatment with buserelin (LHRH A) and tamoxifen (TAM) vs single treatment with each drug alone in premenopausal metastatic breast cancer: preliminary results of EORTC study 10881. *Proc Am Soc Clin Oncol* 1996; **15**: 117a (Abs 132).
16. Boccardo F, Blamey R, Klijn JCM et al.

LHRH-agonist (LHRH-A) + tamoxifen (TAM) versus LHRH-A alone in premenopausal women with advanced breast cancer (ABC): results of a meta-analysis of four trials. *Proc Am Soc Clin Oncol* 1999; **18:** 110a.

17. Klijn J, Blamey R, Boccardo F et al. A new standard treatment for advanced premenopausal breast cancer: a meta-analysis of the combined hormonal agent trialists' group (CHAT). *Eur J Cancer* 1998; **345:** 405.

18. Fisher B, Slack NH. Number of lymph nodes examined and the prognosis of breast carcinoma. *Surg Gynecol Obstet* 1970; **131:** 79–88.

19. McWhirter R. Some factors influencing prognosis in breast cancer. *J Fac Radiol Lond* 1956; **8:** 220–34.

20. Huck P. Artificial menopause as an adjunct to radical treatment of breast cancer. *NZ Med J* 1952; **51:** 364–7.

21. Kennedy BJ, Mielke PW, Fortuny IE. Therapeutic castration versus prophylactic castration in breast cancer. *Surg Gynecol Obstet* 1964; **118:** 524–40.

22. Alrich EM, Liddle HV, Morton CB. Carcinoma of the breast: results of surgical treatment: some anatomic and endocrine consideration. *Ann Surg* 1957; **145:** 779–806.

23. Rennaes S. Prophylactic ovarian irradiation. *Acta Chir Scand* 1960; **266:** 85–90.

24. Cole MP. A clinical trial of an artificial menopause in carcinoma of the breast. In: *Hormones and Breast Cancer*, 5th edn (Namer M, Lalanne CM, eds). Paris: INSERM, 1975: 143–50.

25. Nissen-Meyer R. Ovarian suppression and its supplement by additive hormonal treatment. In: *Hormones and Breast Cancer*, 5th edn (Namer M, Lalanne CM, eds). Paris: INSERM, 1975: 151–8.

26. Ravdin RG, Lewison EF, Slack NH et al. Results of a clinical trial concerning the worth of prophylactic oophorectomy for breast carcinoma. *Surg Gynecol Obstet* 1970; **131:** 1055–64.

27. Meakin JW, Allt WEC, Beale FA et al. Ovarian irradiation and prednisone therapy following surgery and radiotherapy for carcinoma of the breast. *Can Med Assoc J* 1979; **19:** 1221–8.

28. Meakin JW, Hayward JL, Panzarella T et al. Ovarian irradiation and prednisone therapy following surgery and radiotherapy for carcinoma of the breast. *Breast Cancer Res Treat* 1996; **37:** 11–19.

29. Bryant AJS, Weir JA. Prophylactic oophorectomy in operable instances of carcinoma of the breast. *Surg Gynecol Obstet* 1981; **153:** 660–4.

30. Nevinny HB, Nevinny D, Roscoff CB et al. Prophylactic oophorectomy in breast cancer therapy. *Am J Surg* 1969; **117:** 531–6.

31. Meakin JW, Allt WEC, Beale FA et al. Ovarian irradiation and prednisone following surgery and radiotherapy for carcinoma of the breast. *Breast Cancer Res Treat* 1983; **3:** 45–8.

32. Clarke EA, Fetterly JC, Ryan NC. The Ontario Cancer Treatment and Research Foundation Clinical Trial on the comparative effect of ovarian irradiation in carcinoma of the breast in the postmenopausal patient. In: *Treatment of Early Breast Cancer 1: Worldwide Evidence 1985–1990. A Systemic Overview of All Available Randomized Trials of Adjuvant Endocrine and Cytoxic Therapy* (Early Breast Cancer Trialists' Collaborative Group). Oxford: Oxford University Press, 1990.

33. Delozier T, Juret P, Couette JE, Mace-Lesech J. Ovarian irradiation in postmenopausal women with breast cancer and positive axillary nodes. In: *Treatment of Early Breast Cancer 1: Worldwide Evidence 1985–1990. A Systematic Overview of All Available Randomized Trials of Adjuvant Endocrine and Cytoxic Therapy* (Early Breast Cancer Trialists' Collaborative Group). Oxford: Oxford University Press, 1990: 114.

34. Ragaz J, Jackson S, Nilson K et al. Randomized study of locoregional radiotherapy and ovarian ablation in premenopausal patients with breast cancer treated with adjuvant chemotherapy. *Proc Am Soc Clin Oncol* 1988; **7:** 12.

35. The International Breast Cancer Study Group. Late effects of adjuvant oophorectomy and chemotherapy upon premenopausal breast cancer patients. *Ann Oncol* 1990; **1:** 30–5.

36. Early Breast Cancer Trialists' Collaborative Group (EBCTCG). Ovarian ablation in early breast cancer: an overview of the randomized trials. *Lancet* 1996; **348:** 1189–96.

37. Early Breast Cancer Trialists' Collaborative Group (EBCTCG). Treatment of early breast cancer. In: *Treatment of Early Breast Cancer 1: Worldwide Evidence 1985–1990. A Systematic Overview of All Available Randomized Trials of Adjuvant Endocrine and Cytotoxic Therapy* (Early Breast Cancer Trialists' Collaborative Group). Oxford: Oxford University Press, 1990.

38. Early Breast Cancer Trialists' Collaborative Group (EBCTCG). Systemic treatment of early breast cancer by hormonal, cytotoxic or immune therapy: 133 randomized trials involving 31,000 recurrences and 24,000 deaths among 75,000 women. *Lancet* 1992; **339:** 71–85.

39. Early Breast Cancer Trialists' Collaborative Group (EBCTCG). Systemic treatment of early breast cancer by hormonal, cytotoxic, or immune therapy. *Lancet* 1992; **339:** 71–85B.

40. Jakesz R, Hausmaninger H, Samonigg H et al. Comparison of adjuvant therapy with tamoxifen and goserelin vs CMF in premenopausal stage I and II hormone-responsive breast cancer patients: four-year results of Austrian Breast Cancer Study Group (ABCSG) Trial 5. *Proc Am Soc Clin Oncol* 1999; **18:** 67a.

41. Rutqvist LE. Zoladex and tamoxifen as adjuvant therapy in premenopausal breast cancer: a randomized trial by the Cancer Research Campaign (CRC) Breast Cancer Trials Group, the Stockholm Breast Study Group, the South-East Sweden Breast Group & the Gruppo Interdisciplinare Valutazione Interventi in Oncologia (GIVIO). *Proc Am Soc Clin Oncol* 1999; **18:** 67a.

42. Davidson N, O'Neill A, Vukov A et al. Effect of chemohormonal therapy in premenopausal, node (+), receptor (+) breast cancer: an Eastern Cooperative Oncology Group phase III intergroup trial (E5188, INT-0101). *Proc Am Soc Clin Oncol* 1999; **18:** 67a.

43. Howell A, George WD, Crowther D et al. Controlled trial of adjuvant chemotherapy with cyclophosphamide, methotrexate and fluorouracil for breast cancer. *Lancet* 1984; **ii:** 307–11.

44. Pourquier H. The results of adjuvant chemotherapy are predominantly caused by the hormonal changes such therapy induces: In: *Medical Oncology. Controversies in Cancer Treatment* (Van Scoy-Moscher MB, ed). Boston: Hall, 1981: 83–9.

45. Ludwig Breast Cancer Study Group. Adjuvant combination chemotherapy with or without prednisone in premenopausal breast cancer patients with metastases in 1 to 3 axillary lymph nodes: a randomized trial. *Cancer Res* 1985; **45:** 4454–9.

46. Bonadonna G, Valagussa P, DePalo G. The results of adjuvant chemotherapy are predominantly caused by the hormonal changes such therapy induces. In: *Medical Oncology. Controversies in Cancer Treatment* (Van Scoy-Moscher MB, ed). Boston: Hall, 1981: 100–9.

47. Fisher B, Sherman B, Rockette H et al. L-phenyl-alanine mustard (L-PAM) in the management of premenopausal patients with primary breast cancer: lack of association of disease-free survival with depression of ovarian function. *Cancer* 1979; **44:** 847–57.

48. Rubens RD, Knight RK, Fentiman IS et al. Controlled trial of adjuvant chemotherapy with melphalan for breast cancer. *Lancet* 1983; **i:** 839–43.

49. Scottish Cancer Trials Breast Group. Adjuvant ovarian ablation versus CMF chemotherapy in premenopausal women with pathological stage II breast carcinoma: the Scottish trial. *Lancet* 1993; **341:** 1293–8.

50. Fisher B, Brown AM, Dimitrov NV et al. Two months of doxorubicin, cyclophosphamide with and without interval re-induction therapy compared with 6 months vs cyclophosphamide, methotrexate and fluorouracil in positive-node breast cancer patients with tamoxifen-non-responsive tumours: results from the National Surgical Adjuvant Breast and Bowel Project B-15. *J Clin Oncol* 1990; **8:** 1483–96.

51. Levine M, Bramwell V, Pritchard KI et al. A clinical trial of intensive CEF versus CMF in premenopausal women with node positive breast cancer. *Proc Am Soc Clin Oncol* 1995; **14:** 103.

52. Fisher B, Redmond C, Brown A et al. Adjuvant chemotherapy with and without tamoxifen in the treatment of primary breast cancer: 5 year results from the National Surgical Adjuvant Breast and Bowel Project trial. *J Clin Oncol* 1986; **4:** 459–71.

53. Ingle JN, Krook JE, Green SJ et al. Randomized trial of bilateral oophorectomy versus tamoxifen in premenopausal women with metastatic breast cancer. *J Clin Oncol* 1986; **4:** 178–85.

54. Buchanan RB, Blamey RW, Durrant KR et al. A randomized comparison of tamoxifen with surgical oophorectomy in premenopausal patients with advanced breast cancer. *J Clin Oncol* 1986; **4:** 1326–30.

55. Sawka CA, Pritchard KI, Shelley WE et al. A randomized crossover trial of tamoxifen versus ovarian ablation for metastatic breast cancer in premenopausal women: a report of the National Cancer Institute of Canada Clinical Trials Group (NCIC CTG Trial MA.1). *Breast Cancer Res Treat* 1997; **44:** 211–15.

56. Crump M, Sawka CA, DeBoer G et al. An individual patient-based meta-analysis of tamoxifen versus ovarian ablation as first line endocrine therapy for premenopausal women with metastatic breast cancer. *Breast Cancer Res Treat* 1997; **44:** 201–10.

57. Hoogstraten B, Fletcher WS, Gad-el-Mawla N et al. Tamoxifen and oophorectomy in the treatment of recurrent breast cancer. *Cancer Res* 1982; **4:** 4788–791.

58. Kaufmann M, Jonat W, Abel U. Adjuvant chemo

and endocrine therapy alone or in combination in premenopausal patients (GABG Trial 1). *Rec Results Cancer Res* 1989; **115:** 118–25.

59. Kaufmann M, Jonat W, Kleeberg UR. Goserelin, a depot gonadotropin-releasing hormone agonist in the treatment of premenopausal patients with metastatic breast cancer. *J Clin Oncol* 1989; **7:** 1113–19.

60. Kaufmann M, Jonat W, Schachner-Wunschmann E. The depot GnRH analogue goserelin in the treatment of premenopausal patients with metastatic breast cancer – a 5 year experience and further endocrine therapies. *Onkologie* 1991; **14:** 22–30.

61. Blamey RW, Jonat W, Kaufmann M. Goserelin. Depot in the treatment of premenopausal advanced breast cancer. *Eur J Cancer* 1992; **28A:** 810–14.

62. Blamey RW, Jonat W, Kaufmann M. Survival data relating to the use of goserelin depot in the treatment of premenopausal advanced breast cancer. *Eur J Cancer* 1993; **29A:** 1498.

63. West CP, Baird DT. Suppression of ovarian activity by Zoladex depot (ICI 118 630), a long acting luteinizing hormone releasing hormone agonist analogue. *Clin Endocrinol* 1987; **26:** 213–20.

64. Gallen M, Alonso MC, Ojeda B et al. Randomized multicentre trial comparing two different time-spans of adjuvant tamoxifen therapy (ATT) in women with operable node positive breast cancer. *Proc Am Soc Clin Oncol* 1994; **13:** 76.

65. Swedish Breast Cancer Cooperative Group. Randomized trial of 2 versus 5 years of adjuvant tamoxifen in postmenopausal early-stage breast cancer. *Proc Am Soc Clin Oncol* 1996; **15:** 126.

66. Colditz GA, Willett WC, Stampfer MJ. Menopause and the risk of coronary heart disease in women. *N Engl J Med* 1987; **316:** 1105–10.

67. Knoweldon J, Buhr AJ, Dunbar O. Incidence of fractures in persons over 35 years of age: a report to the MRC working party on fractures in the elderly. *Br J Prev Soc Med* 1964; **18:** 130–41.

68. Paterson R, Russell MH. Clinical trials in malignant disease. Part II – Breast cancer: value of irradiation of the ovaries. *J Faculty Radiologists* 1959; **10:** 130–33.

69. Nissen-Meyer R. Ovarian suppression and its supplement by additive hormonal treatment. In: *Hormones and Breast Cancer* (ed. Namer M, Lalanne CM). Paris: INSERM, 1975: 151–58.

70. Nissen-Meyer R. The role of prophylactic castration in the therapy of human mammary cancer. *Eur J Cancer* 1967; **3:** 395–403.

71. Ludwig Breast Cancer Study Group. Chemotherapy with or without oophorectomy in high risk premenopausal patients with operable breast cancer. *J Clin Oncol* 1985; **13:** 1059–67.

72. Kaufmann M, Jonat W, Blamey R, Schumacher M. The Zebra Study: Zoladex (Goserelin) versus CMF as adjuvant therapy in the management of node positive stage II breast cancer in pre/peri-menopausal women aged 50 years or less. *Proc Am Soc Clin Oncol* 1998; **17:** 151a (Abs 577).

73. Jonat W. Zoladex versus CMF adjuvant therapy in pre/peri-menopausal breast cancer: Tolerability and amenorrhea comparisons. *Proc Am Soc Clin Oncol* 2000; **19:** 87a (Abs 333).

74. Roche H, Kerbrat P, Bonneterre J et al. Complete hormonal blockade versus chemotherapy in premenopausal early-stage breast cancer patients (pts) with positive hormone-receptor (HR+) and 1–3 node positive (N+) tumor: Results of the FASG 06 Trial. *Proc Am Soc Clin Oncol* 2000; **19:** 72a (Abs 279).

75. Ejlertsen B, Dombernowski P, Mouridsen HT et al. Comparable effect of ovarian ablation (OA) and CMF chemotherapy in premenopausal hormone receptor positive breast cancer patients (PRP). *Proc Am Soc Clin Oncol* 1999; **18:** 66a (Abs 248).

76. Boccardo F, Rubagotti F, Amoroso D et al. Cyclophosphamide, methotrexate, and fluorouracil versus tamoxifen plus ovarian suppression as adjuvant treatment of estrogen receptor-positive pre-perimenopausal breast cancer patients: results of the Italian Breast Cancer Adjuvant Study Group 02 randomized trial. boccardo@hp380.ist.unige.it *J Clin Oncol* 2000; **18:** 2718–27.

77. Love RR, Mohsin SK, Havighurst T, Allred CC. Overexpression of Her-2 neu as a prognostic factor and as a predictive factor for response to adjuvant combined endocrine therapy in premenopausal Vietnamese women with operable breast cancer. *Breast Cancer Res Treat* 2000; **69:** 223 (Abs 220).

3

Pharmacology, biology, and clinical use of triphenylethylenes

Jenny Chang, Richard M Elledge

CONTENTS • Introduction • Tamoxifen • Newer triphenylethylenes • Summary

INTRODUCTION

Breast cancer is the most common cancer in women in the Western world. Because most breast cancer is dependent on estrogen for growth, reducing estrogen levels through oophorectomy, hypophysectomy, or adrenalectomy may cause cancer to regress. The need for these surgical procedures has been reduced by the introduction of tamoxifen, the first triphenylethylene that acts as an antiestrogen by inhibiting the binding of estrogen to the estrogen receptor (ER). Tamoxifen was approved by the US Food and Drug Administration in 1977 for the treatment of women with advanced breast cancer, and several years later for the adjuvant treatment of primary breast cancer.[1]

TAMOXIFEN

Pharmacology and biology

Pharmacologic and pharmacokinetic properties

The compound administered to patients is *trans*-tamoxifen, since this isomer has higher affinity for estrogen receptors than does its *cis*

isomer.[2] ER is a nuclear transcription factor present in normal breast epithelium and other tissue types, and is overexpressed in 60–70% of breast cancers. *Trans*-tamoxifen has not only antiestrogenic but also estrogenic properties, depending on the species, tissue, and receptor type.[3] Therefore, tamoxifen may be more properly referred to as a selective ER modulator because of these diverse activities. The molecular basis of these properties is poorly understood, but the estrogen-agonist activity of tamoxifen may explain its favorable effects on bone and serum lipid concentrations and its ability to stimulate the endometrium. The estrogen-antagonistic activity in breast tissue accounts for its ability to inhibit tumor growth.

The major metabolites of tamoxifen in humans are *N*-desmethyltamoxifen and *trans*-4-hydroxytamoxifen; the affinity of the latter for ER is equivalent to that of 17β-estradiol.[4] The dimethylaminoethoxy side-chain and the *trans* configuration are crucial for the antiestrogenic activity of tamoxifen;[2] the more highly estrogenic *cis* metabolites and metabolites without the side chain have been found in breast tumors, but their importance are unclear.

Tamoxifen is readily absorbed after oral administration.[2] It is excreted in a biphasic fashion after an initial half-life of 7–14 days, permitting once-daily administration.[2] The usual dose is 20 mg/day. In long-term treatment, the steady-state concentrations of tamoxifen and its metabolites in serum remain constant for as long as 10 years; reduced bioavailability is not a cause of acquired resistance to tamoxifen. Tamoxifen can be detected in the serum for several weeks and in the tumor tissue for several months after treatment is discontinued.[5] Tamoxifen undergoes extensive metabolism in the liver and is excreted predominantly in the feces. Tamoxifen increases the action of warfarin by competing with its metabolizing enzyme cytochrome P450 3A4, a circumstance that can lead to potentially life-threatening bleeding.[6] Therefore, patients receiving tamoxifen should be given less warfarin and clotting times should be closely monitored.

Endocrine effects

Postmenopausal women have low serum estrogen and progesterone concentrations and high serum luteinizing hormone (LH) and follicle-stimulating hormone (FSH) concentrations. In these women, tamoxifen may reduce gonadotropin secretion, although this effect may be variable.[7] In premenopausal women, it slightly increases gonadotropin secretion.[8] Estrogen levels may also rise in premenopausal women, sometimes twofold over pretreatment levels. However, despite this increase, tamoxifen maintains its therapeutic effect in premenopausal women.[9]

Mechanisms of action

The antitumor effects of tamoxifen are thought to be due to its antiestrogenic activity, mediated by competitive inhibition of estrogen binding to the ER. As a consequence, tamoxifen inhibits the expression of estrogen-regulated genes, including growth factors and angiogenic factors secreted by the tumor, resulting in a block in G_1 phase of the cell cycle and thus slowing proliferation. Tumors may then regress because of the altered balance between cellular proliferation and ongoing cell loss. Tamoxifen may also

directly induce apoptosis.[10] The weak estrogen-agonist activity of tamoxifen may be due to the ability of tamoxifen-bound receptor to bind estrogen response elements (EREs) on target genes, and to promote transcription through constitutively active AP-1 sites. After binding a ligand such as estradiol or tamoxifen, the ER dimerizes with another receptor monomer to activate the complex and to facilitate the binding of the receptor dimer to the EREs of target serum. Recent studies suggest that ligand-bound ER can affect gene transcription. For instance, ER can interact with other transcription factors such as the AP-1 transcription factor complex to augment or inhibit the expression of genes regulated by these proteins.[11] This interaction with AP-1 family members could partially explain the 'crosstalk' between estrogen and polypeptide growth factor transcription pathways.

Clinical use of tamoxifen

Adjuvant treatment of invasive breast cancer

Tamoxifen is effective treatment for breast cancer, and recent studies of early-stage breast cancer have confirmed that tamoxifen when given as adjuvant treatment can prevent or delay breast cancer recurrence.[9] However, it may be difficult to distinguish cases in which surgery alone is curative from those in which micrometastases are present and which therefore may require adjuvant therapy. Nevertheless, postoperative therapy with tamoxifen reduces the risk of recurrence and prolongs survival in women with operable breast cancer in whom the tumors are confined to the breast or to the axillary lymph nodes.[9] Its benefit in terms of lowering the odds of recurrence and death is limited to women whose tumors express ER and/or progesterone receptor (PgR).[9] This benefit increases with increasing receptor level (Table 3.1). The benefit of tamoxifen is also dependent on length of treatment, and progressively increases from 1 to 5 years (Table 3.1). Some studies have indicated that more than 5 years is not additionally

Table 3.1 Meta-analysis of trials of adjuvant tamoxifen therapy in women with breast cancer, according to estrogen receptor (ER) status and duration of therapy[a]

Duration of therapy	No. of women	No. of events averted each year	
		Recurrence	Death
1 year:			
ER-negative	1591	0[b]	0[b]
ER-positive	3352	1 in 5	1 in 7
2 years:			
ER-negative	5145	0[b]	0[b]
ER-positive	8635	1 in 3 or 4	
5 years:			
ER-negative	922	0[b]	0[b]
ER-positive	5869	1 in 2	1 in 3 or 4

[a]Data from the Early Breast Cancer Trialists' Collaborative Group.
[b]The data cannot exclude the possibility that occasionally a woman might benefit.

beneficial, and may even be detrimental,[12,13] while others have not confirmed this observation.[14]

More than 37 000 women with operable breast cancer were enrolled in 55 randomized clinical trials of adjuvant therapy with tamoxifen before 1990, providing a large database of findings on long-term follow-up. These results were summarized recently in an update of the meta-analysis conducted by the Early Breast Cancer Trialists' Collaborative Group (EBCTCG).[9] These data indicated that tamoxifen was associated with significant reduction in recurrence and death after a median follow-up of about 10 years. The annual reductions in recurrence and death with tamoxifen as compared with placebo were 26% and 14%, respectively. This means that, each year, about 1 of every 4 recurrences and 1 of every 6 deaths can be delayed or averted with tamoxifen treat-ment. These gains are substantially greater in women with tumors expressing ERs and in women treated for about 5 years.[9]

In women with ER-positive tumors, tamoxifen therapy results in statistically significant reductions in the odds of recurrence and death. Tamoxifen results in a 50% annual reduction in the recurrence rate and a 28% annual reduction in the death rate. This implies that half of the recurrences and more than a fourth of the deaths each year may be averted by tamoxifen treatment. These benefits are greater in women whose tumors have very high concentrations of ERs.[9]

The ER level should be measured in all cases of breast cancer. This may be done by ligand-binding assay or by immunohisto-chemical analysis. The interpretation of data on ER is complicated by the lack of consistency among the cut-off values chosen by various laboratories to define ER-negative results. Those with detectable but low concentrations of ERs may explain why tamoxifen was found to be beneficial in women with so-called 'ER-negative' tumors in some trials.[15] Other data suggest that tumors with any detectable level of ERs – even 1% of cells staining positive – should be considered positive.[16] Similarly, using immunohistochemical analysis, some laboratories include tumors in which 10% or even 20% of cells contain ERs as those designated as 'ER-negative'. Unless those laboratories have correlated their cut-offs with clinical follow-up data, many women may be misclassified as having ER-negative tumors, and thus may not be offered potential beneficial tamoxifen treatment.

It was originally hypothesized more than 20 years ago that PgR expression might be a better indicator of tumor endocrine responsiveness than ER alone, since its presence suggests that ER was not only present but functional.[17] In fact, the ER-negative/PgR-positive tumor phenotype does not occur frequently, and only about 5% of tumors are of this type. Tumors with this phenotype demonstrate a response rate of about 20–40%.[18] Therefore, ER- and PgR-positive tumors should be considered good candidates for tamoxifen therapy. In cases of metastatic breast cancer, the presence of PgR indicates a greater likelihood of response to tamoxifen than its absence,[19,20] but a finding of PgR receptors is less useful in selecting women for adjuvant therapy with this drug.[9]

Preclinical studies suggest that tamoxifen is primarily cytostatic, and therefore prolonged therapy may be more effective than short periods of treatment.[21] Two North American trials comparing tamoxifen treatment for 5 or 10 years,[12,14] and a Scottish trial comparing tamoxifen for 5 years with indefinite treatment[13] have been published, showing no additional benefit with prolonged therapy. However, in the Eastern Cooperative Oncology Group (ECOG) trial, a subset analysis did suggest that more than 5 years of tamoxifen may be beneficial in ER-positive, premenopausal, node-positive women.[14] This data is tentative and based on a post hoc analysis of a small number of patients. Thus, overall, there is no convincing data that treatment lasting longer than 5 years was beneficial. In addition, in the National Surgical Adjuvant Breast and Bowel Project (NSABP) study, there was a trend towards a detrimental effect after treatment for more than 5 years.[12] On the basis of these results, it is now reasonable to recommend that tamoxifen be given for 5 years. A large randomized trial, the ATLAS trial, is now underway to more definitely assess the effects of tamoxifen for more than 5 years.

Ductal carcinoma in situ

Women with ductal carcinoma in situ have a very low risk of death from breast cancer.[22] The mainstay of treatment is surgery – either a simple mastectomy or lumpectomy with or without breast irradiation. A large study evaluating the role of tamoxifen in patients who received a combination of lumpectomy and radiation therapy has shown that tamoxifen was effective in the prevention of invasive breast cancer.[23] At 5 years of follow-up, there was a 4% decrease in the number of events in tamoxifen-treated patients as compared with placebo. The reduction in events included the incidence of contralateral breast cancer as well as ipsilateral breast cancer. There was no significant difference in survival in these two groups of patients.

Benefits according to age or menopausal status

The 1992 meta-analysis suggested that tamoxifen might be of little benefit in younger women.[15] However, in this earlier analysis, many women with ER-negative tumors were included and the duration of treatment was usually for 1 or 2 years. The more recent meta-analysis has shown that women less than 50 years old benefit from tamoxifen as much as older women, and even women younger than 40 have reduced rates of recurrence and death (Table 3.2). These data suggest that tamoxifen inhibits the proliferation of breast cancer cells even in the presence of estrogen.

Table 3.2 Meta-analysis of results of adjuvant tamoxifen therapy for 5 years in women with ER-positive breast cancer, according to age[a]

Age (year)	No. of women	No. of events averted each year	
		Recurrence	Death
<40	1327	1 in 2 or 3	1 in 3 or 4
40–49	1327	1 in 2 or 3	1 in 3 or 4
50–59	2536	1 in 2 or 3	1 in 3 or 4
60–69	3174	1 in 2 or 3	1 in 3 or 4
≥70	390	1 in 2 or 3	1 in 3 or 4

[a]Data from the Early Breast Cancer Trialists' Collaborative Group.

Benefits in women with and without axillary lymph node metastases

The recent meta-analysis demonstrates similar reductions of the rates of recurrences and death for both node-negative and node-positive cancers.[9] While some have suggested continuing tamoxifen beyond 5 years for women with node-positive disease because of a greater risk of relapse, the similar efficacy in node-positive and -negative groups, and the evidence that tamoxifen for more than 5 years in node-negative women may be detrimental, makes this practice questionable outside the context of a clinical trial.

Benefits in elderly women

In many older women, the presence of concurrent illness complicates the identification of optimal local and systemic treatments. However, tamoxifen is beneficial in women 70 years of age and older (Table 3.2).[9] The reduction in rates of recurrence is substantial, and these women tolerate the drug well. In elderly women, tamoxifen may not be an adequate substitute for definitive surgical treatment, since trials comparing tamoxifen alone as primary therapy versus tamoxifen plus surgery demon-

strate a higher local failure rate with tamoxifen alone.

Tamoxifen in combination with adjuvant chemotherapy

Because of the benefits both of adjuvant tamoxifen and of adjuvant chemotherapy, trials were initiated to assess the benefits of these treatments given together in premenopausal women – most showed that the combination therapy offered little benefit.[24,25] However, many of these trials included women who were ER-negative or whose ER status was unknown, and in some cases tamoxifen was only given for 1–2 years. In the meta-analysis of 5 years of treatment of women with ER-positive tumors, tamoxifen plus chemotherapy was superior to the same chemotherapy given alone – not only women 50 years and older but also younger women[9] (Table 3.2).

Given the established benefits of tamoxifen in postmenopausal women, deciding whether or not to add chemotherapy to tamoxifen is an important issue. Given the advantage in terms of disease-free survival found in the 1992 meta-analysis and in several large individualized trials,[9,26] an argument may be made for treating higher-risk postmenopausal women with both chemotherapy and tamoxifen. However, the small therapeutic gains must be weighed against the additional toxicities associated with chemotherapy[27] and individualized decisions regarding risk-to-benefit ratio must be considered.

Treatment of metastatic breast cancer

While objective response rates for chemotherapy in the treatment of metastatic disease are higher, the duration of response is usually short and treatment is associated with considerable toxicity. Treatment of women with steroid receptor-positive metastatic breast cancer with tamoxifen has lower toxicity and cost. Response to tamoxifen, when prolonged stable disease is included, has a clinical benefit rate equal to or greater than that of chemotherapy. It has traditionally been thought that women with more indolent disease (a disease-free interval lasting more than 2 years after initial surgery, soft tissue, bone, nodular, and lung metastases) had the best response to tamoxifen. This is because these patients are more commonly receptor-positive. The critical determinant of likelihood of response is ER status. More recent evidence indicates that those with visceral or liver metastases are just as likely to respond as those with metastases in other areas.[19] Women should be treated sequentially after initial response with multiple endocrine therapies until the tumors no longer respond, at which point chemotherapy is then indicated. Overall, about 30% of women treated with tamoxifen had objective regression of tumor for an average of 12 months, and in another 20% the disease remained stable for at least 6 months.[28] In total, about half of all women with ER-positive tumors receive some benefit from tamoxifen, as compared with only about 5% of tumors in which ERs cannot be detected.

Resistance

New or acquired resistance limits the efficacy of tamoxifen in many patients with breast cancer. Although the mechanisms that underlie primary or acquired tamoxifen resistance are not definitively understood, several possibilities exist. Some tumors become hormone-independent despite the presence of ERs; in others, tumors that are initially ER-positive become ER-negative over time. Yet, at least two-thirds of the tumors that become resistant to tamoxifen continue to express ER, and many of these regress when second-line hormonal therapy is initiated.[28]

In some patients, the disease not only progresses during tamoxifen therapy but actually becomes stimulated by tamoxifen. Tamoxifen-stimulated growth explains the withdrawal response that occurs with some patients when the drug is stopped because of tumor regression.[29] Other mechanisms of tamoxifen resistance include the presence of variant ERs, altered expression of other transcription factors that interact with ERs, and 'crosstalk' between ERs and other growth factor signal transduction pathways.[3,29]

Ancillary benefits

Cardiovascular benefits

In women with breast cancer, some individualized trials of adjuvant therapy have suggested that non-breast-cancer-related deaths may be reduced by tamoxifen treatment, while others have not.[12] This reduction appears to be largely due to a decrease in deaths from cardiovascular causes.[30] Serum concentrations of total cholesterol and low-density lipoproteins are reduced by tamoxifen. This drug may also inhibit atherosclerosis by directly affecting the metabolism of low-density lipoproteins in the arteries. However, the meta-analysis did not confirm a reduction in the incidence of non-cancer-related deaths.[9] In the NSABP P1 trial, in which tamoxifen was compared with placebo for breast cancer prevention, no reduction in cardiac events or death was observed. It may be that any beneficial effect of reduction by tamoxifen is offset by the changes that promote clotting or atheroma formation.[31]

Changes in bone mineral density

In postmenopausal women, long-term tamoxifen treatment increases the bone density of the axial skeleton and the appendicular skeleton.[32] In premenopausal women, however, tamoxifen may decrease the bone mineral density, perhaps by antagonizing the more potent activity of endogenous estrogen.[33]

Prevention of contralateral breast cancer and of breast cancer in women with high risk

Tamoxifen reduces the incidence of contralateral breast cancer. Individual trials and the updated meta-analysis from the EBCTCG indicated that there is a nearly 50% reduction in the risk of contralateral breast cancer after 5 years of treatment.[9,34] These results have provided a rationale for the trials assessing tamoxifen for the prevention of breast cancer in women at risk of the disease. Results from one of the studies, a prevention trial of long-term tamoxifen therapy involving over 13 000 women at increased risk of breast cancer, have shown a 45% reduction in the incidence of breast cancer with tamoxifen when compared with placebo (85 versus 154 cases).[31] According to these findings, tamoxifen for prevention might be considered for women at high risk, but extrapolation of these results to other women is unwarranted. Benefits of tamoxifen for prevention are balanced against risks of endometrial cancer and clotting, especially in postmenopausal women.

Toxicity

Tamoxifen is usually very well tolerated by most patients with breast cancer. In the early trials for adjuvant therapy, fewer than 5% of patients withdrew from therapy because of toxicity.

Menopausal symptoms

The most common adverse events of tamoxifen are menopausal symptoms, and these are more common in premenopausal women. At least 50% of women treated with tamoxifen report hot flashes – but so do 20–40% of women given placebo. Vaginal discharge and irregular menses are also more common in women treated with tamoxifen when compared with placebo.[35]

Embolic and hematologic effects

An increased incidence of thromboembolism has been attributed to tamoxifen in some studies, both in healthy women[31] and when tamoxifen is combined with chemotherapy.[36] This complication occurs in about 1% of postmenopausal patients given tamoxifen for 5 years, and deaths due to thromboembolism have been reported.[31] The risk of thrombosis appears to be decreased in women who are less than 50 years old.[31]

Endometrial and other cancers

The most serious adverse effect of tamoxifen may be its carcinogenic potential. Tamoxifen is experimentally genotoxic and in some strains of rats may cause liver cancers. High levels of stable DNA adducts have been found by postlabeling with phosphorus-32 in rat livers, although in humans there is no apparent increase in adduct formation in liver or endometrial tissue obtained from women on tamoxifen.[37,38] In women treated for breast cancer, the clinical data at present indicate no evidence of increased risk of liver or other cancers (apart from cancer of the endometrium) in those receiving tamoxifen at 20 mg/day.[31] At 40 mg/day, the Scandinavian Adjuvant Trial indicates a possible increase in the risk of gastrointestinal tumors,[39] although this has not been substantiated in any other trial.

More serious is an increased risk in endometrial cancer, similar to that in women receiving estrogen-replacement therapy. This may be related to tamoxifen's estrogenic activity rather than being a direct carcinogenic effect.[35] Nearly all reported endometrial cancers have been in postmenopausal women. In a large 5-year trial of tamoxifen, the annual hazard rate was 1.7 per 1000 women – a relative risk of 2.2 as compared with the population-based rates of endometrial cancer.[35] This translates into a 1% increase in endometrial cancer risk in postmenopausal women taking 5 years of tamoxifen. Most of these cancers are of low grade and stage, similar to that associated with estrogen therapy. In the most recent meta-analysis, the incidence of endometrial cancer was increased and the risk of mortality from endometrial cancer was slightly increased, especially with prolonged treatment.[9]

Miscellaneous effects

There have been sporadic case reports of eye problems associated with tamoxifen medication. Very high doses of tamoxifen (180 mg/day or more) are associated with a characteristic retinopathy and keratopathy. At lower doses, one report indicated evidence of a non-specific retinopathy in 4 of 63 patients that has not been confirmed in other controlled studies.

Acute hepatic toxicity and agranulocytosis have been reported as anecdotal events, the significance of which remains in doubt.

Summary of the clinical use of tamoxifen

Tamoxifen significantly reduces the risk of recurrence and death from breast cancer when given as adjuvant therapy, and it provides effective palliation for patients with advanced breast cancers. It is indicated for both pre- and postmenopausal women who have ER-positive invasive breast cancer. Tamoxifen is also the initial hormonal therapy of choice for postmenopausal women with hormone-receptor-positive metastatic breast cancer, and it is used as either first- or second-line therapy in younger women. It is generally well tolerated and safe, but the risk of endometrial cancer and clotting events is increased. The possible beneficial effects of tamoxifen on bone density and the risk of contralateral breast cancer are added benefits. Increasing data are becoming available on its role in the prevention of breast cancer in women at high risk of the disease.

NEWER TRIPHENYLETHYLENES

Toremifene

Pharmacology and biology

Toremifene is extensively metabolized in animals and humans, with a terminal elimination half-life of 5 days.[40,41] It shows weak estrogen-like properties in the postmenopausal patients. LH and FSH are depressed and sex hormone-binding globulin (SHBG) is increased.[42] Like tamoxifen, toremifene produces estrogen-like effects on the histology of the postmenopausal endometrium.[43]

Clinical use

The initial phase I studies show that toremifene is well tolerated, with activity and minimal toxicity in breast cancer patients.[42] Several phase II trials of toremifene have been reported in postmenopausal patients with advanced disease who have not received prior hormonal or cytotoxic chemotherapy.[44,45] In 46 previously untreated patients with ER-positive metastatic disease, Valavaara et al[44] reported a 63% objective response rate (complete response rate 37%, partial response rate 26%) with toremifene 60 mg/day orally. Responses were observed in soft tissue and visceral sites of disease. Toxicity was mild, with hot flashes occurring in 22% of patients. Gunderson et al[45] reported a 48% response rate in a group of 23 patients with advanced disease, 20 of whom had received no prior therapy. The median duration of response was approximately 14 months. Hot flashes were reported in approximately half of the patients.

In a comparative study of toremifene versus tamoxifen, 648 previously untreated, hormone-receptor-positive or -unknown, metastatic breast cancer patients were randomized between tamoxifen 20 mg/day orally or two different doses of toremifene at 60 or 200 mg/day orally.[46] Tamoxifen produced a response rate of 19% and a median survival of 32 months. Toremifene produced a response rate of 21% at the 60 mg dose and 23% at the 200 mg dose. The median survival of toremifene-treated patients was 38 months (60 mg/day) and 30 months (200 mg/day). The median time to disease progression was not statistically different between the treatment arms. Furthermore, quality-of-life assessments were not different between the arms. Toxicity was mild in all patients, but toremifene-treated patients experienced less nausea (26% versus 37%). The data from this large trial support the use of toremifene as an alternative first-line therapy to tamoxifen in hormone-receptor-positive postmenopausal patients with advanced disease.

Toremifene appears to exhibit significant cross-resistance to tamoxifen, since response rates to toremifene after tamoxifen therapy are low. The largest study was a multicenter phase II trial, in which 102 peri- or postmenopausal women with metastatic breast cancer who failed tamoxifen received toremifene 200 mg/day.[47] Patients in this trial were heavily pretreated, with 65% having failed chemotherapy and 22% having failed two or more hormonal therapies. Forty-nine percent of patients had visceral dominant disease. The objective response rate was 5%, with only two patients achieving complete response. An additional 23% of patients maintained stable disease for a median of 8 months.

Droloxifene

Pharmacology and biology
Droloxifene is rapidly absorbed and excreted, and does not appear to be accumulated like tamoxifen or toremifene. Steady-state levels were achieved rapidly within 5 hours.[48] Droloxifene causes a dose-related decrease in LH and FSH in postmenopausal women.[49]

Clinical use
There have been numerous clinical trials evaluating droloxifene in patients with metastatic breast cancer. The majority of patients on these trials have been previously treated with chemotherapy and/or hormone therapy. The daily dose of droloxifene ranges from 20 to 300 mg. The response rate ranges from 0% to 17%, with most responses occurring in peri- or postmenopausal patients. Trials evaluating different doses of droloxifene have not convincingly demonstrated a dose–response effect.[50–53]

The largest clinical trial involving patients with metastatic breast cancer treated with droloxifene has been updated.[52] This phase II study compares droloxifene in doses of 20, 40,

and 100 mg/day in postmenopausal women with metastatic, inoperable recurrent, or advanced primary breast cancer who had not received hormonal therapy. Of 369 patients randomized, 292 were eligible and 268 assessable for response. Response rates were 30% in the 20 mg group, 47% in the 40 mg group, and 44% in the 100 mg group. Those responses occurred within 2 months of stopping therapy. In all trials reported, droloxifene has been extremely well tolerated, with the most common toxicities cited being hot flashes, fatigue, and nausea.

Idoxifene

Pharmacology and biology
Idoxifene has an initial half-life of 15 hours and a terminal half-life of 23.3 days (i.e. three times greater than tamoxifen). Idoxifene also causes modest decreases in LH and FSH but no increase in SHBG.[54] A large randomized phase III trial of idoxifene versus tamoxifen has been closed because preliminary data indicated an increased incidence of endometrial polyps and uterine prolapse with idoxifene, with no significant difference in efficacy. The further development of this drug has been terminated by the sponsor.

Clinical use
Results of a phase I clinical trial in which 20 patients with advanced breast cancer (ER-positive or ER-unknown) treated with one of four dose levels of idoxifene have been reported.[54] The majority of patients previously received tamoxifen, second-line hormone therapy, and chemotherapy. Responses were observed in 14% of patients; an additional 29% of patients had stable disease for 1.4–14 months. Toxicity was mild and not dose-related.[54]

SUMMARY

The successful development of tamoxifen has created opportunities for the development of new drugs that could be applied throughout medicine. Triphenylethylene derivatives with antiestrogenic properties are currently being developed with the possibility of different therapeutic roles. Direct comparison of these compounds is difficult, and there remain significant gaps in our knowledge about the efficacy and long-term safety of these new agents. In the future, new antiestrogens with more favorable toxicity profiles may be developed, and they should be tested against tamoxifen as the gold standard of therapy in terms of both efficacy and acceptable adverse toxicity profile in breast cancer patients.

REFERENCES

1. Jordan VC. The development of tamoxifen for breast cancer therapy. In: *Long-Term Tamoxifen Treatment for Breast Cancer* (Jordan VC, ed). Madison: University of Wisconsin Press, 1994: 3–26.
2. Langan FSM, Jordan VC, Frits NF et al. Clinical pharmacology and endocrinology of long-term tamoxifen therapy. In: *Long-Term Tamoxifen Treatment for Breast Cancer* (Jordan VC, ed). Madison: University of Wisconsin Press, 1994.
3. Osborne CK, Elledge RM, Fuqua SAW. Estrogen receptors in breast cancer therapy. *Sci Med* 1996; **3**: 32–41.
4. Buckley M-T, Goa KL. Tamoxifen: a reappraisal of its pharmacodynamic and pharmacokinetic properties, and therapeutic use. *Drugs* 1989; **37**: 451–90.
5. Lien EA, Solheim E, Ueland PM. Distribution of tamoxifen and its metabolites in rat and human tissues during steady-state treatment. *Cancer Res* 1991; **51**: 4837–44.
6. Lodwick R, McConkey B, Brown AM. Life threatening interaction between tamoxifen and warfarin. *BMJ* 1987; **295**: 1141.
7. Jordan VC, Fritz NF, Langan-Fahey SM et al. Alteration of endocrine parameters in premenopausal women with breast cancer during long-term adjuvant therapy with tamoxifen as the single agent. *J Natl Cancer Inst* 1991; **83**: 1488–91.
8. Ravdin PM, Fritz NF, Tormey DC, Jordan VC. Endocrine status of premenopausal node-positive breast cancer patients following adjuvant

chemotherapy and long-term tamoxifen. *Cancer Res* 1988; **48**: 1026–9.
9. Early Breast Cancer Trialists' Collaborative Group (EBCTCG). Tamoxifen for early breast cancer: an overview of the randomized trials. *Lancet* 1998; **351**: 1451–67.
10. Ellis PA, Saccani-Jotti G, Clarke R et al. Induction of apoptosis by tamoxifen and ICI 182780 in primary breast cancer. *Int J Cancer* 1997; **72**: 608–13.
11. Webb P, Lopez GN, Uht RM. Tamoxifen activation of the estrogen receptor stroke AP-1 pathway: potential origin for the cell-specific estrogen-like effects of antiestrogen. *Mol Endocrinol* 1995; **9**: 443–56.
12. Fisher B, Dignam J, Bryant J et al. Five years versus more than five years of tamoxifen therapy for breast cancer patients with negative lymph nodes and estrogen receptor-positive tumors. *J Natl Cancer Inst* 1996; **88**: 1529–42.
13. Stewart HJ, Forrest AP, Everington D et al. Randomised comparison of 5 years of adjuvant tamoxifen with continuous therapy for operable breast cancer: the Scottish Cancer Trials Breast Group. *Br J Cancer* 1996; **74**: 297–9.
14. Tormey DC, Gray R, Falkson HC et al. Post-chemotherapy adjuvant tamoxifen therapy beyond five years in patients with lymph node-positive breast cancer. *J Natl Cancer Inst* 1996; **88**: 1828–33.
15. Early Breast Cancer Trialists' Collaborative Group (EBCTCG). Systemic treatment of early breast cancer by hormonal, cytotoxic or immune therapy: 133 randomised trials involving 31,000 recurrences and 24,000 deaths among 75,000 women. *Lancet* 1992; **339**: 1–15, 71–85.
16. Clark GM, Harvey JM, Osborne CK, Allred DC. Estrogen receptor status determined by immunohistochemistry is superior to biochemical ligand-binding assay for evaluating breast cancer patients. *Proc Am Soc Clin Oncol* 1997; **16**: 129a.
17. Horwitz KB, McGuire WL, Pearson OH, Segaloff A. Predicting response to endocrine therapy in human breast cancer: a hypothesis. *Science* 1975; **189**: 726–7.
18. Osborne CK, Yochmowitz MG, Knight WAI, McGuire WL. The value of estrogen and progesterone receptors in the treatment of breast cancer. *Cancer* 1980; **46**: 2884–8.
19. Ravdin PM, Green S, Dorr TM et al. Prognostic significance of progesterone receptor levels in

estrogen receptor-positive patients with metastatic breast cancer treated with tamoxifen: results of a prospective Southwest Oncology Group study. *J Clin Oncol* 1992; **10:** 1284–91.

20. Elledge RM, Green S, Pugh RP et al. Estrogen receptor (ER) and progesterone receptor (PgR) by ligand-binding assay compared with ER, PgR, and pS2 by immuno-histochemistry in predicting response to tamoxifen in metastatic breast cancer: a Southwest Oncology Group Study. *Int J Cancer* 2000; **89:** 111–17.

21. Osborne CK, Coronado E, Robinson JP. Human breast cancer in the athymic nude mouse: cytostatic effects of long-term antiestrogen therapy. *Eur J Cancer Clin Oncol* 1987; **23:** 1189–96.

22. Morrow M, Schnitt SJ, Harris JR. Ductal carcinoma is situ. In: *Diseases of the Breast* (Harris JR, Lippman ME, Morrow M, Hellman S, eds). Philadelphia: Lippincott-Raven, 1996.

23. Fisher B, Dignam J, Wolmark N et al. Tamoxifen in treatment of intraductal breast cancer: National Surgical Adjuvant Breast and Bowel Project B-24 randomised controlled trial. *Lancet* 1999; **353:** 1986–7.

24. Boccardo R, Rubagotti A, Bruzzi P et al. Chemotherapy versus tamoxifen versus chemotherapy plus tamoxifen in node-positive, estrogen receptor-positive breast cancer patients: results of a multicenter Italian study. *J Clin Oncol* 1990; **8:** 1310–20.

25. Tormey DC, Gray R, Gilchrist K et al. Adjuvant chemohormonal therapy with cyclophosphamide, methotrexate, 5-fluorouracil, and prednisone (CMFP) or CMFP plus tamoxifen compared with CMF for premenopausal breast cancer patients: an Eastern Cooperative Oncology Group trial. *Cancer* 1990; **65:** 200–6.

26. Fisher B, Redmond C, Legault-Poisson S et al. Postoperative chemotherapy and tamoxifen compared with tamoxifen alone in the treatment of positive-node breast cancer patients age 50 years and older with tumors responsive to tamoxifen: results from the National Surgical Adjuvant Breast and Bowel Project B-16. *J Clin Oncol* 1990; **8:** 1005–18.

27. Goldhirsch A, Gelman RS, Gelber RD, Castiglione M. Treatment of breast cancer in elderly patients. *Lancet* 1990; **336:** 564.

28. Saez RA, Osborne CK. Hormonal treatment of advanced breast cancer. In: *Breast Cancer* (Kennedy BJ, ed). New York: Alan R Liss, 1989.

29. Wiebe VJ, Osborne CK, Fuqua SAW, DeGregorio MW. Tamoxifen resistance in breast cancer. *Crit Rev Oncol Hematol* 1993; **14:** 173–88.

30. McDonald CC, Steward HJ. Fatal myocardial infarction in the Scottish Adjuvant Trial. The Scottish Breast Cancer Committee. *Br J Cancer* 1991; **303:** 435–7.

31. Fisher B, Costantino J, Wickerham DL et al. Tamoxifen for prevention of breast cancer: report of the National Surgical Adjuvant Breast and Bowel Project P-1 study. *J Natl Cancer Inst* 1998; **90:** 1371–88.

32. Love RR, Mazess RB, Barden HS et al. Effects of tamoxifen on bone mineral density in postmenopausal women with breast cancer. *N Engl J Med* 1992; **326:** 852–6.

33. Powles TJ, Hickish T, Kanis JA et al. Effects of tamoxifen on bone mineral density measured by dual-energy x-ray absorptiometry in healthy premenopausal and postmenopausal women. *J Clin Oncol* 1996; **14:** 78–84.

34. Skoog L, Wilking N, Humla S et al. Estrogen and progesterone receptors and modal DNA value in tumor cells obtained by fine-needle aspiration from primary breast carcinomas during tamoxifen treatment. *Diagn Oncol* 1991; **1:** 282–7.

35. Fisher B, Costantino J, Redmond C et al. Endometrial cancer in tamoxifen-treated breast cancer patients: findings from the National Surgical Adjuvant Breast and Bowel Project (NSABP) B-14. *J Natl Cancer Inst* 1994; **86:** 527–37.

36. Pritchard KI, Paterson AH, Paul NA et al. Increased thromboembolic complications with concurrent tamoxifen and chemotherapy in a randomized trial of adjuvant therapy for women with breast cancer. *J Clin Oncol* 1996; **14:** 2731–7.

37. Martin EA, Rich KJ, White IN et al. ^{32}P-postlabelled DNA adducts in liver obtained from women treated with tamoxifen. *Carcinogenesis* 1995; **16:** 1651–4.

38. Carmichael PL, Ugwumadu AH, Neven P et al. Lack of genotoxicity of tamoxifen in human endometrium. *Cancer Res* 1996; **56:** 1475–9.

39. Rutqvist LE, Johanson H, Signomklao IU et al. Adjuvant tamoxifen therapy for early stage breast cancer and second primary malignancies. Stockholm Breast Cancer Study Group. *J Natl Cancer Inst* 1995; **87:** 645–51.

40. Antila M, Valavaara R, Kivinen S et al. Pharmacokinetics of toremifene. *J Steroid Biochem* 1990; **36:** 249–52.

41. Kangas L. Biochemical and pharmacological

effects of toremifene metabolites. *Cancer Chemother Pharmacol* 1990; **27:** 8–12.

42. Hamn JT, Tormey DC, Kholer PC et al. Phase I study of toremifene in patients with advanced cancer. *J Clin Oncol* 1991; **9:** 2036–41.

43. Tomas E, Kauppila A, Blanco G et al. Comparison between the effects of tamoxifen and toremifene on the uterus in postmenopausal breast cancer patients. *Gynecol Oncol* 1995; **59:** 261–6.

44. Valavaara R, Pyrhonen S, Heikkinen M et al. Toremifene, a new antiestrogenic treatment of advanced breast cancer. Phase II study. *Eur J Cancer* 1988; **24:** 785–90.

45. Gunderson S. Toremifene, a new antiestrogenic compound in the treatment of advanced breast cancer. Phase II study. *Eur J Cancer* 1990; **24:** 785–90.

46. Hayes DF, Van Zyl JA, Hacking A et al. Randomized comparison of tamoxifen and two separate doses of toremifene in postmenopausal patients with metastatic breast cancer. *J Clin Oncol* 1995; **113:** 2556–66.

47. Vogel CL, Shemano I, Schoenfelder J et al. Multicenter phase II efficacy trial of toremifene in tamoxifen-refractory patients with advanced breast cancer. *J Clin Oncol* 1993; **11:** 345–50.

48. Grill HJ, Pollow K. Pharmacokinetics of drolox- ifene and its metabolites in breast cancer patients. *Am J Clin Oncol* 1991; **14**(Suppl 2): s21–9.

49. Geisler J, Ekse D, Hosch S, Lonning PE. Influence of droloxifene (3-hydroxytamoxifen), 40 mg daily, on plasma gonadotrophins, sex hormone binding globulin and estrogen levels in post-menopausal breast cancer patients. *J Steroid Biochem Mol Biol* 1995; **55:** 193–5.

50. Bellmunt J, Sole L. European early phase II dose finding study of droloxifene in advanced breast cancer. *Am J Clin Oncol* 1991; **14:** 536–9.

51. Haarstad H, Gundersen S, Wist E et al. Droloxifene – a new anti-estrogen. A phase II study in advanced breast cancer. *Acta Oncol* 1992; **31:** 425–8.

52. Rausching W, Pritchard KI. Droloxifene, a new antiestrogen: its role in metastatic breast cancer. *Breast Cancer Res Treat* 1994; **31:** 83–94.

53. Buzdar AU, Kau S, Hortobagyi GN et al. Phase I trial of droloxifene in patients with metastatic breast cancer. *Cancer Chemother Pharmacol* 1994; **33:** 313–16.

54. Coombes RC, Haynes BP, Dowsett M et al. Idoxifene: report of a phase I study in patients with metastatic breast cancer. *Cancer Res* 1995; **55:** 1070–4.

4

Selective estrogen receptor modulators (SERMs)

Anthony Howell, Stephen RD Johnston

INTRODUCTION

Ever since evidence emerged that human breast carcinomas may be associated with estrogen, attempts have been made to block or inhibit estrogen's biological effects as a therapeutic strategy for women with breast cancer. Estrogen has important physiological effects on the growth and function of hormone-dependent reproductive tissues, including normal breast epithelium, uterus, vagina, and ovaries, as well as preserving bone mineral density and reducing the risk of osteoporosis, protecting the cardiovascular system by reducing cholesterol levels, and modulating cognitive function and behaviour. Thus a strategy to block or reduce estrogen function in an attempt to treat/prevent breast cancer could have a severe impact on a woman's health by interfering with normal estrogen-regulated tissues.

For over 50 years, synthetic antiestrogens have been developed as treatment for estrogen receptor (ER)-positive breast cancer. The synthetic estrogen diethylstilbestrol and the triphenylethylene derivative trichlorophenylethylene were the first hormonal compounds to be used clinically that interacted with the estrogen receptor, with efficacy in advanced breast cancer.[1-3] Tamoxifen is now the most widely used and tested drug in breast cancer, and is now recognized to significantly improve survival as adjuvant therapy in early breast cancer,[4,5] as well as reducing the incidence of breast cancer in healthy women at risk of the disease.[6] Despite concerns about unfavourable antiestrogenic effects on healthy tissues, paradoxically it was discovered that tamoxifen acted as an estrogen on bone, blood lipids and the endometrium.[7] In the adjuvant setting, the increased risk of endometrial cancer due to the use of tamoxifen has been perceived as small in relation to the substantial benefit from reduction in breast-cancer-related events.[8] However, both in adjuvant and metastatic therapy with tamoxifen, breast epithelial cells and established tumours adapt to chronic antiestrogen exposure and develop resistance to tamoxifen, which may relate to the partial agonist effect of tamoxifen in stimulating tumour growth (reviewed by Osborne and Fuqua[9] and by

Johnston[10]). Experimental models have shown that novel antiestrogens devoid of agonist effects can antagonize tamoxifen-stimulated growth,[11] and, treatment of hormone-sensitive tumours, may delay the emergence of resistance. This generated the hope that better agents with an improved antiestrogen/estrogen profile may overcome this form of resistance and improve further on the efficacy of tamoxifen in treating breast cancer.

The ability of separate antiestrogens to have alternative effects on various estrogen-regulated targets led to the use of the term selective estrogen receptor modulators (SERMs) to describe this class of drugs. High-dose estrogens have not been considered as SERMs until recently, but it is clear that these agents also have antiestrogenic effects on tumours and estrogenic effects on the breast and endometrium for example. It is now possible to develop SERMs ranging from full estrogen agonists to pure antagonists with different effects in separate target tissues. As such, SERMs offer the potential to treat and prevent a number of conditions, ranging from osteoporosis, menopausal symptoms, cardiovascular disease, and breast/endometrial cancer. This chapter reviews the development of SERMs in breast cancer, addressing in particular the limitations of tamoxifen that this has attempted to overcome, and the clinical data available to date with regard to each of the SERM compounds.

HIGH-DOSE ESTROGENS – THE FIRST SERMs

Testosterone was the first additive systemic therapy for breast cancer, but this was rapidly followed by high-dose estrogens, particularly diethylstilbestrol[1–3] and ethinylestradiol.[12] Several other estrogens have been used, including dienestrol,[13] conjugated equine estrogens,[14,15] and estradiol diproprionate.[16]

In randomized trials, DES or ethinylestradiol were generally equivalent to triphenylethylene antiestrogens, although the studies were very small by modern standards[12] (Table 4.1). The 20-year results of the largest study of this type have been reported.[17] The response rates were non-significantly higher for DES compared with tamoxifen, and there was a survival advantage for the patients treated with DES. Importantly, responses were seen to both agents at crossover, suggesting a degree of non-cross-resistance between these two classes of SERMs (Table 4.2).

Table 4.1 Summary of clinical trials comparing estrogen and antiestrogen therapy for advanced breast cancer

Treatment[a]	No. of patients	Antiestrogen	Estrogen
Tam vs EE_2 (Beex, 1981)[111]	63	10/33 (33%)	9/29 (31%)
Naf vs EE_2 (Heuson, 1975)[112]	98	15/49 (31%)	7/49 (14%)
Tam vs DES (Ingle, 1981)[113]	143	23/69 (33%)	30/74 (41%)
Tam vs DES (Paschold, 1981)[114]	37	3/16 (19%)	4/11 (36%)
Tam vs DES (Stewart, 1980)[115]	72	9/29 (31%)	6/27 (22%)
Tam vs EE_2 (Matelski, 1985)[12]	43	10/19 (53%)	6/24 (25%)

[a]Tam, tamoxifen; EE_2, ethinylestradiol; Naf, nafoxidine; DES, diethylstilbestrol.

Table 4.2 Diethylstilbestrol (5 mg three times daily) versus tamoxifen (20 mg once daily) in first-line treatment for advanced breast cancer[17]

	Tamoxifen	Diethylstilbestrol
No. of patients	69	74
CR	6 (9%)	8 (11%)
PR	17 (25%)	23 (31%)
CR + PR	23 (34%)	31 (42%)
MDR	9.9	11.8
5-year survival rate	16%	35%
Median survival	2.4 years	3.0 years
Second response	5/16 (31%)	6/28 (21%)

CR, complete response; PR, partial response; MDR, median duration of response (months).

We have studied the effectiveness of DES in a group of 30 patients with advanced breast cancer after a median of four previous endocrine therapies.[18] Twenty nine percent of patients obtained clinical benefit for a median duration of 49 weeks, indicating the usefulness of this 'old' type of SERM treatment. In general, large doses of DES (5 mg three times daily) and ethinylestradiol (3 mg once daily) have been used, leading to greater toxicity compared with triphenylethylenes. It might be possible to use treatments giving lower serum concentrations, which may be less toxic and lead to the reestablishment of this type of SERM therapy to provide additional choice of treatment. In this regard, Stoll[19] showed that responses in advanced breast cancer could be obtained with the doses of hormones used in the contraceptive pill.[19]

NOVEL SERMs – POTENTIAL ADVANTAGES FOR BREAST CANCER

An understanding of how the triphenylethylene antiestrogen tamoxifen interacts with ER has allowed novel SERMs to be synthesized that possess an improved antiestrogenic/estrogenic profile. These drugs have been developed with the aim of retaining both the antagonist activity of tamoxifen within the breast and its agonist profile in bone and the cardiovascular system, yet at the same time eliminating unwanted agonist effects on the gynaecological tract, in particular the uterus. Non-steroidal SERMs fall into two broad categories: those that are structurally similar to the triphenylethylene structure of tamoxifen, and those that are structurally different and more closely related to the benzothiophene structure of raloxifene (Figure 4.1). A third class of antiestrogen includes the steroidal antiestrogen (fulvestrant, ICI 182,780, Faslodex), which is a structural derivative of estradiol with a long hydrophobic side-chain at the 7α position (Figure 4.1).[20] Pharmacologically, these latter compounds are pure antiestrogens that not only impair ER dimerization but also induce ER degradation,[21,22] and thus act as potent antiestrogens in all tissues, including the breast, uterus, and probably bone.

Each of the SERMs demonstrated pharmacological or pharmacodynamic benefit over tamoxifen in various preclinical studies, and as a

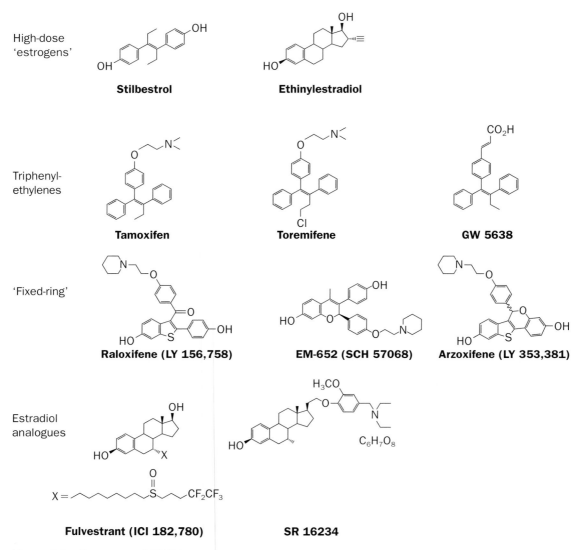

Figure 4.1 Structures of SERMs.

consequence had a profile that supported their clinical development in women with advanced breast cancer in the hope of producing a more effective and beneficial antiestrogen. The potential preclinical advantage for these SERMs included greater potency due to enhanced affinity for ER, greater efficacy compared with tamoxifen against breast cancer in vitro or in vivo, and reduced risk of toxicity compared with tamoxifen on end organs such as the liver and endometrium (Table 4.3). If resistance to tamoxifen occurs in part due to the agonist effects of the drug stimulating tumour regrowth,[9,10,23] then SERMs would be expected to either be active against tamoxifen-resistant tumours or delay the emergence of resistance. In the clinic, this profile would be manifest either as a superior response rate or as a delay in the emergence of resistance during long-term therapy. As such, one might expect to see evidence of activity for SERMs in phase II studies in tamoxifen-resistant breast cancer, or alternatively an increased duration of clinical response or time to disease progression compared with tamoxifen in randomized phase III trials as first-line therapy for ER-positive hormone-sensitive breast cancer (Table 4.3). The progress to date with each SERM compound is reviewed below – in particular, with regard to recent data from clinical trials of SERMs in women with either tamoxifen-resistant or hormone-sensitive breast cancer.

TAMOXIFEN-LIKE TRIPHENYLETHYLENE SERMs

Of the triphenylethylene derivatives, clinical data from phase II/III clinical trials in women

with advanced breast cancer have been published with three triphenylethylene tamoxifen-like compounds (toremifene, droloxifene, and idoxifene). For each one, preclinical data that had suggested an improved SERM profile compared with tamoxifen led to their clinical development with the hope that these may prove safer or more effective antiestrogens for the treatment of breast cancer.

Toremifene

Toremifene's only structural difference compared with tamoxifen relates to a single chlorine atom at position 4 (Figure 4.1), and the pharmacological profiles of the two drugs are similar.[24,25] Unlike tamoxifen, toremifene was found not to be hepatocarcinogenic in preclinical models,[26,27] which in part may relate to an

---

Table 4.3 The ideal profile of a novel SERM in comparison with tamoxifen

Preclinical

- Greater binding affinity for ER
- Ability to antagonize estrogen-dependent growth of breast cancer cells in vitro
- Equal or greater inhibition of hormone-dependent xenograft growth in vivo
- Activity against tamoxifen-dependent (resistant) tumours
- Delayed emergence of antiestrogen resistance in vivo
- Reduced agonist effects in uterotrophic assays
- Lack of stimulation of endometrial cancer cells in vitro/in vivo
- Lack of DNA-adduct formation
- Prevention of bone loss in ovariectomized animals

Clinical

- Activity in hormone-sensitive breast cancer, at least equivalent to that of tamoxifen
- Increase in time – to disease progression compared with tamoxifen
- Activity in tamoxifen-resistant breast cancer
- Improved side-effect profile (i.e. less hot flushes)
- No endometrial thickening/hyperplasia/cancer risk
- Preservation of bone mineral density
- Reduction in serum cholesterol

inability of toremifene compared with tamoxifen to induce DNA adducts in the rat liver.[28] Toremifene had a similar relative binding affinity (RBA) for ER compared with tamoxifen, and inhibited the growth of ER-positive breast cancer cells in vitro[29] and hormone-dependent breast cancer xenograft growth in vivo.[30] However, like tamoxifen, toremifene had estrogenic effects on both endometrial cells and the uterus in vivo,[31,32] although it had slightly reduced estrogenic effects on bone.[33] Toremifene was developed, therefore, as an alternative to tamoxifen that may have less genotoxic potential, and as such could be a safer antiestrogen for breast cancer treatment.

High-dose toremifene (120–240 mg) has been investigated in five phase II studies as second-line therapy in a total of 260 patients with tamoxifen-resistant breast cancer. These patients had failed to respond to tamoxifen for advanced disease, had progressed after an initial response, or had relapsed on adjuvant tamoxifen. In the largest study of 102 patients who had been treated with 200 mg toremifene daily, the overall objective response rate was only 5% (95% confidence interval (CI) = 3–7%), with an additional 23% of patients who had stable disease for a median of 7.8 months, although the authors felt that the latter could relate to slow progression of an intrinsically indolent tumour.[34] Responses were more likely in those patients who had previously responded to tamoxifen for advanced disease. In the second study, 56 patients with tamoxifen-refractory breast cancer were treated with toremifene 240 mg daily.[35] Objective responses were seen in only 2 patients (4%; 95% CI = 0.5–14%), with stable disease for more than 5 months in 9 patients, with activity again more likely in previous tamoxifen responders. In the third study in 51 patients with tamoxifen-refractory disease, a higher objective response rate of 14% was seen, with an additional 19% patients having stable disease for more than 6 months.[36] However, the two other smaller studies found no responders to 240 mg toremifene in tamoxifen-refractory patients;[37,38] one of these was a randomized study against tamoxifen

with prospective crossover at progression on each antiestrogen.[38] Thus, while occasional tamoxifen-refractory patients may have an objective response to toremifene (especially if they had responded to tamoxifen previously), cross-resistance probably exists between the two drugs.[39]

As first-line therapy in hormone-sensitive advanced breast cancer, five phase II studies in a total of 175 patients showed objective response rates of 48–68% with toremifene in doses of 60–240 mg daily, with a suggestion that higher response rates occurred with the 240 mg dose (reviewed by Karlsson et al[27]). Low-dose (20 mg) toremifene was associated with a response rate of only 21% in an additional small study, and was not investigated further.[40] Subsequently, there have been five large phase III randomized controlled trials published that have compared toremifene (40–60 mg) versus tamoxifen (20–40 mg) as first-line endocrine therapy in advanced breast cancer (Table 4.4).[41–46] The response rate to toremiphene in these larger multicentre studies was lower than in the phase II studies, ranging from 21% to 38%. In all of these studies, toremifene showed equivalent efficacy to tamoxifen for objective response rate, stable disease, time to disease progression, and overall survival (Table 4.4). In addition, two of these studies randomized patients between 60 mg toremifene or higher doses (200/240 mg), and found no significant difference in efficacy.[43,45] There was no difference in drug-related toxicities, and both toremifene and tamoxifen were well tolerated. A recent meta-analysis of 1421 patients from these trials showed a similar response rate for toremifene compared with tamoxifen (24% versus 25.3%), with no significant difference in time to disease progression (hazard ratio 0.98; 95% CI = 0.87–1.11) or overall survival (hazard ratio 0.98; 95% CI = 0.83–1.15).[46]

Any potential difference in carcinogenicity that had been identified in preclinical studies was not evaluated in any of these studies, and is probably of relatively little clinical significance in advanced breast cancer. However, at

Table 4.4 Summary of clinical efficacy data from the randomized phase III trials of toremifene (40–60 mg/day) versus tamoxifen (20–40 mg/day) as first-line endocrine treatment of advanced breast cancer in postmenopausal women (ER status positive or unknown)

Study	Toremifene			Tamoxifen		
	No. of patients	ORR (%)	TTP (months)	No. of patients	ORR (%)	TTP (months)
Hayes et al[42]	221	21	5.6	215	19	5.8
Pyrhonen et al[43]	214	31	7.3	201	37	10.2
Gershanovich et al[44]	157	21	4.9	149	21	5.0
Nomura et al[41]	62	24	5.1	60	27	5.1
Milla-Santos et al[45]	106	38	11.9	111	32	9.2
Meta-analysis[46,a]	725	24.0	4.9	696	25.3	5.3

ORR, objective response rate, including complete and partial responses; TTP, median time to disease progression.

[a] The meta-analysis was published in 1999 and included data from the first four trials, together with an unpublished small German study, but did not include the Spanish study,[45] which was only published in 2001.

least two adjuvant studies were subsequently initiated to compare efficacy and in particular long-term tolerability and safety in early breast cancer patients. Preliminary data from approximately 900 postmenopausal node-positive patients after a median follow-up of 3.4 years has been reported, and there were no significant differences in efficacy or tolerability compared with tamoxifen.[47] In particular, the number of subsequent second cancers was similar, although longer follow-up will be needed to see if any differences emerge.

Droloxifene

Structurally, droloxifene is 3-hydroxytamoxifen. It has a tenfold higher RBA for ER compared with tamoxifen.[48] In preclinical studies, droloxifene had several potential advantages over tamoxifen, including a shorter half-life,[49] greater growth inhibition of breast cancer cells

and reduced estrogenicity in the rat uterus,[50] and absence of DNA-adduct formation or carcinogenicity.[51] However, like tamoxifen, it also behaved as an estrogen in bone, preserving bone mineral density.[52]

Early phase I/II studies suggested some efficacy in patients who had received previous tamoxifen.[53,54] A phase II study of droloxifene 100 mg daily in 26 patients who had received previous tamoxifen found a response rate of 15%, with stable disease for more than 6 months in a further 5 (19%) patients.[55] A large randomized dose-finding study of 20, 40, and 100 mg droloxifene in 369 patients as first-line therapy showed objective response rates of 30%, 47%, and 44%, respectively.[56,57] Better response duration and time to disease progression were seen with the two higher doses, and there were no significant drug-related toxicities. Other first-line phase II studies were undertaken, including one study in 39 patients that showed a response rate of 51% (95%

CI = 35–67%) and median time to progression of 8 months.[58] These first-line data suggested a level of efficacy comparable to that expected with tamoxifen, and randomized phase III studies comparing droloxifene versus tamoxifen were initiated. However, droloxifene was found to be less active than tamoxifen, and further development was stopped.[59,60]

Idoxifene

Idoxifene is a SERM that is metabolically more stable than tamoxifen as a result of a pyrrolidino side-chain, with increased binding affinity for ER due to substitution of an iodine atom at the 4 position.[61] Idoxifene inhibited hormone-dependent breast cancer growth, and was more effective than tamoxifen at inhibiting both MCF-7 cell growth in vitro and rat mammary tumour growth in vivo.[62] As a SERM, idoxifene had estrogenic agonist effects on bone.[63] However, reduced agonist activity on breast cancer cells for idoxifene compared with tamoxifen in vivo was suggested by greater inhibition of MCF-7 xenograft growth in the absence of estradiol.[64] Likewise, reduced stimulation of uterine weight was seen in various uterotrophic assays.[62,63] Thus, idoxifene was developed in the hope that the reduced agonist profile in breast and gynaecological tissues would be an advantage over tamoxifen for breast cancer patients.

In a phase I study of idoxifene in 14 patients who had previously received tamoxifen, two patients had a partial response with idoxifene and 3 patients had disease stabilization for more than 6 months.[65] Results from a randomized phase II study showed little evidence of significant clinical activity for idoxifene in tamoxifen-resistant breast cancer.[66] A total of 56 postmenopausal patients with progressive locally advanced/metastatic breast cancer previously treated with tamoxifen 20 mg/day were randomized to idoxifene 40 mg/day or tamoxifen 40 mg/day. Two partial responses (objective response rate 9%) and 2 patients with stable disease were seen with idoxifene; in contrast, no objective responses were seen with higher-dose tamoxifen, although 2 patients had stable disease. In a phase III trial, a total of 220 postmenopausal women with metastatic breast cancer were randomized to receive either idoxifene 40 mg/day or tamoxifen 20 mg/day as first-line endocrine therapy.[67] Prior adjuvant tamoxifen, which had stopped at least 12 months previously, had been received by 21% and 14% of patients, respectively. The objective response rate (complete and partial responses) was 20% (95% CI = 12.7–28.2%) for idoxifene and 19% (95% CI = 12.5–28.2%) for tamoxifen, with a median duration of objective response of 8.1 months for idoxifene and 7.3 months for tamoxifen. In addition, stable disease for 6 months or more was observed in 19% of idoxifene-treated and 29% of tamoxifen-treated patients. Overall, there were no significant differences in time to disease progression or overall survival. Possible drug-related side-effects (i.e. hot flushes) were infrequent (<5%) and similar in incidence between the two groups. In particular, there was no difference in gynaecological adverse events between idoxifene and tamoxifen, although in a parallel osteoporosis programme an increased incidence of uterine prolapse and polyps was reported in idoxifene-treated women. Thus, despite a reduced agonist profile for idoxifene seen in preclinical studies, there appear to be no major differences in terms of clinical efficacy or safety profile between idoxifene and tamoxifen, and further development of the drug was stopped.

Other structural analogues of tamoxifen have been synthesized, including TAT-59 (miproxifene), which has a tenfold higher affinity for ER than tamoxifen and was more effective at inhibiting human breast cancer xenograft growth in vivo.[68,69] However it was equivalent to tamoxifen in a phase III trial, and its further development has been abandoned.[70]

Other tamoxifen-like derivatives in development

GW 5638 (Figure 4.1) is a carboxylic derivative in early clinical development that demonstrated significantly reduced agonist activity on the uterus in ovariectomized rats, yet remained a full agonist in reducing cholesterol and maintaining bone mineral density.[71] CGP 336,156 (lasofoxifene) is a derivative of tetrahydronaphthalene that maintains bone mineral density in animal models,[72] and as such may find an application for prevention of osteoporosis. There are few (if any) published clinical data for any of these compounds in advanced breast cancer.

Clinical efficacy of tamoxifen-like SERMs

From the clinical data following failure of tamoxifen in advanced breast cancer, overall little significant activity has been observed with the first-generation tamoxifen-like SERMs (toremifene, droloxifene, and idoxifene), with a median response rate from all studies of only 5% (range 0–15%) (Table 4.5). The reduced agonist profile seen with droloxifene and idoxifene

in preclinical studies may have been tissue- or cell-specific, and did not appear to manifest itself as any improved efficacy in treating or preventing tamoxifen resistance in patients with breast cancer. If the agonist activity of tamoxifen were a major mechanism for the development of resistance, one might have hoped that SERMs with reduced agonist activity might have resulted in a longer response duration or time to progression. The fact that they did not implies that, unlike the steroidal antiestrogen fulvestrant, these drugs are probably completely cross-resistant with tamoxifen. Perhaps this is not surprising, given the similar tamoxifen-like mechanism of action and structure–function interaction with ER for these triphenylethylene compounds. In contrast, fulvestrant acts by downregulating ER expression,[21,22] and this may explain why the drug appears to have much better activity in tamoxifen-resistant breast cancer than toremifene or idoxifene.[73,74]

Table 4.5 Overall efficacy of tamoxifen-like SERMs in advanced breast cancer: response rate ranges from phase II trials of toremifene, droloxifene and idoxifene in tamoxifen-resistant or hormone-sensitive patients, and from phase III trials in a first-line therapy versus tamoxifen

	Tamoxifen-resistant, phase II		Hormone-sensitive		
	ORR (%)	SD (%)	Phase II ORR (%)	Phase III ORR (%)	Phase II/III TTP (months)
Toremifene	0–14	16–30	21–68	21–38	4.9–11
Droloxifene	15	19	30–51	—	—
Idoxifene	9	9	—	20	6.5
Median	5	18	31		6.9

ORR, objective response rate, including complete and partial responses; SD, percentage of patients with stable disease for 6 months or more: TTP, median time to disease progression.

The definitive test of this hypothesis will be the results of the current first-line trials of fulvestrant, where one may anticipate that time to progression could be prolonged compared with tamoxifen, as has been demonstrated in xenograft models.[20]

As first-line therapy, the combined phase II/III clinical trial data for tamoxifen-like SERMs (toremiphene, droloxifene, and idoxifene) suggest a median response rate of 31% (range 20–68%), with a median time to disease progression of 6.9 months (Table 4.5). In the randomized first-line trials in hormone-sensitive advanced breast cancer, both toremifene and idoxifene were shown to be very similar to tamoxifen in terms of both clinical efficacy and toxicity,[41–45,67] while droloxifene appeared to be inferior.[59] The toxicity profile was the same, including gynaecological effects seen with idoxifene. On the basis of these current data, therefore, it is unlikely that the first-generation triphenylethylene SERMs will replace tamoxifen for advanced breast cancer, since they have failed to show superiority or any significant clinical advantage.

'FIXED-RING' SERMs

Greater optimism has surrounded the profile of second- and third-generation SERMs, in particular the possibility that this may translate into an improved clinical benefit for breast cancer patients. Much of the enthusiasm relates to the fact that these drugs appear to be devoid of any agonist activity in the endometrium, whilst at the same time appearing to be potent antiestrogens in the breast and retaining agonist activity in bone. Structurally, most of these drugs resemble the benzothiophene raloxifene, which is the most extensively studied SERM in this class.

Raloxifene

The binding affinity of raloxifene (Figure 4.1) for ER is similar to that of tamoxifen,[75] and most of the pharmacological data showed similar activity to tamoxifen in terms of inhibiting breast cancer cells in vitro and rat mammary tumour growth in vivo.[76,77] In preclinical models, the drug maintained bone mineral density[78] and reduced total cholesterol,[79] but compared with tamoxifen it had significantly less estrogenic activity on endometrial cells and could inhibit tamoxifen-stimulated endometrial cancer growth in vivo. Raloxifene was subsequently developed, and is now indicated for osteoporosis based on clinical trails that showed prevention of bone loss in postmenopausal women.[80]

While raloxifene was not developed as an antiestrogen for breast cancer, limited data exist on its activity in patients with advanced breast cancer. In a small study in 14 patients who had become resistant to tamoxifen following an initial response, only 1 patient had a minor response when treated with 200 mg raloxifene.[81] In 21 patients with ER-positive metastatic breast cancer treated with raloxifene 150 mg twice daily as first-line therapy, 4 (19%) patients had a partial response for a median duration of 22 months, with an additional 3 (14%) patients showing stable disease.[82] Raloxifene does not appear to relieve vasomotor symptoms such as hot flushes. However, during raloxifene's development for osteoporosis, it was found to significantly reduce the incidence of breast cancer (in particular ER-positive tumours) in postmenopausal women by 76% (95% CI = 56–87%), without any increase in endometrial thickening or risk to the gynaecological tract.[83,84] Because tamoxifen may also reduce breast cancer incidence, although with an increased risk of endometrial cancer and thrombotic events,[6] the current Study of Tamoxifen and Raloxifene (STAR) chemoprevention trial is comparing the effects of raloxifene with tamoxifen. The potential exists that as a SERM raloxifene may reduce breast cancer incidence with a better safety profile compared with tamoxifen, and it is hoped that this trial will clarify for which patients (i.e. at what level of breast cancer risk) benefit will be derived from chemoprevention.

Arzoxifene

Arzoxifene (LY 353381) (Figure 4.1) is a benzothiophene analogue that is a more potent antiestrogen with an improved SERM profile compared with raloxifene.[85] In particular, arzoxifene was a more potent inhibitor of breast cancer cells in vitro than either tamoxifen or raloxifene, and inhibited the growth of mammary tumour xenografts in vivo.[86,87] As a SERM, in preclinical studies, arzoxifene was a more potent agonist on bone and cholesterol metabolism than raloxifene,[88,89] with no evidence of any estrogen-like agonist effects on uterine tissues.[85] In view of these promising data, arzoxifene has entered clinical development for the treatment of breast cancer.

In a phase I study, 32 patients who had received a median of two prior endocrine therapies were treated with arzoxifene in doses ranging from 10 to 100 mg daily.[90] No significant toxicities were seen, and in particular transvaginal ultrasound showed no endometrial thickening following 3 months' therapy. Six patients had stable disease for a median of 7.7 months (range 6–33 months). In a phase II study as first-line therapy, 92 patients were randomized to either 20 or 50 mg arzoxifene daily.[91] Only 95 patients had received tamoxifen previously in the adjuvant setting. There was no difference in response rate (36% versus 34%), clinical benefit rate, which included stable disease (63% versus 64%), or time to disease progression (10.4 months versus 8.9 months). Likewise, toxicities were minor, although 30% of patients reported minor hot flushes. More recently, preliminary results were reported of a further phase II trial that compared both doses in 63 tamoxifen-resistant patients, and separately in 49 patients with hormone-sensitive disease (i.e. first-line therapy).[92] Response rates were low in the tamoxifen-resistant patients (10% for 20 mg, and 3% for 50 mg), all of whom had either relapsed on adjuvant tamoxifen after at least 1 year's therapy or progressed on tamoxifen for advanced disease following an initial response. In contrast, a response rate of 30% was seen with 20 mg arzoxifene in the hormone-sensitive group, with a further 17% having stable disease and an overall median time to progression of 8.3 months. The response rate for the 50 mg dose was somewhat lower (8%), although numbers are small (only 25 patients). Based on all the phase II data, 20 mg arzoxifene has now been taken forward into a large multicentre phase III trial against tamoxifen as first-line therapy.

EM-800

EM-800 is an orally active so-called pure non-steroidal antiestrogen that is a prodrug of the active benzopyrene derivative EM-652 (SCH 57068) (Figure 4.1).[93] The binding affinity of EM-652 for ER is significantly greater than those of estradiol, tamoxifen, raloxifene, and fulvestrant.[94] The prodrug EM-800 is a potent antiestrogen, and was more effective than 4-hydroxytamoxifen and fulvestrant at inhibiting estradiol-induced cell proliferation in breast cancer cells in vitro, and in the absence of estradiol had no agonist effects on growth.[95] In ZR-75-1 xenografts, EM-800 was significantly more effective than tamoxifen at inducing tumour regressions in vivo, and in the absence of estrone antagonized tamoxifen-stimulated tumour growth.[96] In intact mice, EM-800 was 30-fold more potent than tamoxifen at inhibiting uterine weight and reducing uterine/vaginal ER expression.[97] Likewise, EM-800 was devoid of any stimulatory effect on alkaline phosphatase activity (a sensitive marker of estrogenic activity) in Ishikawa endometrial carcinoma cells,[98] while EM-652 had no agonist activity in an immature rat uterotrophic assay.[99] In addition, studies have shown that EM-800 prevented bone loss in the ovariectomized rat[100] and lowered serum cholesterol levels.[93] Interestingly, EM-800 appears to significantly downregulate ER levels both in tumours and in normal estrogen-sensitive tissues in a similar fashion to the steroidal antiestrogen fulvestrant,[97] but its specific agonist effects on bone differentiate it from fulvestrant, which has not been shown to prevent bone loss. As such,

EM-800/EM-652 has a potentially promising SERM profile.

In terms of clinical development, a phase II study of EM-800 (20 or 40 mg) was undertaken in 43 postmenopausal women who had failed tamoxifen in either the metastatic or adjuvant setting.[93,101] There were one complete and five partial responses (response rate 14%), with most of the responses occurring in those who had received at least 3 years adjuvant tamoxifen.[101] An additional 10 (23%) patients had stable disease for more than 6 months. On the basis of these results, a randomized phase III study in patients who had failed tamoxifen was undertaken, comparing the efficacy of EM-800 (20 or 40 mg) with the third-generation aromatase inhibitor anastrozole. At the defined interim review, when over 300 patients had been entered, the efficacy was substantially less than that of anastrozole, and the trial was terminated (C Tendler, personal communication). There are no data at present on the activity of EM-800 in the first-line hormone-sensitive population.

ERA-923

ERA-923 is a novel SERM that appears to have an improved preclinical profile compared with tamoxifen and raloxifene. It is now being evaluated in a randomized dose-finding phase II trial (25 mg versus 100 mg) as second-line therapy in 100 ER-positive patients with tamoxifen-resistant metastatic breast cancer. A similar randomized phase II trial has been proposed in receptor-positive hormone-sensitive metastatic breast cancer as first-line therapy.[102]

Clinical efficacy of 'fixed-ring' SERMs

These new compounds in preclinical models appear to offer a greater increase in potency and tumour growth inhibition, together with an improved SERM profile on other tissues, in comparison with the tamoxifen-like SERMs. At the current time, there are too few clinical data to know whether these potential advantages will translate into beneficial effects for breast cancer patients. However, in tamoxifen-resistant patients, the level of activity reported for raloxifene,[81] arzoxifene,[92] and EM-800[93] are all low (Table 4.6), with a median response rate of 6.5%, which is very similar to that observed with the tamoxifen-like SERMs (Table 4.5). It is probable that activity in first-line will be similar to tamoxifen, since the only phase II data with raloxifene and arzoxifene give a median response rate of 30%, with a median time to progression of 9.4 months (Table 4.6). Results of ongoing phase II/III trials with arzoxifene and ERA-923 are awaited, but to date there is little clinical evidence to suggest that in advanced breast cancer substantial improvements in efficacy will be made over tamoxifen.

CONCLUSION – FUTURE ROLE FOR SERMs IN BREAST CANCER

It is unclear to what extent any preclinical advantages that have been observed for each of these SERMs over tamoxifen may be predictive for clinical outcome in the treatment of advanced breast cancer. So far, the clinical data in advanced breast cancer summarized above are somewhat disappointing for the tamoxifen-like SERMs. Instead, much greater potential may exist either in the adjuvant or chemopreventive setting, where an improved SERM profile on bone, lipid metabolism, and the endometrium will be of maximum benefit. It remains to be seen whether the vasomotor symptoms associated with both tamoxifen and raloxifene are any less frequent with the new SERMs. The dilemma faced by those developing these therapies, however, is the need to demonstrate clinical activity against breast cancer that is at least equivalent to that of tamoxifen. The clinical data outlined above suggest that while there is probably little role for other triphenylethylenes and 'fixed-ring' SERMs following failure of tamoxifen, their efficacy and tolerability in hormone-sensitive advanced breast cancer is probably equivalent

Table 4.6 Overall efficacy of second- and third-generation SERMs in advanced breast cancer: response rate ranges from phase II studies of raloxifene, arzoxifene, and EM-800 in tamoxifen-resistant or hormone-sensitive patients

	Tamoxifen-resistant, phase II		Hormone-sensitive, phase II	
	ORR (%)	SD (%)	ORR (%)	TTP (months)
Raloxifene	0	—	19	—
Arzoxifene	3–10	3–7	30–36	8.3–10.4
EM-800	14	23	—	—
Median	6.5	7	30	9.4

ORR, objective response rate, including complete and partial responses; SD, percentage of patients with stable disease for 6 months or more: TTP, median time to disease progression.

to that of tamoxifen. It is possible that fulvestrant will prove superior to tamoxifen in the first-line comparative phase III trial to be reported in late 2002.[103] Further studies will be needed to determine how it should be integrated into the treatment of advanced breast cancer with the new aromatase inhibitors. It is now clear that the third-generation aromatase inhibitors (i.e. letrozole and anastrozole) are probably superior and better tolerated than tamoxifen,[104,105] but it is possible, given that fulvestrant is at least equivalent to anastrozole in tamoxifen failures, that it might be superior in patients with advanced breast cancer not previously treated with tamoxifen. It also remains to be seen whether the new orally bioavailable pure antiestrogens, SR 16234 and ZK 191703 (Figure 4.1) will have equivalent or superior potency to the intramuscularly given fulvestrant.

In vitro, it is known that breast cancer cells adapt when subjected to long-term estrogen deprivation, remaining ER-positive and becoming hypersensitive to very low concentrations of estradiol.[106] It is conceivable that potent antiestrogens, including SERMs, could be active in this setting, and clinical trials with fulvestrant following aromatase inhibitor failure are in progress.

An alternative role for SERMs could be as adjuvant therapy, either alone or in combination with aromatase inhibitors, thus providing protection to the bone and cardiovascular system while enhancing antitumour efficacy. While it has always been thought that endocrine therapies are better given in sequence than in combination, this has been challenged recently by data in premenopausal ER-positive advanced breast cancer, where combined estrogen deprivation with a luteinizing hormone-releasing hormone (LHRH) agonist and an antiestrogen was superior to either therapy alone, including in terms of overall survival.[107] However, in order to develop SERMs as adjuvant therapy, there seems to be no shortcut to performing some form of clinical efficacy/safety study in advanced breast cancer. Additional evidence of a SERM's biological activity and clinical efficacy could be ascertained from short-term randomized neoadjuvant studies, as undertaken for idoxifene,[108] raloxifene,[109] and fulvestrant.[110] The next five years will be crucial to see whether the latest generation of SERMs have a significant role to play in breast cancer therapy – and more importantly what that role might be.

REFERENCES

1. Haddow A, Watkinson JM, Paterson E. Influence of synthetic oestrogens upon advanced malignant disease. *BMJ* 1944; **ii:** 393–8.
2. Binnie GG. Regression of tumours following treatment with stilboestrol and xray therapy with notes on cases of breast tumour which regressed on stilboestrol alone. *Br J Radiol* 1944; **17:** 42–5.
3. Stilboestrol for advanced breast cancer. A combined investigation. *BMJ* 1944; **ii:** 20–1.
4. Cole MP, Jones CTA, Todd IDH et al. A new antiestrogenic agent for breast cancer. An early appraisal of ICI 46,474. *Br J Cancer* 1971; **25:** 270–5.
5. Early Breast Cancer Trialists' Collaborative Group (EBCTCG). Tamoxifen for early breast cancer; an overview of the randomised trials. *Lancet* 1998; **351:** 1451–67.
6. Fisher B, Costantino JP, Wickerham DL et al. Tamoxifen for the prevention of breast cancer; report of the National Surgical Adjuvant Breast and Bowel Project P-1 study. *J Natl Cancer Inst* 1998; **90:** 1371–88.
7. Jordan VC. The development of tamoxifen for breast cancer therapy. In: *Long-Term Tamoxifen Treatment for Breast Cancer* (Jordan VC, ed). Madison: University of Wisconsin Press, 1994: 3–26.
8. Fisher B, Costantino JP, Redmond CK et al. Endometrial cancer in tamoxifen-treated breast cancer patients; findings from the National Surgical Adjuvant Breast and Bowel Project (NSABP) B-14. *J Natl Cancer Inst* 1994; **86:** 527–37.
9. Osborne CK, Fuqua SAW. Mechanisms of tamoxifen resistance. *Breast Cancer Res Treat* 1994; **32:** 49–55.
10. Johnston SRD. Acquired tamoxifen resistance in human breast cancer; potential mechanisms and clinical implications. *Anticancer Drugs* 1997; **8:** 911–30.
11. Osborne CK, Coronado-Heinsohn EB, Hilsenbeck SG et al. Comparison of the effects of a pure steroidal antioestrogen with those of tamoxifen in a model of human breast cancer. *J Natl Cancer Inst* 1995; **87:** 746–50.
12. Matelski H, Huberman M, Zipoli T et al. Randomised trial of estrogen vs tamoxifen therapy for advanced breast cancer. *Am J Clin Oncol* 1985; **8:** 128–33.
13. Walpole AL, Paterson E. Synthetic oestrogens in mammary cancer. *Lancet* 1949; **ii:** 783.
14. Council on Drugs. Androgens and oestrogens in the treatment of disseminated mammary carcinoma. Retrospective study of 1944 patients. *JAMA* 1960; **172:** 1271–83.
15. Segaloff A, Gordon D, Carabasi RA et al. Hormonal therapy of cancer of the breast VII. Effect of conjugated oestrogens (equine) on clinical course and hormone secretion. *Cancer* 1954; **7:** 758–63.
16. Taylor SG III, Slaughter DP, Smejkal V et al. The effects of sex hormones on advanced carcinoma of the breast. *J Cancer* 1948; **1:** 4.
17. Peethambaram PP, Ingle JN, Suman VJ et al. Randomised trial of stilboestrol vs tamoxifen in postmenopausal women with metastatic breast cancer. An updated analysis. *Breast Cancer Res Treat* 1999; **54:** 117.
18. Lonning PE, Taylor PD, Anker G et al. High-dose estrogen treatment in postmenopausal breast cancer patients heavily exposed to endocrine therapy. *Breast Cancer Res Treat* 2001; **67:** 111–16.
19. Stoll BA. Effect of Lyndiol, an oral contraceptive, on breast cancer. *BMJ* 1967; **i:** 150–3.
20. Wakeling AE. Similarities and distinctions in the mode of action of different classes of anti-oestrogens. *Endocr Rel Cancer* 2000; **7:** 17–28.
21. Dauvois S, Daniellan PS, White R et al. Antiestrogen ICI 164,384 reduces cellular estrogen content by increasing its turnover. *Proc Natl Acad Sci USA* 1992; **89:** 4037–41.
22. Parker MG. Action of pure antiestrogens in inhibiting estrogen receptor function. *Breast Cancer Res Treat* 1993; **26:** 131–7.
23. Howell A, Dodwell D, Anderson H et al. Response after withdrawal of tamoxifen and progestagens in advanced breast cancer. *Ann Oncol* 1992; **3:** 611–17.
24. Robinson SP, Parker CJ, Jordan VC. Preclinical studies with toremiphene as an antitumour agent. *Breast Cancer Res Treat* 1990; **16:** 9–17.
25. DiSalle E, Zaccheo T, Ornati G. Antiestrogenic

and antitumour properties of the new triphenylethylene derivative toremiphene in the rat. *J Steroid Biochem* 1990; **36**: 203–6.

26. Hard GC, Iatropoulos MJ, Jordan K et al. Major differences in the hepatocarcinogenicity and DNA adduct forming ability between toremiphene and tamoxifen in female Crl; cd (BR) rats. *Cancer Res* 1993; **53**: 4534–41.

27. Karlsson S, Hirsimaki Y, Mantyla E et al. A two-year dietary carcinogenicity study of the antiestrogen toremifene in Sprague–Dawley rats. *Drug Chem Toxicol* 1996; **19**: 245–66.

28. White IN, DeMatteis F, Davies A et al. Genotoxic potential of tamoxifen and analogues in female Fischer F344/n rats, DBA/2 and C57BL/6 mice and in human MCL-5 cells. *Carcinogenesis* 1992; **13**: 2197–203.

29. Kangas L, Nieminen A-L, Blanco G et al. A new triphenylethylene compound, Fc-1157a. II. Antitumour effects. *Cancer Chemother Pharmacol* 1986; **17**: 109–13.

30. Robinson SP, Jordan VC. Antiestrogenic action of toremiphene on hormone-dependent, -independent, and heterogenous breast tumour growth in the athymic mouse. *Cancer Res* 1989; **49**: 1758–62.

31. O'Regan RM, Cisneros A, England GM et al. Effects of the antiestrogens tamoxifen, toremifene, and ICI 182,780 on endometrial cancer growth. *J Natl Cancer Inst* 1998; **90**: 1552–8.

32. Tomas E, Kauppila A, Blanco G et al. Comparison between the effects of tamoxifen and toremifene on the uterus in post-menopausal breast cancer patients. *Gynecol Oncol* 1995; **59**: 241–66.

33. Marttunen MB, Hietanen P, Tiitinen A et al. Comparison of effects of tamoxifen and toremifene on bone biochemistry and bone mineral density in postmenopausal breast cancer patients. *J Clin Endocrinol Metab* 1998; **83**: 1158–62.

34. Vogel CL, Shemano I, Schoenfelder J et al. Multicenter phase II efficacy trial of toremiphene in tamoxifen-refractory patients with advanced breast cancer. *J Clin Oncol* 1993; **11**: 345–50.

35. Pyrhonen S, Valavaara R, Vuorinen J, Hajba A. High dose toremifene in advanced breast cancer resistant to or relapsed during tamoxifen treatment. *Breast Cancer Res Treat* 1994; **29**: 223–8.

36. Asaishi K, Tominaga T, Abe O et al. Efficacy and safety of high-dose NK 622 (toremifene citrate) in tamoxifen failed patients with breast cancer. *Gan to Kagaku Ryoho* 1993; **20**: 91–9.

37. Jonsson PE, Malmberg M, Bergljung L et al. Phase II study of high dose toremifene in advanced breast cancer progressing during tamoxifen treatment. *Anticancer Res* 1991; **11**: 873–6.

38. Stenbygaard LE, Herrstedt J, Thomsen JF et al. Toremifene and tamoxifen in advanced breast cancer – a double-blind cross-over trial. *Breast Cancer Res Treat* 1993; **25**: 57–63.

39. Wiseman LR, Goa KL. Toremifene; a review of its pharmacological properties and clinical efficacy in the management of advanced breast cancer. *Drugs* 1997; **54**: 141–60.

40. Valavaara R, Pyrhonen S. Low dose toremifene in the treatment of estrogen receptor positive advanced breast cancer in postmenopausal women. *Curr Ther Res* 1989; **46**: 966–73.

41. Nomura Y, Tominaga T, Abe O et al. Clinical evaluation of NK 622 (toremifene citrate) in advanced or recurrent breast cancer – a comparative study by a double-blind method with tamoxifen. *Jpn J Cancer Chemother* 1993; **20**: 247–58.

42. Hayes DF, Van Zyl JA, Hacking A et al. Randomised comparison of tamoxifen and two separate doses of toremifene in postmenopausal patients with metastatic breast cancer. *J Clin Oncol* 1995; **13**: 2556–66.

43. Pyrhonen S, Valavaara R, Modig H et al. Comparison of toremifene and tamoxifen in post-menopausal patients with advanced breast cancer: a randomised double-blind, the 'Nordic' phase II study. *Br J Cancer* 1997; **76**: 270–7.

44. Gershanovich M, Garin A, Baltina D et al. A phase III comparison of two toremifene doses to tamoxifen in postmenopausal women with advanced breast cancer. *Breast Cancer Res Treat* 1997; **45**: 251–62.

45. Milla-Santos A, Milla L, Rallo L, Solano V. Phase III trial of toremifene vs tamoxifen in hormonodependent advanced breast cancer. *Breast Cancer Res Treat* 2001; **65**: 119–24.

46. Pyrhonen S, Ellman J, Vuorinen J et al. Meta-analysis of trials comparing toremiphene with tamoxifen and factors predicting outcome of antiestrogen therapy in postmenopausal women with breast cancer. *Breast Cancer Res Treat* 1999; **56**: 133–43.

47. Holli K, Valvaara R, Blanco G et al. Toxicity and early survival results of a prospective randomised adjuvant trial comparing toremifene and tamoxifen in node-positive breast cancer. *Proc Am Soc Clin Oncol* 2000; **19:** 87a (Abst 334).

48. Roos WK, Oeze L, Loser R et al. Antiestrogen action of 3-hydroxy-tamoxifen in the human breast cancer cell line MCF-7. *J Natl Cancer Inst* 1983; **71:** 55–9.

49. Eppenberger U, Wosikowski K, Kung W. Pharmacologic and biologic properties of droloxifene, a new antiestrogen. *Am J Clin Oncol* 1991; **141:** S5–14.

50. Loser R, Seibel K, Roos W, Eppenberger U. In vivo and in vitro antiestrogenic action of 3-hydroxytamoxifen, tamoxifen and 4-hydroxytamoxifen. *Eur J Cancer Clin Oncol* 1985; **21:** 985–90.

51. Hasmann M, Rattel B, Loser R. Preclinical data for droloxifene. *Cancer Lett* 1994; **84:** 89–95.

52. Ke H, Simmons HA, Pierie CM et al. Droloxifene, a new estrogen antagonist/agonist, prevents bone loss in ovariectomised rats. *Endocrinology* 1995; **136:** 2435–41.

53. Stamm H, Roth R, Almendral A et al. Tolerance and efficacy of the antiestrogen droloxifene in patients with advanced breast cancer. *J Steroid Biochem* 1987; **28**(Suppl): 1085.

54. Brietbach GP, Moous V, Bastert G et al. Droloxifene; efficacy and endocrine effects in treatment of metastatic breast cancer. *J Steroid Biochem* 1987; **28**(Suppl): 1095.

55. Haarstad H, Gundersen S, Wist E et al. Droloxifene – a new antiestrogen. *Acta Oncol* 1992; **31:** 425–8.

56. Bruning PF. Droloxifene, a new antioestrogen in postmenopausal advanced breast cancer: preliminary results of a double-blind dose-finding phase II trial. *Eur J Cancer* 1992; **28A:** 1404–7.

57. Rausching W, Pritchard KI. Droloxifene, a new antiestrogen; its role in metastatic breast cancer. *Breast Cancer Res Treat* 1994; **31:** 83–94.

58. Haarstad H, Lonning P, Gundersen S et al. Influence of droloxifene on metastatic breast cancer as first-line endocrine treatment. *Acta Oncol* 1998; **37:** 365–8.

59. Dhingra K. Antiestrogens; tamoxifen, SERMs and beyond. *Invest New Drugs* 1999; **17:** 285–311.

60. Lien EA, Lonning PE. Selective oestrogen receptor modifiers (SERMs) and breast cancer therapy. *Cancer Treat Rev* 2000; **26:** 205–27.

61. McCague R, Leclerq G, Legros N et al. Derivatives of tamoxifen; dependence of antiestrogenicity on the 4-substituent. *J Med Chem* 1989; **32:** 2527–33.

62. Chander SK, McCague R, Luqmani Y et al. Pyrrolidino-4-iodotamoxifen and 4-iodotamoxifen, new analogues of the antiestrogen tamoxifen for the treatment of breast cancer. *Cancer Res* 1991; **51:** 5851–8.

63. Nuttall ME, Bradbeer JN, Stroup GB et al. A novel selective estrogen receptor modulator prevents bone loss and lowers cholesterol in ovariectomise rats and decreases uterine weight in intact rats. *Endocrinology* 1998; **139:** 5224–34.

64. Johnston SRD, Riddler S, Haynes BP et al. The novel antioestrogen idoxifene inhibits the growth of human MCF-7 breast cancer xenografts and reduces the frequency of acquired antiestrogen resistance. *Br J Cancer* 1997; **75:** 804–9.

65. Coombes RC, Haynes BP, Dowsett M et al. Idoxifene: report of a phase I study in patients with metastatic breast cancer. *Cancer Res* 1995; **55:** 1070–4.

66. Johnston SRD, Gumbrell L, Evans TRJ et al. A phase II randomised double-blind study of idoxifene (40 mg/d) vs. tamoxifen (40 mg/d) in patients with locally advanced/metastatic breast cancer resistant to tamoxifen (20 mg/d). *Proc Am Soc Clin Oncol* 1999; **18:** 109 (Abst 413).

67. Johnston SRD, Gorbunova V, Lichinister M et al. A multicentre double-blind randomised phase III trial of idoxifene versus tamoxifen as first-line endocrine therapy for metastatic breast cancer. *Proc Am Soc Clin Oncol* 2001; **20:** 29a (Abst 113).

68. Toko T, Sugimoto Y, Matsuo E et al. TAT-59, a new triphenylethylene derivative with antitumour activity against hormone-dependent tumors. *Eur J Cancer* 1990; **26:** 397–404.

69. Iiono Y, Takai Y, Ando T et al. A new triphenylethylene derivative TAT-59; hormone receptors, insulin-like growth factor 1 and growth suppression of hormone dependent MCF-7 tumours in athymic mice. *Cancer Chemother Pharmacol* 1994; **34:** 372–6.

70. Nomura Y, Nakajima M, Tominaga T et al. Late phase II study of TAT-59 (miproxifene phosphate) in advanced or recurrent breast cancer patients (a double blind comparative study with tamoxifen citrate). *Gan to Kagaku Ryoho* 1998; **25:** 1045–63.

71. Wilson TM, Norris JD, Wagner BL et al. Dissection of the molecular mechanism of action

of GW5638, a novel estrogen receptor ligand, provides insights into the role of estrogen receptor in bone. *Endocrinology* 1997; **138**: 3901–11.

72. Ke HZ, Paralkar VM, Grasser WA et al. Effects of CP-336,156, a new non-steroidal estrogen agonist/antagonist, on bone, serum cholesterol, uterus and body composition in rat models. *Endocrinology* 1998; **139**: 2068–76.

73. Howell A, DeFriend D, Robertson J et al. Response to a specific antiestrogen (ICI182,780) in tamoxifen-resistant breast cancer. *Lancet* 1995; **345**: 29–30.

74. Robertson JFR, Howell A, DeFriend D et al. Duration of remission to ICI182,780 compared to megestrol acetate in tamoxifen-resistant breast cancer. *Breast* 1997; **6**: 186–9.

75. Black LJ, Jones CD, Folcone JF. Antagonism of estrogen action with a new benzothiophene-derived antiestrogen. *Life Sci* 1983; **32**: 1031–6.

76. Moulin R, Merand Y, Poirier D. Antiestrogenic properties of keoxifene, *trans*-4-hydroxytamoxifen and ICI 164,384, a new steroidal antiestrogen, in ZR-75-1 human breast cancer cells. *Breast Cancer Res Treat* 1989; **14**: 65–76.

77. Gottardis MM, Jordan VC. The antitumor action of keoxifene (raloxifene) and tamoxifen in the *N*-nitromethylurea-induced rat mammary carcinoma model. *Cancer Res* 1987; **47**: 4020–4.

78. Jordan VC, Robinson SP. Species specific pharmacology of antiestrogens; role of metabolism. *Fed Proc* 1987; **46**: 1870–4.

79. Balfour JA, Goa KL. Raloxifene. *Drugs Aging* 1998; **12**: 335–41.

80. Delmas PD, Bjarnason NH, Mitlak BH et al. Effects of raloxifene on bone mineral density, serum cholesterol concentrations, and uterine endometrium in postmenopausal women. *N Engl J Med* 1997; **337**: 1641–7.

81. Buzdar A, Marcus C, Holmes F et al. Phase II evaluation of LY156758 in metastatic breast cancer. *Oncology* 1988; **45**: 344–5.

82. Gradishar WJ, Glusman JE, Vogel CL et al. Raloxifene HCL, a new endocrine agent, is active in estrogen receptor positive (ER+) metastatic breast cancer. *Breast Cancer Res Treat* 1997; **46**: 53 (Abst 209).

83. Cummings SR, Eckert S, Krueger KA et al. The effect of raloxifene on risk of breast cancer in postmenopausal women: results from the Multiple Outcomes of Raloxifene Evaluation (MORE) randomised trial. *JAMA* 1999; **281**: 2189–97.

84. Cauley JA, Norton L, Lippman ME et al. Continued breast cancer risk reduction in postmenopausal women treated with raloxifene: 4-year results from the MORE trial. *Breast Cancer Res Treat* 2001; **65**: 125–34.

85. Sato M, Turner CH, Wang TY et al. A novel raloxifene analogue with improved SERM potency and efficacy in vivo. *J Pharmacol Exp Ther* 1998; **287**: 1–7.

86. Fuchs-Young R, Iversen P, Shelton P et al. Preclinical demonstration of specific and potent inhibition of mammary tumour growth by new selective estrogen receptor modulators (SERMs). *Proc Am Assoc Cancer Res* 1997; **38**: A3847.

87. Johnston SRD, Riddler S, Detre S, Dowsett M. Dose-dependent inhibition of MCF-7 breast cancer xenograft growth with LY353381, a novel selective estrogen receptor modulator (SERM). *Proc Am Assoc Cancer Res* 2000; **41**: 25 (Abst 164).

88. Sato M, Zeng GQ, Rowley E et al. LY353381 × HCL; an improved benzothiophene analog with bone efficacy complementary to parathyroid hormone-(1-34). *Endocrinology* 1998; **139**: 4642–51.

89. Rowley E, Adrian MD, Bryant H et al. The new SERM LY353381 × HCL has advantages over estrogen, tamoxifen, and raloxifene in reproductive and non-reproductive tissues of aged ovariectomised rats. *Proc Am Soc Bone Min Res* 1997; A490.

90. Munster PN, Buzdar A, Dhingra K et al. Phase I study of a third generation selective estrogen receptor modulator LY353381 × HCL in metastatic breast cancer. *J Clin Oncol* 2001; **19**: 2002–9.

91. Baselga J, Llombart-Cussat A, Bellet M et al. Double-blind randomised phase II study of a selective estrogen receptor modulator in patients with locally advanced or metastatic breast cancer. *Breast Cancer Res Treat* 1999; **57**: A25.

92. Buzdar A, O'Shaughnessy J, Hudis C et al. Preliminary results of a randomised double-blind phase II study of the selective estrogen receptor modulator (SERM) arzoxifene in patients with locally advanced or metastatic breast cancer. *Proc Am Soc Clin Oncol* 2001; **20**: 45a (Abst 178).

93. Labrie F, Labrie C, Belanger A et al. EM-652 (SCH 57068), a third generation SERM acting as a pure antiestrogen in the mammary gland and endometrium. *J Steroid Biochem Mol Biol* 1999; **69**: 51–84.

94. Martel C, Provencher L, Li X et al. Binding characteristics of novel antiestrogens to the rat uterine estrogen receptors. *J Steroid Biochem Mol Biol* 1998; **64:** 199–205.

95. Simard J, Labrie CL, Belanger A et al. Characterisation of the effects of the novel non-steroidal antiestrogen EM-800 on basal and estrogen-induced proliferation of T47-D, ZR-75-1 and MCF-7 human breast cancer cells in vitro. *Int J Cancer* 1997; **73:** 104–12.

96. Couillard S, Gutman M, Labrie C et al. Comparison of the effects of the antiestrogens EM-800 and tamoxifen on the growth of human breast ZR-75-1 cancer xenografts in nude mice. *Cancer Res* 1998; **58:** 60–4.

97. Luo S, Martel C, Sourla A et al. Comparative effects of 28-day treatment with the new anti-estrogen EM-800 and tamoxifen on estrogen-sensitive parameters in intact mice. *Int J Cancer* 1997; **73:** 381–91.

98. Simard J, Sanchez R, Poirier D et al. Blockade of the stimulatory effect of estrogens, OH-tamoxifen, OH-toremifene, and raloxifene on alkaline phosphatase activity by the antiestrogen EM-800 in human endometrial adenocarcinoma Ishikawa cells. *Cancer Res* 1997; **57:** 3494–7.

99. Johnston SRD, Detre S, Riddler S, Dowsett, M. SCH 57068 is a selective estrogen receptor modulator (SERM) without uterotrophic effects compared with either tamoxifen or raloxifene. *Breast Cancer Res Treat* 2000; **64:** A163.

100. Martel C, Picard S, Richard V et al. Prevention of bone loss by EM-800 and raloxifene in the ovariectomised rat. *J Steroid Biochem Mol Biol* 2000; **74:** 45–56.

101. Labrie F, Champagne P, Labrie C et al. Response to the orally active specific antiestrogen EM-800 (SCH-57070) in tamoxifen-resistant breast cancer. *Breast Cancer Res Treat* 1997; **46:** 53 (Abst 211).

102. Greenberger L, Komm B, Miller C et al. Pre-clinical pharmacology profile of a new selective estrogen receptor modulator (SERM), ERA-923, for the treatment of ER-positive breast cancer. *Breast Cancer Res Treat* 2000; **64:** 52 (Abst 166).

103. Howell A, Osborne CK, Morris C et al. ICI 182780 (Faslodex): development of a novel, pure, antioestrogen. *Cancer* 2000; **89:** 817–25.

104. Bonneterre J, Thurlimann B, Robertson JFR et al. Anastrozole versus tamoxifen as first-line therapy for advanced breast cancer in 688 post-menopausal women: results of the tamoxifen or

arimidex randomised group efficacy and tolerability study. *J Clin Oncol* 2000; **18:** 3748–57.

105. Mouridsen H, Gershanovich M, Sun Y et al. Superior efficacy of letrozole (Femara) versus tamoxifen as first-line therapy for post-menopausal women with advanced breast cancer: results of a phase III study of the International Letrozole Breast Cancer Group. *J Clin Oncol* 2001; **19:** 2596–606.

106. Masamura S, Santner SJ, Heitjan DF, Santen RJ. Estrogen deprivation causes estradiol hypersensitivity in human breast cancer cells. *J Clin Endocrinol Metab* 1995; **80:** 2918–25.

107. Klijn JGN, Blamet RW, Boccardo F et al. Combined tamoxifen and luteinising hormone-releasing hormone (LHRH) agonist versus LHRH agonist alone in premenopausal advanced breast cancer: a meta-analysis of four randomised trials. *J Clin Oncol* 2001; **19:** 343–53.

108. Dowsett M, Dixon JM, Horgan K et al. Antiproliferative effect of idoxifene in a placebo-controlled trial in primary human breast cancer. *Clin Cancer Res* 2000; **6:** 2260–7.

109. Dowsett M, Lu Y, Hills M et al. Effect of raloxifene on Ki67 and apoptosis. *Breast Cancer Res Treat* 1999; **57:** 31.

110. DeFriend D, Howell A, Nicholson RI et al. Investigation of a new pure antiestrogen (ICI 182,780) in women with primary breast cancer. *Cancer Res* 1995; **54:** 408–14.

111. Beex L, Pieters G, Smals A et al. Tamoxifen versus ethinylestradiol in the treatment of post-menopausal women with advanced breast cancer. *Cancer Treat Reports* 1981; **65:** 179–85.

112. Heuson JC, Engelsman E, Blank-van der Wijst J et al. Comparative trial of nafoxidene and ethinyloestradiol in advanced breast cancer: an EORTC study. *BMJ* 1975; **ii:** 711–3.

113. Ingle JN, Ahmann DL, Green SJ et al. Randomized clinical trial of diethylstilboestrol versus tamoxifen in postmenopausal women with advanced breast cancer. *NEJM* 1981; **304:** 16.

114. Paschold EH, Slatkoff ML, Muss HB et al. Hormonal therapy of advanced breast cancer–efficacy and toxicity of diethylstilboestrol (DES) versus tamoxifen. *Proc Am Assoc Cancer Res* 1981; **22:** (Abs 380).

115. Stewart HJ, Forrest AP, Gunn JM et al. The tamoxifen trial—a double-blind comparison with stilboestrol in postmenopausal women with advanced breast cancer. *Eur J Cancer* 1980; (Suppl 1): 83.

5

Fulvestrant (ICI 182,780, Faslodex): A 'pure' antiestrogen

Anthony Howell, John FR Robertson

CONTENTS • Introduction • New antiestrogens • Fulvestrant: mode of action • Preclinical studies • Clinical studies • Pharmacokinetics • Phase III data • Conclusions

INTRODUCTION

The term 'antiestrogen' encompasses all agents that antagonize the physiologic effects of the female hormone estrogen or 17β-estradiol. Tamoxifen is a non-steroidal, triphenylethylene-based, antiestrogen (Figure 5.1), with tissue-specific estrogenic (agonist) and antiestrogenic (antagonist) activity, and has been the antiestrogen of choice in the clinic for over 25 years. Its biological effects are mediated primarily by inhibiting the actions of estrogen mediated through its binding to the estrogen receptor (ER).[1] The antiestrogenic activity of tamoxifen in the breast has established it as the standard for the treatment of all stages of breast cancer in postmenopausal women. Tamoxifen given for different durations in an adjuvant setting has been associated with an up to 47% reduction in the risk of contralateral breast cancer,[2] and a 45% reduction in invasive cancer in patients with ductal carcinoma in situ.[3] Furthermore, the prospective evaluation of tamoxifen for the prevention of cancer in high-risk women in the National Surgical Adjuvant Breast and Bowel Project (NSABP)-P1 breast cancer prevention

study[4] showed tamoxifen to reduce the relative risk of invasive cancer by 49% in all age groups. Although these observations have not been confirmed in two European studies, tamoxifen has been approved by the US Food and Drug Administration (FDA) for breast cancer prevention in high-risk individuals.[5]

Long-term tamoxifen treatment is associated with at least two other clinical benefits normally associated with endogenous systemic estrogen. These are the maintenance of bone density[6,7] and the lowering of circulating low-density lipoprotein cholesterol,[8] with a beneficial effect on cardiovascular disease,[5,9] both of which are issues of importance to perimenopausal and postmenopausal women. However, tamoxifen is also associated with a slight increase in the risk of endometrial cancer[4,9,10] and as yet unsubstantiated concerns over other second malignancies.[11] These observations are of particular concern when tamoxifen is used in an adjuvant setting, since these patients may be receiving therapy for up to 5 years. Tamoxifen is also associated with a tumour-stimulatory effect, sometimes seen as a transient flare at the start of treatment,[12] and,

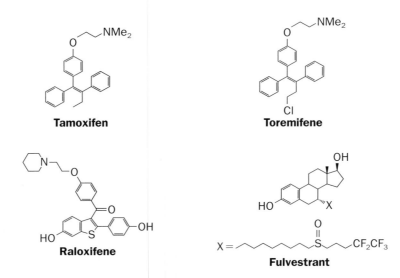

Figure 5.1 Chemical structures of three different non-steroidal antiestrogens and fulvestrant.

perhaps most importantly, the acquisition of 'tamoxifen resistance', where tamoxifen no longer inhibits tumour growth – and in some cases actually promotes it.[13] Antiestrogen therapy is also associated with an increased incidence of thromboembolic phenomena, including deep vein thrombosis, pulmonary embolism, and possibly cerebrovascular events.[14,15] The most common serious adverse event with tamoxifen is thromboembolism.[4] However, despite these negative aspects of tamoxifen therapy, the benefits for the treatment and prevention of breast cancer are considered to substantially outweigh the risks.

The success of tamoxifen in the treatment of breast cancer has proved invaluable in the search for, and development of, new antiestrogens that selectively retain the favourable estrogenic and antiestrogenic properties of tamoxifen. It is the standard against which all new endocrine therapies, including third-generation aromatase inhibitors, are being and will be measured, in well-established pre-clinical and clinical settings as summarized in Table 5.1.

NEW ANTIESTROGENS

The last decade has seen an upsurge in the activity invested in the search for the successor to tamoxifen. The strategies employed have included the chemical modification of tamoxifen, either by altering the side-chains to produce new tamoxifen analogues such as toremifene[16] (Figure 5.1), idoxifene,[17] droloxifene,[18] and TAT-59,[19,20] or by altering the non-steroidal triphenylethylene ring structure of tamoxifen to produce new non-steroidal ring structures such as the benzothiophene derivative raloxifene[21,22] (Figure 5.1) and the benzopyran derivative EM-800.[23] These non-steroidal antiestrogens have all been classified as selective estrogen receptor modulators (SERMs) and exhibit mixed tissue-dependent agonist/antagonist activity. None of these non-steroidal antiestrogens have yet shown any significant advantage over tamoxifen in clinical trials in terms of either efficacy or tolerance.[24] Also, the possibility of cross-resistance between most of these agents and tamoxifen may limit their potential usefulness in the treatment of

---

Table 5.1 Preclinical and clinical assessment of new antiestrogens

Preclinical in vitro and in vivo assessments
- Estrogen receptor (ER) binding
- ERα and ERβ transcriptional activation
- Tumour antagonism
- Estrogenic activity in breast and uterus
- Activity against tamoxifen-resistant cell lines
- Estrogenic activity on bone and serum lipids
- Mechanism of ER activation (coactivators, corepressors, and ligand-independent activity)

Clinical assessment
- Activity as first-line therapy
- Activity in tamoxifen-resistant tumours
- Activity as neoadjuvant and adjuvant therapy
- Activity in prevention
- Side-effect profile
- Scheduling relative to aromatase inhibitors

---

advanced disease following adjuvant tamoxifen therapy[24] (see Chapters 3, 4, 10). Indeed, all of the triphenylethylene tamoxifen analogues, with the exception of toremifene, have been withdrawn from development for the treatment of breast cancer.

Another avenue has been to produce steroidal analogues of estrogen with a bulky side-chain at either the 7α position[25–28] or the 11β position[29] of estradiol, which are completely lacking in agonist activity. These agents have been termed 'pure' antiestrogens, and include ICI 164,384, fulvestrant (Faslodex, formerly ICI 182,780), and RU 58668. The most advanced of these in terms of both preclinical and clinical evaluation is fulvestrant (Figure 5.1).[28] Two other oral pure antiestrogens (SR 16234) and ZK 191703) are in late preclinical/early clinical development.

FULVESTRANT: MODE OF ACTION

Fulvestrant is one of two steroidal antiestrogens with pure antiestrogenic activity developed from a series of 7α-alkyl analogues of estradiol.[28] ICI 164,384 has been studied extensively in a preclinical setting, but it is the more potent fulvestrant that is being actively studied in clinical trials in patients with breast cancer.[25,26]

Fulvestrant is distinguishable from tamoxifen and other SERMs both pharmacologically and in terms of its molecular activity. Although both classes of agent mediate their effects through the ER, they differ significantly in their downstream effects (Table 5.2). Binding of estradiol and the non-steroidal antiestrogens to the estrogen-binding sites of the ER initiates a series of events, which include dissociation of heat-shock proteins and ER dimerization. Dimerization facilitates the binding of the ER to specific DNA estrogen response elements (EREs) in the vicinity of estrogen-regulated genes.[30,31] Many proteins interact with the receptor to act as corepressors or coactivators, whilst, to further complicate matters, at least 50 transcriptional activating factors modulate the effects of estrogen on the target gene.[32,33] There are at least two ERs, α and β,[34-36] which have different tissue distributions. Both ERs contain two activating functions, AF-1 and AF-2, both of which are active when estrogen binds to the receptors. Both activating functions are inactivated when the benzothiophene derivative raloxifene binds to the ER, but only one (AF-2) is inactivated when tamoxifen binds to the ER. The latter scenario leads to incomplete attenuation of transcription, with the AF-1 domain allowing selective gene expression to occur.

Thus, the partial agonist activity of tamoxifen is attributed, in part, to its inability to inactivate AF-1.

The activity of the steroidal antiestrogens such as fulvestrant is different (Table 5.2). The steroidal antiestrogens bind to the ER, but, because of their long bulky side-chains at the 7α and 11β positions, receptor dimerization appears to be sterically hindered.[37] There is evidence that ER turnover is increased and nuclear localization is disrupted, with a concomitant reduction in the number of detectable ER molecules in the cell both in vitro and in vivo.[38] This is in marked contrast to the stable or increased levels of ER expression associated

---

Table 5.2 Modes of action of estradiol, tamoxifen, and fulvestrant following binding to the estrogen receptor (ER)

Estradiol
1. The natural ligand estradiol (E_2) binds to the ER with high affinity and dissociates hsp90
2. The E_2-ER complex homodimerizes and localizes preferentially in the cell nucleus
3. E_2-ER homodimer binds to the estrogen response element (ERE) in the promoter region of estrogen-sensitive genes
4. Activation of transcription by ER involves two transcription activation functions, AF-1 and AF-2, of the ER and transcriptional coactivators to stimulate the activity of RNA polymerase II (RNA pol II)

Tamoxifen (SERM)
1. Tamoxifen (T) binds to ER with low affinity compared with estradiol and dissociates hsp90.
2. The T–ER complex homodimerizes and translocates to the cell nucleus. AF-1 but not AF-2 is active.
3. The T–ER dimer binds to the ERE in the promoter region of estrogen-sensitive genes
4. Transcription of estrogen-responsive gene(s) is attenuated because AF-2 is inactive and the T–ER complex attenuates coactivator binding; partial agonist activity results because AF-1 in the T–ER complex remains active.

Fulvestrant (SERD)
1. Fulvestrant (F) binds to ER with high affinity and dissociates hsp90
2. Rapid degradation of ER is triggered by binding
3. There is a reduced rate of dimerization and nuclear localization of the F–ER complex
4. There is reduced binding of F–ER to the ERE
5. There is no transcription of estrogen-responsive genes; since AF-1 and AF-2 are inactive, no co-activators are recruited

with tamoxifen and its analogues. In vitro and in vivo studies suggest that as a consequence of ER 'downregulation', ER-mediated transcription is completely attenuated since fulvestrant inactivates both AF-1 and AF-2, and this leads to complete suppression of the expression of estrogen-dependent genes. Thus, not only is fulvestrant described as a pure antiestrogen, it is now also described as a selective estrogen receptor downregulator (SERD).

PRECLINICAL STUDIES

The preclinical characteristics of fulvestrant, which define this compound as a 'pure' antiestrogen devoid of estrogen-like activity, have been extensively reviewed,[28,39,40] and provided the first evidence that fulvestrant may offer a potential therapeutic advantage over tamoxifen. These include an affinity for the ER approximately a 100 times that of tamoxifen, the specific absence of estrogen-like activity on the uterus both in vitro and in vivo, and the capacity to completely block the stimulatory activities of both estrogens and antiestrogens with partial agonist activity, such as tamoxifen. For example, in the rat uterus, in contrast to estradiol and tamoxifen, fulvestrant did not induce genes such as calbindin D, IGF-I, VEGF, and c-fos, and, when administered prior to estradiol or tamoxifen, completely blocked the induction of these genes by these agents.[24] Moreover, fulvestrant does not block the uptake of [³H]estradiol in the brain, suggesting that fulvestrant does not cross the blood–brain barrier[41] and therefore in humans may not cause the hot flushes associated with the nonsteroidal antiestrogens. The preclinical animal data on the effects of fulvestrant on bone density are conflicting, with reports of reduced cancellous bone volume in one study[42] and no effect on overall density in another,[43] and are being investigated further. The absence of estrogenic activity has important consequences for the development of resistance, which is a major concern during tamoxifen therapy. In vitro studies demonstrate that tamoxifen-resis-

tant cell lines remain sensitive to growth inhibition by fulvestrant,[44–46] while cells resistant to fulvestrant exhibit cross-resistance to tamoxifen.[47] Also, tamoxifen-resistant tumours remain sensitive to fulvestrant in vivo.[48] Preclinical studies in nude mice show that fulvestrant suppresses the growth of established MCF-7 xenografts for twice as long as tamoxifen and delays the onset of tumour growth for longer than tamoxifen.[48] Taken collectively, these data suggest that fulvestrant is a more effective estrogen antagonist than tamoxifen, and able to produce a longer response in the animal model. Moreover, other animal studies confirm the complete absence of uterine-stimulating activity and show that fulvestrant blocks the uterotrophic action of tamoxifen.[27] In ovariectomized, estrogen-treated monkeys, the extent of involution of the endometrium was similar in animals treated with fulvestrant compared with withdrawal of estrogen.[39] Overall, these data indicate that the mode of action and the preclinical effects of fulvestrant are distinct from those of tamoxifen and the newer SERMs, and support the concept that fulvestrant represents a novel type of antiestrogen with clinical potential and implications for the endocrine management of breast cancer in terms of the sequencing of steroidal and non-steroidal antiestrogen therapies.

CLINICAL STUDIES

Data regarding the clinical potential of fulvestrant in patients with breast cancer are encouraging. Administration of a short-acting propylene glycol–based formulation of fulvestrant at doses of 6 or 18 mg daily by intramuscular injection for one week, to postmenopausal breast cancer patients prior to surgery resulted in a reduction in proliferation, as measured by Ki67 labelling index, and a reduction or absence of expression of ER and progesterone receptor (PgR) in ER-positive tumours.[26] Treatment with fulvestrant also resulted in a clinically significant reduction in expression of the estrogen-regulated gene pS2, but this was unrelated to tumour ER status. Similar experiments with tamoxifen had produced no change in ER expression, slightly increased PgR expression, and reduction in the Ki67 labelling index after a median 21 days of treatment.

Although fulvestrant reduced ER expression to almost undetectable levels, no other changes suggestive of an endocrine-insensitive phenotype were observed.[24] This, coupled with the absence of changes in Ki67 in ER-negative tumours treated with fulvestrant, suggests that the effect is the result of antagonism of estrogen at the ER level. This antiestrogenic effect has been confirmed in a study in premenopausal patients scheduled for hysterectomy for benign gynaecological disease who were randomized to receive either seven consecutive daily doses of the short-acting formulation of fulvestrant or observation prior to surgery. No increase in endometrial thickness was observed in the fulvestrant-treated patients,[49] and there was also significantly lower ER expression in the myometrium of the treated group.[50]

In a much larger preoperative study, the antitumour effects of single-dose long-acting fulvestrant were compared with those of tamoxifen in postmenopausal primary breast cancer patients prior to surgery.[51] In this study, 201 patients were randomized to receive fulvestrant over a range of doses (50, 125, or 250 mg) administered, intramuscularly, or tamoxifen administered orally at a dose of 20 mg/day, or matching tamoxifen placebo for 14–21 days prior to surgery. A dose-dependent reduction in the levels of ER expression was observed across all three doses of fulvestrant compared with placebo. Also, when the fulvestrant dose normally used clinically (250 mg) was compared with tamoxifen, there was a significantly greater reduction in ER index for fulvestrant. A dose-dependent reduction in PgR expression was also observed following fulvestrant treatment, which was greater for all three doses of fulvestrant than for tamoxifen, which actually resulted in stimulation of PgR expression.[51] At all three doses fulvestrant reduced proliferation. These data once again provide evidence that fulvestrant acts as an ER downregulator

with clear antiestrogenic and antiproliferative activity.[51] Furthermore, the effect on PgR provides evidence of a more complete blockade of this ER-dependent pathway compared with tamoxifen, which increases PgR levels as a result of its partial agonist activity.[51]

The clinical efficacy of fulvestrant was demonstrated in a small phase II trial in 19 patients with tamoxifen-refractory disease who received a long-acting monthly intramuscular injection, starting with 100 mg in the first month and increasing to 250 mg for the second and subsequent months in the absence of local and systemic toxicity. Thirteen patients achieved a clinical benefit, with a median duration of 25 months, with seven patients demonstrating a partial response (PR) and six patients stable disease (SD).[25,52] These data clearly confirmed the lack of cross-resistance with tamoxifen observed in preclinical studies. Furthermore, luteinizing hormone (LH) and follicle-stimulating hormone (FSH) levels rose after the patients were removed from tamoxifen, but then plateaued – suggesting that there is no effect of fulvestrant on the pituitary–hypothalamic axis. Hot flushes and sweats were not induced, and no negative effects were observed on the liver, brain, or genital tract – suggesting that fulvestrant might have fewer side-effects in terms of menopausal symptoms than tamoxifen. Thus, fulvestrant at the drug concentrations used in this study was effective as a second-line antiestrogen therapy, supporting a mechanism of action distinct from tamoxifen. In addition, this phase II study clearly indicated that fulvestrant was well tolerated. Also, comparison with a well-matched historical control group of patients treated with the progestin megestrol acetate suggested a longer duration of response for patients receiving fulvestrant: 26 months versus 14 months (Figure 5.2).[53]

PHARMACOKINETICS

The pharmacokinetics of multiple-dose fulvestrant administration were assessed in the phase II trial described above[25] and more recently in a

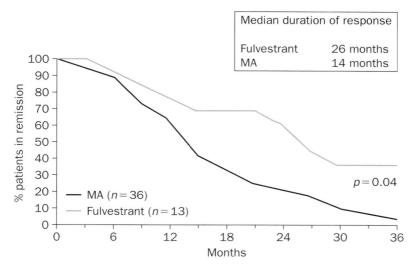

Figure 5.2 Duration of response for fulvestrant versus the progestin megestrol acetate (MA) in patients with tamoxifen-resistant breast cancer.[53] Reproduced from Robertson JFR, Howell A, De Friend DJ et al. Duration of remission to ICI 182,780 compared to megestrol acetate in tamoxifen resistant breast cancer. *Breast Cancer Res Treat* 1997; **6:** 186–9, with permission from Churchill Livingstone (Harcourt Heath Sciences).

subset of patients enrolled in a phase III trial.[54] In the phase II trial, peak levels of fulvestrant occurred at a median of 8–9 days after dosing and then declined, but were still above the projected therapeutic threshold at day 28.[25] Mean C_{max} (which occurred on day 7) increased from 10.5 ng/ml during the first month to 12.6 ng/ml at month 6. The area under the curve (AUC) increased by 47% at 6 months, suggesting some drug accumulation. In addition, the pharmacokinetic properties of single-dose fulvestrant were investigated in two multicentre randomized trials in postmenopausal patients with either primary[55] or advanced[56] breast cancer and are reviewed elsewhere.[57] Significantly, the administration regimen $(1 \times 5 \, \text{ml}$ or $2 \times 2.5 \, \text{ml}$ intramuscular injections) did not appear to alter the pharmacokinetic profile of fulvestrant.[56]

PHASE III DATA

The phase II second-line and preoperative trials reported above provided the initiative for two phase III studies – one in North America and one in Europe, Australia, and South Africa (ROW) – which compared the efficacy and tolerability of fulvestrant (250 mg) administered once monthly with those of the third-generation aromatase inhibitor anastrozole (1 mg) administered orally once daily, in postmenopausal women whose disease had progressed on or after prior adjuvant endocrine therapy.[58,59] The vast majority (>96%) of patients, across both trials, had received prior tamoxifen therapy. The North American trial was a double-blind trial and recruited patients from 83 centres in the USA and Canada, whilst the second trial, was an open-label study conducted principally in Europe, recruiting patients from 82 centres. In the North American and ROW trials, 400 and 451 patients respectively were analysed for efficacy. The primary endpoint in both trials was time to disease progression, with secondary endpoints across both trials including objective response, duration of response, time to death, tolerability, quality of life, and pharmacokinetics.

The median time to disease progression was numerically longer with fulvestrant compared with anastrozole for both the North American (5.4 months versus 3.4 months) and ROW (5.5 months versus 5.1 months) trials, but was not statistically significant in either trial. The objective response rates were not significantly different in either trial: 17.5% for both arms in the North American trial and 20.7% versus 15.7% for fulvestrant and anastrozole, respectively, in the ROW trial. In responding patients, the median durations of response to fulvestrant and anastrozole were 19.3 months and 10.5 months respectively in the North American trial and 14.3 months and 14.0 months respectively in the ROW trial. The clinical benefit rates (defined as complete and partial responses and disease stabilization lasting for 24 weeks or more) for fulvestrant versus anastrozole were 42.2% versus 36.1% in the North American trial and 44.6% versus 45.0% in the ROW trial. In both trials, the most frequently reported adverse events were gastrointestinal disturbances (e.g. nausea, vomiting, constipation, and diarrhoea): 53.4% and 39.7% of patients suffered from at least one gastrointestinal disturbance in the North American and ROW trials, respectively. Overall, the incidence of adverse events was similar for the recipients of anastrozole and fulvestrant in both trials. The withdrawal rates in the fulvestrant and anastrozole groups were low in both trials, with 2.5% versus 2.6% of patients withdrawing owing to an adverse event in the North American trial and 3.2% versus 2.2% of patients withdrawing owing to an adverse event in the ROW trial.[58,59] Thus, in both studies, fulvestrant was at least as effective as the aromatase inhibitor anastrozole, with a longer duration of response in the North American trial, confirming fulvestrant as an effective treatment in postmenopausal patients with advanced breast cancer recurring or progressing even after tamoxifen therapy.

Fulvestrant was also well tolerated, and is the first antiestrogen reported to be at least as effective as a new-generation aromatase inhibitor. This is of particular significance in light of the fact that two trials comparing anastrozole with tamoxifen in the first-line treatment of breast cancer have shown anastrozole to be superior to tamoxifen – both in terms of time to progression and in terms of a lower incidence of thromboembolic events and vaginal bleeding.[60,61]

CONCLUSIONS

Fulvestrant is the first in a new class of antiestrogen to enter clinical practice, and is currently being investigated in phase III trials versus tamoxifen. Its mode of action (Table 5.2) and clinical efficacy and side-effect profile (Table 5.3) are distinct from those of tamoxifen, and preliminary data from two phase III studies

Table 5.3 Summary of clinical efficacy and side-effect profiles of fulvestrant and tamoxifen

Clinical activity	Tamoxifen	Fulvestrant
Prevention	+	ND
Neoadjuvant	+	+
Advanced disease	+	+
Tamoxifen-resistant	0	+
Agonist activity on uterus	+	−
Bone density	+	?
Lipids	↓	=
Blood–brain barrier	+	NT

ND, not determined; ↓, favourable change; =, no change; NT, not tested.

show it to be as effective as the third-generation aromatase inhibitor anastrozole as a second-line endocrine therapy in postmenopausal patients who have failed on prior tamoxifen therapy.[58,59]

It is well recognized that patients whose disease progresses after responding to tamoxifen can achieve further responses with third-generation steroidal (exemestane) and non-steroidal (anastrozole and letrozole) aromatase inhibitors, and these are currently being investigated as first-line therapy in metastatic, adjuvant, and neoadjuvant settings. Fulvestrant is also being investigated in these clinical settings. Thus, not only does fulvestrant provide an alternative to tamoxifen, it also offers the opportunity of a further response, at least equivalent to that of anastrozole, in patients who have failed on tamoxifen as well as showing potential as a follow-on therapy after tamoxifen in an adjuvant setting. The results of the ongoing phase III clinical trials are awaited, particularly those comparing fulvestrant with tamoxifen as first-line treatment in advanced disease.

REFERENCES

1. Cole MP, Jones CTA, Todd IDH. A new anti-oestrogenic agent in late breast cancer. An early clinical appraisal of ICI 164,474. *Br J Cancer* 1996; **25**: 270–5.

2. Early Breast Cancer Trialists' Collaborative Group (EBCTCG). Tamoxifen for early breast cancer: an overview of the randomised trials. *Lancet* 1998; **351**: 1451–67.

3. Wolmark N, Colangelo L, Wieand S. National Surgical Adjuvant Breast and Bowel Project trials in colon cancer. *Semin Oncol* 2001; **28**: 9–13.

4. Fisher B, Costantino JP, Wickerham DL et al. Tamoxifen for prevention of breast cancer: report of the National Surgical Adjuvant Breast and Bowel Project P-1 study. *J Natl Cancer Inst* 1998; **90**: 1371–88.

5. Chlebowski RT, Collyar DE, Somerfield MR et al. American Society of Clinical Oncology technology assessment on breast cancer risk reduction strategies: tamoxifen and raloxifene. *J Clin Oncol* 1999; **17**: 1939–55.

6. Love RR, Mazess RB, Barden HS et al. Effects of tamoxifen on bone mineral density in post-menopausal women with breast cancer. *N Engl J Med* 1992; **326**: 852–6.

7. Bilmoria MM, Jordan VC, Morrow M. Additional benefits of tamoxifen for post-menopausal patients. In: *Tamoxifen: A Guide for Clinicians and Patients* (Jordan VC, ed). Huntington, NY: PRR, 1996: 75–89.

8. Love RR, Newcomb A, Wiebe DA et al. Effects of tamoxifen therapy on lipid and lipoprotein levels in postmenopausal patients with node-negative breast cancer. *J Natl Cancer Inst* 1990; **82**: 1327–32.

9. Love RR, Wiebe DA, Newcomb PA et al. Effects of tamoxifen on cardiovascular risk factors in postmenopausal women. *Ann Intern Med* 1991; **115**: 860–4.

10. Fisher B, Costantino JP, Redmond CK et al. Endometrial cancer in tamoxifen-treated breast cancer patients: findings from the National Surgical Adjuvant Breast and Bowel Project (NSABP) B-14. *J Natl Cancer Inst* 1994; **86**: 527–37.

11. Jordan VC, Morrow M. Should clinicians be concerned about the carcinogenic potential of tamoxifen? *Eur J Cancer* 1994; **11**: 1714–21.

12. Plotkin D, Lechner JJ, Jung WE et al. Tamoxifen flare in advanced breast cancer. *JAMA* 1978; **240**: 2644–6.

13. Howell A, Dodwell DJ, Anderson H et al. Response after withdrawal of tamoxifen. *Ann Oncol* 1992; **3**: 611–17.

14. Hendrick A, Subramanian VP. Tamoxifen and thromboembolism. *JAMA* 1980; **243**: 514–15.

15. Lipton A, Harvey HA, Hamilton RW. Venous thrombosis as a side effect of tamoxifen treatment. *Cancer Treat Rep* 1984; **68**: 887–9.

16. Kangas L, Nieminen A, Blanco G et al. A new triphenylethylene compound, Fc-1157a. II. Antitumor effects. *Cancer Chemother Pharmacol* 1986; **17**: 109–13.

17. Chander SK, McCague R, Luqmani Y et al. Pyrrolidino-4-iodotamoxifen and 4-iodotamoxifen, new analogues of the antiestrogen tamoxifen for the treatment of breast cancer. *Cancer Res* 1991; **51**: 5851–8.

18. Loser R, Seibel K, Eppenberger U. No loss of estrogenic or anti-estrogenic activity after demethylation of droloxifene (3-OH-tamoxifen). *Int J Cancer* 1985; **36**: 701–3.

19. Toko T, Sugimoto Y, Matsuo K et al. TAT-59, a new triphenylethylene derivative with anti-tumor activity against hormone-dependent tumors. *Eur J Cancer* 1990; **26**: 397–404.

20. Toko T, Shibata J, Nukatsuka M et al. Antiestrogenic activity of DP-TAT-59, an active metabolite of TAT-59 against human breast cancer. *Cancer Chemother Pharmacol* 1997; **39:** 390–8.

21. Palkowitz AD, Glasebrook AL, Thrasher KJ et al. Discovery and synthesis of [6-hydroxy-3-[4-[2-(1-piperidinyl)ethoxy]phenoxy]-2-(4-hydroxy-phenyl)]benzo[*b*]thiophene: a novel, highly potent, selective estrogen receptor modulator. *J Med Chem* 1997; **40:** 1407–16.

22. Clemens JA, Bennett DR, Black LJ et al. Effects of a new antiestrogen, keoxifene (LY156758), on growth of carcinogen-induced mammary tumors and on LH and prolactin levels. *Life Sci* 1983; **32:** 2869–75.

23. Gauthier S, Caron B, Cloutier J et al. (*S*)-(+)-4-[7-(2,2-dimethyl-1-oxopropoxy)-4-methyl-2-[4-[2-(1-piperidinyl)-ethoxy]phenyl]-2*H*-1-benzopyran-3-yl]-phenyl 2,2-dimethylpropanoate (EM-800): a highly potent, specific, and orally active non-steroidal antiestrogen. *J Med Chem* 1997; **40:** 2117–22.

24. Howell A, Osborne CK, Morris C et al. ICI 182,780 (Faslodex): development of a novel, 'pure' antiestrogen. *Cancer* 2000; **89:** 817–25.

25. Howell A, DeFriend DJ, Robertson JF et al. Pharmacokinetics, pharmacological and anti-tumour effects of the specific anti-oestrogen ICI 182780 in women with advanced breast cancer. *Br J Cancer* 1996; **74:** 300–8.

26. DeFriend DJ, Howell A, Nicholson RI et al. Investigation of a new pure antiestrogen (ICI 182780) in women with primary breast cancer. *Cancer Res* 1994; **54:** 408–14.

27. Wakeling AE, Dukes M, Bowler J. A potent specific pure antiestrogen with clinical potential. *Cancer Res* 1991; **51:** 3867–73.

28. Wakeling AE, Bowler J. ICI 182,780, a new antioestrogen with clinical potential. *J Steroid Biochem Mol Biol* 1992; **43:** 173–7.

29. Van de Velde P, Nique F, Planchon P et al. RU 58668: further in vitro and in vivo pharmacological data related to its antitumoral activity. *J Steroid Biochem Mol Biol* 1996; **59:** 449–57.

30. McGregor JI, Jordan VC. Basic guide to the mechanisms of antioestrogen action. *Pharmacol Rev* 1998; **50:** 151–96.

31. Beato M, Chalepakis G, Schauer M et al. DNA regulatory elements for steroid hormones. *J Steroid Biochem* 1989; **32:** 737–47.

32. Webb P, Nguyen P, Shinsako J et al. Estrogen receptor activation function 1 works by binding to p160 coactivator proteins. *Mol Endocrinol* 1998; **12:** 1605–18.

33. Johnston SR, Lu B, Scott GK et al. Increased activator protein-1 DNA binding and c-jun NH_2-terminal kinase activity in human breast tumors with acquired tamoxifen resistance. *Clin Cancer Res* 1999; **5:** 251–6.

34. Kuiper GG, Gustafsson JA. The novel estrogen receptor-β subtype: potential role in the cell- and promoter-specific actions of estrogens and anti-estrogens. *FEBS Lett* 1997; **410:** 87–90.

35. Katzenellenbogen BS, Korach KS. A new actor in the estrogen receptor drama – enter ERβ. *Endocrinology* 1997; **138:** 861–2.

36. Mosselman S, Polman J, Dijkema R. ERβ: identification and characterization of a novel human estrogen receptor. *FEBS Lett* 1996; **392:** 49–53.

37. Parker MG. Action of 'pure' antiestrogens in inhibiting estrogen receptor action. *Breast Cancer Res Treat* 1993; **26:** 131–7.

38. Pink JJ, Jordan VC. Models of estrogen receptor regulation by estrogens and antiestrogens in breast cancer cell lines. *Cancer Res* 1996; **56:** 2321–30.

39. Dukes M, Miller D, Wakeling AE et al. Antiuterotrophic effects of a pure antioestrogen, ICI 182,780: magnetic resonance imaging of the uterus in ovariectomized monkeys. *J Endocrinol* 1992; **135:** 239–47.

40. Dukes M, Waterton JC, Wakeling AE. Antiuterotrophic effects of the pure antioestrogen ICI 182,780 in adult female monkeys (*Macaca nemestrina*): quantitative magnetic resonance imaging. *J Endocrinol* 1993; **138:** 203–10.

41. Wade GN, Blaustein JD, Gray JM et al. ICI 182,780: a pure antiestrogen that affects behaviors and energy balance in rats without acting in the brain. *Am J Physiol* 1993; **265:** R1392–8.

42. Gallagher A, Chambers TJ, Tobias JH. The estrogen antagonist ICI 182,780 reduces cancellous bone volume in female rats. *Endocrinology* 1993; **133:** 2787–91.

43. Wakeling AE. The future of pure antioestrogens in clinical breast cancer. *Breast Cancer Res Treat* 1993; **25:** 1–9.

44. Coopman P, Garcia M, Brunner N et al. Anti-proliferative and anti-estrogenic effects of ICI 164,384 and ICI 182,780 in 4-OH-tamoxifen-resistant human breast-cancer cells. *Int J Cancer* 1994; **56:** 295–300.

45. Brunner N, Frandsen TL, Holst-Hansen C et al.

MCF7/LCC2: a 4-hydroxytamoxifen resistant human breast cancer variant that retains sensitivity to the steroidal antiestrogen ICI 182,780. *Cancer Res* 1993; **53:** 3229–32.

46. Hu XF, Veroni M, De Luise, M et al. Circumvention of tamoxifen resistance by the pure anti-estrogen ICI 182,780. *Int J Cancer* 1993; **55:** 873–6.

47. Brunner N, Boysen B, Jirus S et al. MCF7/LCC9: an antiestrogen-resistant MCF-7 variant in which acquired resistance to the steroidal antiestrogen ICI 182,780 confers an early cross-resistance to the nonsteroidal antiestrogen tamoxifen. *Cancer Res* 1997; **57:** 3486–93.

48. Osborne CK, Coronado-Heinsohn EB, Hilsenbeck SG et al. Comparison of the effects of a pure steroidal antiestrogen with those of tamoxifen in a model of human breast cancer. *J Natl Cancer Inst* 1995; **87:** 746–50.

49. Thomas EJ, Walton PL, Thomas NM et al. The effects of ICI 182,780, a pure anti-oestrogen, on the hypothalamic-pituitary-gonadal axis and on endometrial proliferation in pre-menopausal women. *Hum Reprod* 1994; **9:** 1991–6.

50. Dowsett M, Howell R, Salter J et al. Effects of the pure anti-oestrogen ICI 182780 on oestrogen receptors, progesterone receptors and Ki67 antigen in human endometrium in vivo. *Hum Reprod* 1995; **10:** 262–7.

51. Robertson JFR, Nicholson R, Anderson E et al. The anti-tumour effects of single-dose long-lasting Faslodex (ICI 182,780) compared with tamoxifen in postmenopausal primary breast cancer patients treated before surgery. *Breast Cancer Res Treat* 2000; **59:** 99.

52. Howell A, DeFriend D, Robertson J et al. Response to a specific antioestrogen (ICI 182780) in tamoxifen-resistant breast cancer. *Lancet* 1995; **345:** 29–30.

53. Robertson JFR, Howell A, De Friend DJ et al. Duration of remission to ICI 182,780 compared to megestrol acetate in tamoxifen resistant breast cancer. *Breast Cancer Res Treat* 1997; **6:** 186–9.

54. Robertson J, Harrison M. ICI 182,780 (Faslodex) (FAS) 250 mg monthly intramuscular (i.m.) injec-

tion shows consistent PK during long-term dosing in postmenopausal women with advanced breast cancer (ABC). *Proc Am Assoc Cancer Res* 2001; **42:** 856.

55. Robertson J, Nicholson R, Gee JM et al. The pharmacokinetics of single dose Faslodex (TM) (ICI 182,780) in postmenopausal primary breast cancer – relationship with estrogen receptor down regulation. *Proc Am Soc Clin Oncol* 2000; **19:** (Abst 362).

56. Robertson JFR. A comparison of single-dose pharmacokinetics of Faslodex (fulvestrant) 250 mg when given as either one × 5 ml intramuscular injection or two × 2.5 ml injections in postmenopausal women with advanced breast cancer. *Breast Cancer Res Treat* 2000; **64:** 53 (Abst 172).

57. Curran M, Wiseman L. Fulvestrant. *Drugs* 2001; **61:** 807–13.

58. Howell A, Robertson JFR, Quaresma-Albano J et al. Comparison of efficacy and tolerability of fulvestrant (Faslodex™) with anastrazole (Arimidex™) in post-menopausal women with advanced breast cancer (ABC) – preliminary results. *Breast Cancer Res Treat* 2000; **64:** 27.

59. Osborne CK, Pippen J, Jones SE et al. Faslodex (ICI 182,780) shows longer duration of response compared with Arimidex (anastrozole) in post-menopausal (PM) women with advanced breast cancer (ABC). Preliminary results of a phase III North American trial. *Breast Cancer Res Treat* 2001; **65:** 261.

60. Nabholtz JM, Buzdar A, Pollak M et al. Anastrozole is superior to tamoxifen as first-line therapy for advanced breast cancer in post-menopausal women: results of a North American multicenter randomized trial. Arimidex Study Group. *J Clin Oncol* 2000; **18:** 3758–67.

61. Bonneterre J, Thurlimann B, Robertson JF et al. Anastrozole versus tamoxifen as first-line therapy for advanced breast cancer in 668 post-menopausal women: results of the Tamoxifen or Arimidex Randomized Group Efficacy and Tolerability study. *J Clin Oncol* 2000; **18:** 3748–57.

6

Aromatase inhibitors in breast cancer

Wei Yue, Gil Mor, Fred Naftolin, Robert Pauley, Woo-Shin Shim, Harold A Harvey, Richard J Santen

INTRODUCTION

Epithelial cells of the normal breast undergo dynamic changes during various events in a woman's life, such as puberty, the follicular and luteal phases of the menstrual cycle, pregnancy, and menopause. The coordinated interaction of growth factors and steroid hormones regulates the proliferation and differentiated function of epithelial and stromal cells in the normal mammary gland. The key growth factors are insulin-like growth factor I (IGF-I), prolactin, insulin, the fibroblast growth factor (FGF) family of growth factors, and growth hormone, while the major steroid hormones are estradiol, progesterone, and testosterone.[1]

In the induction of breast cancer, estrogens appear to play a predominant role. These sex steroids are believed to initiate and promote the process of breast carcinogenesis by enhancing the rate of cell division and reducing the time available for DNA repair. An emerging new concept is that estrogens can be metabolized to catechol-estrogens and then to quinones that directly damage DNA. These two processes – estrogen-receptor-mediated genomic effects on proliferation and receptor-independent genotoxic effects of estrogen metabolites – can act in an additive or synergistic fashion to cause breast cancer.[2]

The breast cancers that arise in patients can be divided into hormone-dependent and hormone-independent subtypes.[3] The role of estrogens as modulators of mitogenesis overrides the influence of other factors in the hormone-dependent subtype. These sex steroids stimulate cell proliferation directly by increasing the rate of transcription of early-response genes such as c-*myc* and indirectly through stimulation of growth factors that are produced largely in response to estrogenic regulation.[4]

Based upon the concept that estrogen is the proximate regulator of cell proliferation, two general strategies were developed for treatment of hormone-dependent breast cancer: blockade of estrogen receptor action and inhibition of estradiol biosynthesis. Antiestrogens such as tamoxifen bind to the estrogen receptor and interfere with transcription of estrogen-induced genes involved in regulating cell proliferation. Clinical trials showed tamoxifen to be effective in inducing objective tumor regressions and to be associated with minimal side-effects and toxicity. The second strategy, blockade of estradiol biosynthesis, was demonstrated to be feasible using the steroidogenesis inhibitor aminoglutethimide, which produced tumor regressions equivalent to those observed with tamoxifen.[3] However, side-effects from aminoglutethimide were considerable and its effects on several steroidogenic enzymes required concomitant use of a glucocorticoid.[3] Consequently, tamoxifen became the preferred first-line endocrine agent with which to treat advanced breast cancer. However, the clinical efficacy of aminoglutethimide focused attention upon the need to develop more potent, better tolerated, and more specific inhibitors of estrogen biosynthesis.

INHIBITION OF ESTRADIOL BIOSYNTHESIS

Multiple enzymatic steps are involved in the biosynthesis of estradiol and could potentially be used as targets for inhibition. These include cholesterol side-chain cleavage, 3β-ol dehydrogenase-$\Delta^{4,5}$-isomerase, 17α-hydroxylase, 17β-hydroxysteroid dehydrogenase, estrone sulfatase, and aromatase. The ideal strategy would be to block the synthesis of estrogen without inhibiting production of other important steroids or the need to use pharmacological amounts of progestins or glucocorticoids. For this reason, blockade of the terminal step in estradiol biosynthesis, catalyzed by the enzyme aromatase, is considered a more specific and

therefore preferable strategy. Several pharmaceutical companies sought to develop potent aromatase inhibitors designed to specifically block estrogen biosynthesis without altering glucocorticoid and mineralocorticoid synthesis.

PHYSIOLOGY AND REGULATION OF AROMATASE

Aromatase is a cytochrome P450 enzyme that catalyzes the rate-limiting step in estrogen biosynthesis, namely the conversion of androgens to estrogens.[5–8] Two major androgens, androstenedione and testosterone, serve as substrates for aromatase. The aromatase enzyme consists of a complex containing a cytochrome P450 protein as well as the flavoprotein NADPH cytochrome P450 reductase.[5] The gene coding for the cytochrome P450 protein (P450 AROM) exceeds 70 kb and is the largest of the cytochrome P450 family.[5] The cDNA of the aromatase gene contains 3.4 kb and encodes a polypeptide of 503 amino acids with a molecular weight of 55 kDa. Approximately 30% homology exists with other cytochrome P450 proteins. Because its overall homology to other members of the P450 superfamily is low, aromatase belongs to a separate gene family designated CYP19.

Transcription of the aromatase gene is highly regulated.[7] The first exon of the aromatase gene is transcribed into aromatase message but not translated into protein. There exist nine alternative first exons that can initiate the transcription of aromatase. Each of these alternate exons contain upstream DNA sequences that can either enhance or silence the transcription of aromatase. Different tissues utilize specific alternate exons to initiate transcription. For example, the placenta utilizes alternate exon I.1, the testis alternate exon II, adipose tissue I.3 and I.4, and brain If. Regulatory macromolecules that interact with upstream elements of these alternate exons markedly stimulate the rate of transcription of the aromatase gene. Thus each tissue can regulate the amount of aromatase transcribed in a highly specific manner.[5]

Aromatase is expressed in many organs, including ovary, placenta, hypothalamus, liver, muscle, adipose tissue, and breast cancer itself. Aromatase catalyzes three separate steroid hydroxylations that are involved in the conversion of androstenedione to estrone or testosterone to estradiol. The first two give rise to 19-hydroxy and 19-aldehyde structures, and the third, although still controversial, probably also involves the C-19 methyl group with release of formic acid.[9] This enzymatic action results in the conversion of the A-ring of the steroid molecule to a benzene ring, giving an aromatic structure – hence the term 'aromatization'.

In the premenopausal state, the major source of aromatase and of its substrates is the ovary. However, extraglandular aromatization of adrenal substrates in peripheral sites such as fat, liver, and muscle also contributes substantially to the estrogen pool in the early follicular and late luteal phases of the menstrual cycle. In the postmenopausal state, the ovary loses its complement of aromatase enzyme, although it does continue to secrete androstenedione. The adrenal subsumes the primary role of providing substrate for aromatase by directly secreting testosterone and androstenedione. In addition, dehydroepiandrosterone and its sulfate are secreted by the adrenal and converted into the aromatase substrates androstenedione and testosterone in peripheral tissues. The major source of the aromatase enzyme in postmenopausal women is peripheral tissues, particularly fat and muscle.

AROMATIZATION IN SITU IN BREAST TISSUE

Recent studies have identified an additional important site of estrogen production, namely breast tissue itself. Two-thirds of breast carcinomas contain aromatase and synthesize biologically significant amounts of estrogen locally in the tumor.[10–12] Proof of local estradiol synthesis includes measurement of tumor aromatase activity by radiometric or product isolation assays, by immunohistochemistry, by demonstration of aromatase messenger RNA in tissue, and by aromatase enzyme assays performed on cells isolated from human tumors and grown in cell culture. The expression of aromatase is highest in the stromal compartment of breast tumors,[11] but is present in epithelial cells as well. In breast tissue surrounding the tumors, pre-adipocyte fibroblasts contain aromatase activity that can be detected by biochemical assay or immunohistochemical staining.[11,12] Aromatase is also present in normal breast tissue, as documented by immunohistochemistry, by demonstration of aromatase message, and by enzyme assays of cultured cells.[13,14]

To test the relative importance of in situ aromatization versus uptake of estrogen from plasma, one of the authors (WY) of this chapter established a xenograft model of aromatase-transfected MCF-7 cells in nude mice.[15] To assess the role of estradiol uptake from plasma, we utilized steroid-filled Silastic implants to 'clamp' plasma estradiol concentrations at desired levels in oophorectomized animals. Examination of in situ synthesis involved administration of the aromatase substrate androstenedione, with measurement of tumor estradiol levels and tumor size as a biologic endpoint. To validate the model, we first established that peripheral tissues could not synthesize estradiol. Thus, the estradiol detected in breast tumors had to originate either from in situ aromatization or from uptake of estrogen from plasma. The Silastic 'clamp' method allowed us to simulate plasma estrogen levels that normally circulate in postmenopausal women. With these experimental strategies, we evaluate the relative importance of in situ aromatization versus the uptake mechanism in regulating tumor tissue estradiol levels and on the growth of breast tumors.

Sex hormone-binding globulin (SHBG), to which about 40% of circulating estradiol is tightly bound in the human, is not present in mouse plasma. Consequently, the Silastic implant that maintains plasma estradiol concentration at estimated levels of 5 pg/ml results in levels equivalent to the physiological estradiol concentration of postmenopausal women.

Our results have shown that the concentration of estradiol in the tumor tissue was significantly increased to a greater extent by in situ aromatization than by uptake. Consistent with the higher tissue estradiol concentration produced by in situ aromatization, tumor growth was maximally stimulated by estrogen synthesized in situ when compared with that taken up from clamped levels of plasma estradiol produced by the Silastic implant (Figure 6.1). Taken together, these studies support the importance of in situ estrogen production by breast tumors, and suggest that aromatase inhibitors in patients must be sufficiently potent to block intratumoral aromatase.

To further explore the biological function of breast tissue aromatase, we utilized an immunohistochemical method to determine whether aromatase-expressing cells have an increased level of progesterone receptor (PgR). Since PgR is an estrogen receptor (ER)-regulated gene, we would expect that tissues making more estradiol through aromatase would have higher levels of PgR. We selected tumors from women older than 50 years as a means of identifying those likely to have come from postmenopausal women. These tumors were then examined for the presence of aromatase, ER, and PgR. Samples were only selected for further study if all three were positive. The rationale for selecting ER-positive tumors was that any estrogen formed through aromatase could only act if the ER were present. The rationale for selecting PgR-positive tumors was that the presence of this receptor suggested that the ERs present in the tissue were biologically functional. Finally, only tumors that were aromatase-positive would be expected to form estradiol in situ and to stimulate PgR content. Tumours meeting the triple criteria of ER, PgR, and aromatase positivity were selected sequentially from the most recent samples collected to those obtained many years ago. This reduced the possibility that antigenic recognition would deteriorate over time.

Using these criteria, we selected and exam-

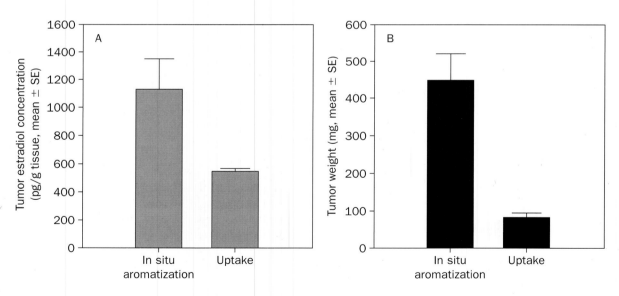

Figure 6.1 Comparison of the effect of estradiol synthesized inside tumors (in situ aromatization) with that concentrated in breast by an endocrine mechanism (uptake). Both tissue estradiol concentration (A) and tumor growth (B) were examined. Aromatase-transfected MCF-7 cells were inoculated into ovariectomized nude mice. The animals were injected with androstenedione (0.1 mg/day) to test in situ aromatization or received Silastic implants that provided 5 pg/ml of plasma estradiol concentration (uptake). Tumor tissue estradiol concentration and tumor weight were measured 8 weeks later.

ined 36 breast tumor specimens from over 1200 formalin-fixed tumors available to us from the Michigan Cancer Foundation tumor bank. We used the intensity of staining with specific antibodies to semiquantitate the amount of aromatase and PgR present in tumor tissue. Preliminary studies examined the intensity of staining versus the age of the sample. We found no deterioration of staining intensity as a function of the age of the sample, and concluded that no deterioration in recognition sites occurred over time.

We wished to test the hypothesis that locally synthesized estradiol would stimulate the amount of PgR contiguous to the aromatase-positive cells. Unfortunately, we detected no correlation between expression of aromatase and PgR in the 36 individual human tumors

(Figure 6.2). The difficulties inherent in examining local effects of estradiol in tissue make interpretation of these negative results difficult. For example, one would expect that the estradiol made in an aromatase-positive cell would stimulate the expression of the PgR in a surrounding cell. However, for this to occur, the surrounding cells must contain ERs. In various portions of an individual tumor, the surrounding cells may or may not be ER-positive, even though the tumor overall is ER-positive. Our analysis examined the entire tumor and not focal areas. Consequently, we may easily have missed an association that occurred at a focal level. We recognized at the outset that only a positive correlation between aromatase level and PgR content would be meaningful.

A potentially important biologic phenomenon

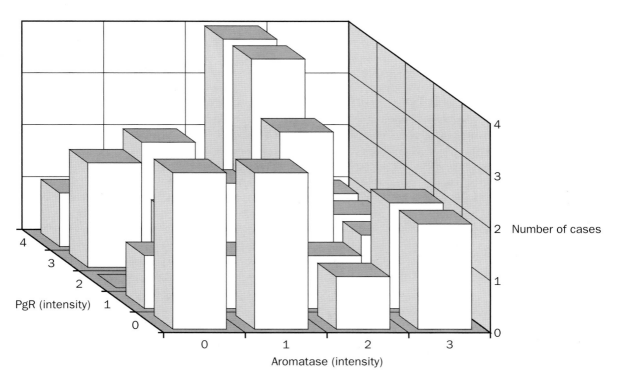

Figure 6.2 Expression of aromatase and progesterone receptor (PgR) in 36 human breast tumors from postmenopausal women. Tumors for evaluation were selected on the basis of staining positively for estrogen receptor (ER). Aromatase and PgR were detected by an immunohistochemical method using specific antibodies. Contents of aromatase and PgR were semiquantitated by scoring on a scale of 0 to 4+. Data show no correlation between aromatase and PgR ($p =$ NS).

is the regulation of the amount of aromatase in benign and malignant breast tissue. Breast tissue aromatase can be regulated by several enhancers of aromatase transcription.[5–7] Dexamethasone, phorbol esters, cyclic AMP, interleukin-6, and prostaglandins can all stimulate aromatase transcription in cultured breast cancer cells, and specifically in the stromal components. Interestingly, products secreted by epithelial cells in the breast tumors appear to stimulate aromatase in the stroma and provide a means for autoregulation of tumor growth through estrogen production. A rather novel means of regulation of aromatase levels has also been described – stabilization of the degradation of the enzyme.[16] Aromatase inhibitors bind to the active site of the enzyme and, through mechanisms not completely understood, prevent proteolysis of the aromatase protein. Each of these mechanisms may enhance the amount of aromatase in tumor tissue and increase the need for very potent aromatase inhibitors.

DEVELOPMENT OF AROMATASE INHIBITORS

The first aromatase inhibitors were discovered some three decades ago, and included aminoglutethimide and testololactone.[3] Testololactone was not very potent as an inhibitor, while aminoglutethimide blocked several P450-mediated enzymatic reactions and was associated with troublesome side-effects. On the other hand, aminoglutethimide appeared to be quite effective in causing tumor regressions in patients with breast cancer. For this reason, pharmaceutical companies and individual investigators focused upon developing more potent and specific inhibitors. Second- and third-generation inhibitors were developed with 10 to 10 000-fold greater potency than aminoglutethimide and greater specificity (Figures 6.3 and 6.4). The half-lives of the inhibitors increased with synthesis of more potent inhibitors. The third-generation aromatase inhibitors are capable of decreasing the levels of circulating estrogens to a greater extent than the first- and second-generation inhibitors in postmenopausal women with hormone-dependent breast cancer. Hypothetically, these highly potent agents could also reduce levels of intratumoral aromatase activity to a greater extent than the earlier inhibitors, but this has not yet been examined.

PHARMACOLOGIC CLASSIFICATION OF AROMATASE INHIBITORS

A convenient classification divides inhibitors into mechanism-based or 'suicide' inhibitors (type I) and competitive inhibitors (type II).[17] Suicide inhibitors initially compete with natural substrates (i.e. androstenedione and testos-

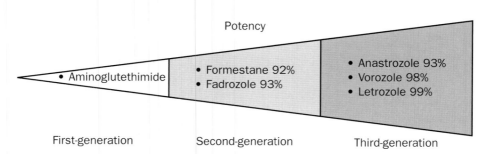

Figure 6.3 Diagrammatic representation of the potency of aromatase inhibitors as reflected by the isotopic kinetic method for determining the degree of aromatase inhibition. The percentage conversion of androstenedione to estrone is measured isotopically, correcting for losses of estrone by giving [^{14}C]estrone tracer. The values indicated represent percentage inhibition of total body aromatase.

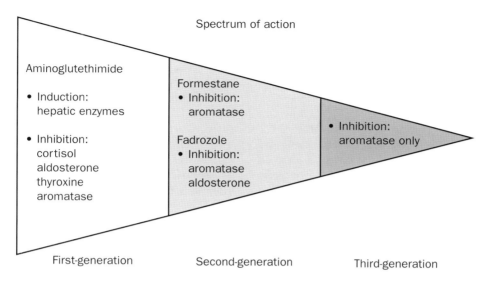

Figure 6.4 Diagrammatic representation of the spectrum of action of first- through third-generation aromatase inhibitors. With the development of newer inhibitors, the spectrum of action narrows. The third-generation aromatase inhibitors act exclusively on the aromatase enzyme and do not appear to exert additional effects.

terone) for binding to the active site of the enzyme. The enzyme then specifically acts upon the inhibitor to yield reactive alkylating species that form covalent bonds at or near the active site of the enzyme. Through this mechanism, the enzyme is irreversibly inactivated. Competitive inhibitors, on the other hand, bind reversibly to the active site of the enzyme and prevent product formation only as long as the inhibitor occupies the catalytic site. Whereas mechanism-based inhibitors are exclusively steroidal in type, competitive inhibitors consist of both steroidal and non-steroidal compounds.[17]

METHODS USED TO DEMONSTRATE AROMATASE INHIBITION

The standard method to study aromatase inhibitors in patients is to measure either plasma or urinary estrogen by radioimmunoassay. Early studies demonstrated 50–80% inhibition of plasma or urinary estrone or estradiol.[3] Another method involves measurement of each estrogen metabolite in urine, with calculation of the total aromatized product. This technique provides results similar to those from measurements of urinary estrone or estradiol.[18] Using these plasma or urinary methods, each agent appeared to suppress estrogen levels to concentrations approaching the sensitivity of the radioimmunoassays used. To gain greater specificity and sensitivity, investigators utilized the isotopic kinetic technique of Siiteri et al to measure total body aromatase.[19–22] This required administration of [^{3}H]androstenedione and [^{14}C]estrone to patients under steady-state conditions and measurement of radiochemically pure [^{3}H]estrone and [^{3}H]estradiol.[22] The [^{14}C]estrone allowed correction for losses during multiple purification steps. Using this technique, the degree of inhibition with various inhibitors ranged from 90% to 99%.

From these observations, it was recognized that more sensitive plasma assays of estradiol were needed. One approach was the use of the plasma estrone sulfate assay, since basal levels of this conjugate in postmenopausal women are tenfold higher than the levels of unconjugated estrone and estradiol.[23,24] With this measurement, suppression to 85% of basal values was observed with most inhibitors. Finally, an ultra-sensitive bioassay of plasma estradiol that was 50- to 100-fold more sensitive than radioim-munoassay was developed.[25] Surprisingly, with this assay, one could demonstrate suppression to levels of estradiol of 0.05–0.07 pg/ml, concentrations substantially lower than the 2–5 pg/ml suppressed levels detected by radioimmunoassay (Figure 6.5). As observed with the use of other highly sensitive plasma hormone assays (e.g. for LH, FSH, TSH, and growth hormone), the levels measured under basal conditions and during suppression with these assays are much lower than with insensitive radioimmunoassays. This probably reflects the fact that insensitive assays are measuring a substantial fraction of 'blank' or non-specific assay artifact. With the use of highly sensitive assays, this artifactual measurement is eliminated and the actual values measured are much

lower. Thus, with the ultrasensitive estradiol bioassay, the basal levels in postmenopausal women average 1–3 pg/ml (versus 5–20 pg/ml with radioimmunoassay).[25] During development of the second- and third-generation aromatase inhibitors, each of these methods has been used to demonstrate the magnitude of suppression of enzymatic activity. For these measurements, the isotopic kinetic technique is considered the 'gold standard', since it is highly sensitive and allows comparison among various inhibitors (Figure 6.3).

FIRST-GENERATION AROMATASE INHIBITORS

The first aromatase inhibitor to be widely used in the treatment of metastatic breast cancer in postmenopausal women was amino-glutethimide.[3,26] Isotopic kinetic studies demonstrated a 90–95% inhibition of aromatase activity.[22] Plasma estrone and estradiol levels and urinary estrogens fell by 50–80% in response to this aromatase inhibitor. An addition effect, described by Lonning and co-workers,[27] was acceleration of the metabolism of estrogen sulfate. This effect resulted in further lowering of free estrogen levels in plasma and in urine. With further study of amino-glutethimide, multiple metabolic effects were demonstrated, including inhibition of 11β-hydroxylase, aldosterone synthase, and thyroxine synthesis, as well as induction of enzymes metabolizing synthetic glucocorticoids and aminoglutethimide itself.[3]

When aminoglutethimide was combined with a corticosteroid such as hydrocortisone, the regimen produced durable clinical responses in 30–50% of patients.[3,26] This approach, however, had several important drawbacks. First, aminoglutethimide was associated with troublesome side-effects, including drowsiness, skin rash, and ataxia. Secondly, standard doses of 1000 mg daily of amino-glutethimide could also inhibit other cytochrome P450-mediated steroid hydroxylations, particularly those involving the choles-

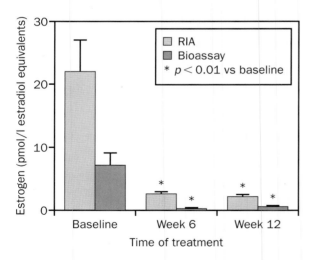

Figure 6.5 Inhibition of plasma estrogen levels as assessed by radioimmunoassay and by an ultrasensitive recombinant DNA-based bioassay.[21] Basal estradiol levels are approximately threefold lower when measured by the ultrasensitive assay. During administration of the aromatase inhibitor, levels fall to 0.05–0.07 pg/ml as assessed by the ultrasensitive assay and to 2–5 pg/ml with the standard radioimmunoassay.

terol side-chain cleavage enzymes.[3,28] This non-selectivity for aromatase led to inhibition of the biosynthesis of cortisol and aldosterone and also of thyroid hormone. This necessitated co-administration of the glucocorticoid hydrocortisone and, in about 5% of patients, thyroxine.

Four randomized controlled clinical trials compared aminoglutethimide in combination with hydrocortisone with tamoxifen in advanced breast cancer.[29-32] The antiestrogen tamoxifen and the inhibitor of estrogen biosynthesis aminoglutethimide/hydrocortisone produced similar rates of objective disease regression and duration of response.[3,29] Tamoxifen produced far fewer side-effects than did aminoglutethimide/hydrocortisone. Crossover responses to aminoglutethimide/ hydrocortisone in patients relapsing on tamoxifen were substantial, ranging from 25% to 50%, and 36% in the largest randomized study.[29] In marked contrast, patients initially treated with aminoglutethimide/hydrocortisone responded less frequently when crossed-over to tamoxifen (19%).[29] With development of better aromatase inhibitors, aminoglutethimide is now of historical interest only.

SECOND-GENERATION AROMATASE INHIBITORS

Fadrozole

Fadrozole inhibits aromatase with a K_i of 0.19 nM (versus 600 nM for aminoglutethimide).[33] Cholesterol side-chain cleavage activity is minimal, but C-11 hydroxylase inhibitory effects are observed in vitro at high drug concentrations. Initial dose-seeking studies conducted in patients demonstrated effective aromatase inhibition at doses of 1.8–4.0 mg daily.[33] A phase II study then compared doses of 0.6 mg three times daily, 1 mg twice daily, and 2 mg twice daily. Maximal suppression of plasma and urinary estrogens occurred at a dose of 1.0 mg twice daily and minimal effects on cortisol secretion were observed. Basal cortisol and adrenocorticotropic hormone (ACTH) levels were unaffected and cortisol levels

increased appropriately after exogenous synthetic ACTH (Cortrosyn) administration in all patients. Basal levels of aldosterone also remained stable following administration of all three drug doses. However, Cortrosyn-stimulated aldosterone levels were significantly blunted at all three doses.[34] Based on several phase II trials, toxicity attributed to this agent was mild and consisted mainly of nausea, anorexia, fatigue, and hot flashes.

Two large multicenter phase III trials in the USA compared fadrozole hydrochloride with megestrol acetate in 672 patients who had received only tamoxifen as prior hormonal therapy.[35,36] Final clinical results show that there were no significant differences between the two treatment arms of the trials with respect to time to progression, objective response rates, response duration, or overall survival. In these two trials, responses to megestrol acetate were somewhat lower than expected from previous studies, with objective response rates of 11% and 13% respectively. Randomized patients receiving fadrozole experienced objective responses of 11% and 16%, which did not differ significantly from these with megestrol. Stable disease for more than 6 months occurred in 25% of patients receiving fadrozole and 20% taking megestrol acetate.

Two trials compared fadrozole with tamoxifen.[37,38] In the first, 1 mg twice daily of fadrozole was compared with 20 mg daily of tamoxifen in 212 postmenopausal patients with metastatic breast cancer. Response rates to tamoxifen (27%) and to fadrozole (20%) did not differ significantly, nor did response durations (20 months versus 15 months). However, tamoxifen achieved a significantly longer time to treatment failure (8.5 months versus 6 months; $p < 0.05$). In the second study, fadrozole was compared with tamoxifen as first-line therapy in a randomized, controlled trial conducted in South Africa. Response rates to tamoxifen were 48% versus 43% with fadrozole ($p = NS$). However, response duration was significantly longer with tamoxifen (median duration not reached versus 343 days; $p < 0.009$), as was overall survival (34 months for tamoxifen versus 26 months for fadrozole; $p < 0.046$).

Taken together, these studies demonstrate that fadrozole may be inferior to tamoxifen in efficacy and no better tolerated than megestrol acetate. Based upon these findings, the second-generation aromatase inhibitor fadrozole would likely find its place as third-line therapy. Fadrozole has been approved for the treatment of advanced breast cancer in postmenopausal women in Japan. This agent is not likely to be further developed in the USA, since both anastrozole and letrozole appear to be more potent and more selective aromatase inhibitors.

Careful analysis of the fadrozole/megestrol acetate trials raises the concern that responses to endocrine therapies appeared to be less frequent than observed in prior studies. For example, a randomized comparison of the first-generation aromatase inhibitor aminoglutethimide with surgical adrenalectomy demonstrated response rates of 40–50% in patients previously treated with tamoxifen.[39] Other studies with megestrol acetate as second-line therapy demonstrated response rates ranging from 30% to 50%. Several possibilities could explain the low response rates. In recent studies, more stringent criteria have been used than in previous trials. For example, recalcification of mixed lytic/blastic metastases was previously considered objective evidence of partial response. Such lesions are now considered non-assessable, non-measurable disease. External review of cases probably also increases the stringency of assessment. It should be noted that in a previous study comparing tamoxifen alone versus tamoxifen and fluoxymestrone, the objective response rate for tamoxifen alone was only 10%.[40] These considerations lead to the conclusion that one can only compare new agents with established ones such as tamoxifen and assess the relative differences between them. It is inappropriate to compare the percentage of objective responses with those observed in historical controls.

Formestane

Formestane (4-hydroxyandrostenedione, 4-OHA) is a structural analog of androstenedione and is thus a highly specific aromatase inhibitor. It was the first steroidal suicide-type (type I) aromatase inhibitor to enter clinical trials, and is now commercially available in Europe. Using the in vitro placental aromatase assay system, formestane was shown to be 60-fold more potent than aminoglutethimide $K_i = 4.1$ μM). Extensive studies revealed no estrogenic, anti-estrogenic, or antiandrogenic properties.[41] However, transformation to 4-hydroxytestosterone occurs and androgenic effects can be demonstrated under certain circumstances.[42]

Formestane has been studied extensively in Europe in postmenopausal women with breast cancer. Data from four phase II clinical trials of formestane demonstrated a 33% objective regression rate of breast cancer in postmenopausal patients previously treated with multiple endocrine therapies. Toxicity included six patients with sterile abscesses due to intramuscular injections, two of which were of sufficient severity to warrant discontinuation of therapy. No androgenic effects were observed.[43]

Höffken and colleagues[44] conducted a large trial of formestane in postmenopausal women. Patients initially received 500 mg intramuscularly every 2 weeks for 6 weeks and then 250 mg every 2 weeks thereafter. Of 86 evaluable patients, there were 2 complete and 19 partial remissions (24%) and 26 with disease stabilization (30%). Studies of the degree of aromatase inhibition using isotopic kinetic techniques demonstrate that formestane is not as effective as the third-generation inhibitors in blocking estrogen production (Figure 6.3). For this reason, it is unlikely that this agent will compete successfully with the newer inhibitors.

THIRD-GENERATION AROMATASE INHIBITORS

Anastrozole

Anastrozole is a potent and selective benzyltriazole derivative.[45,46] Studies in women demonstrated suppression of plasma estrogen to levels approaching assay sensitivity.[47]

Anastrozole produces no effects on aldosterone, cortisol, or thyroxine synthesis.[47] The estimated elimination half-life in humans is 32.2 hours.

Anastrozole was the first aromatase inhibitor to be approved in the USA for the management of advanced breast carcinoma in postmenopausal women. This approval was based on the results of two pivotal trials that together accrued a total of 764 patients randomized to receive either oral anastrozole 1 mg daily or anastrozole 10 mg daily or megestrol acetate 40 mg four times a day.[45] These patients had metastatic disease that was progressing following therapy with tamoxifen given either in the adjuvant setting or as first-line endocrine therapy for metastatic disease. Patients in the three arms of the trial had similar prognostic characteristics, including age, ER status, disease-free interval, and sites of metastases. Results from these important trials showed similar overall rates of response to either dose of anastrozole or to megestrol acetate. No statistically significant dose response differences were observed between the 1 mg and 10 mg daily dosages. The rates of overall objective response of 10.3% and 8.9% were also surprisingly low – probably for reasons discussed above. Overall responses including complete and partial objective response rates and stabilization of disease of greater than 6 months averaged 35%. It should be noted that recent studies have demonstrated that disease stabilization for greater than 6 months is a meaningful clinical parameter, since patients experiencing this response survive equally as long as patients undergoing partial objective response.[48–50] Patients with complete or partial objective responses or stable disease survive longer than those with disease progression.

In initial reports, the third-generation aromatase inhibitor anastrozole was considered superior to megestrol acetate because it was better tolerated. It was associated with less undesirable weight gain and dyspnea and fewer thromboembolic events when compared with megestrol acetate.[45] Since there were no differences between the two doses of anastrozole, the drug was approved at a dose of 1 mg daily.

With further maturity of this trial, anastrozole 1 or 10 mg daily conferred a survival advantage compared with the progestin (median of 26.7 months versus 22.5 months)[51] (Table 6.1). The 2-year survival rate was 56.1% for the group of patients receiving anastrozole 1 mg, compared with 46.3% for patients treated with megestrol acetate. The demonstration that anastrozole has superior efficacy with respect to overall survival and reduced side-effects versus megestrol acetate suggests that the aromatase inhibitor should be used as second-line therapy in preference to megestrol acetate.

Letrozole

The second aromatase inhibitor to gain approval in the USA with the indication for management of postmenopausal women with metastatic breast cancer was letrozole, a potent non-steroidal competitive aromatase inhibitor.[52–55] This agent possesses considerable selectivity for aromatase. In preclinical studies, letrozole caused inhibition of aldosterone production in vitro only at concentrations 10 000 times higher than those required for inhibition of estrogen production. Letrozole is a highly potent and selective aromatase inhibitor. When administered orally to adult female rats at a dose of 1 mg/kg/day for 14 days, letrozole decreases uterine weight to that observed after a surgical ovariectomy. At doses greater than 1000 times higher than the concentration required to cause a 50% inhibition of the aromatase enzyme, letrozole does not significantly suppress either aldosterone or corticosterone in rats. Letrozole also causes significant regression of DMBA-induced rat mammary tumors.[54]

Clinical studies in normal healthy volunteers as well as dose-seeking phase I trials in postmenopausal women with advanced breast cancer showed that letrozole in an oral dose as small as 0.25 mg daily caused maximal suppression of plasma and urinary estrogens. A highly sensitive recombinant DNA-based estradiol bioassay was used to assess estradiol levels in one of these studies.[25] The levels of estradiol

Table 6.1 Comparison of third-generation aromatase inhibition with progestin therapy

Response parameters	MA vs vorozole[59]			MA vs anastrozole (1 mg)[51]			MA vs letrozole (2.5 mg)[52]		
	MA	Vorozole	p	MA	Anastrozole	p	MA	Letrozole	p
Overall survival	28.7 months	26 months	NS	22.5 months	26.7 months	0.02	21.5 months	25.3 months	0.15
Objective response rates (CR + PR)	7.6%	10.5%	NS	12.2%	12.6%	NS	16.4%	23.6%	0.04
Clinical benefit (CR + PR + stable > 6 months)	NR	NR	—	40.2%	42.3%	—	32%	35%	NS
Time to progression	3.6 months	2.7 months	NS	5 months	5 months	NS	5.5 months	5.6 months	0.07
Number in study	452			764			551		

MA, megestrol acetate; NS, not significant; CR, complete response; PR, partial response; NR, not reported.

were decreased by 95% to levels of 0.05–0.07 pg/ml as detected by this assay (Figure 6.5). This observation underscores the limitation of standard radioimmunoassays for detection of estradiol levels in patients given highly potent aromatase inhibitors.

Additional studies established the fact that letrozole was quite selective for the inhibition of aromatase, since, over a wide dose range, there were no significant changes in the levels of gonadotropins, ACTH, cortisol, aldosterone, or thyroid-stimulating hormone (TSH).[55,56] Early trials of letrozole in heavily pretreated post-menopausal women with metastatic breast cancer demonstrated both clinical efficacy and lack of significant toxicity.[57]

Approval of this agent was based on the results of two large multicenter, randomized trials similar in design to the studies involving anastrozole.[52,53] In a pivotal trial,[52] 551 post-menopausal women with metastatic breast carcinoma progressing after treatment with tamoxifen were randomized to receive letrozole 0.5 mg daily, letrozole 2.5 mg daily, or standard doses of megestrol acetate (Tables 6.1 and 6.2). The women in the three treatment groups were comparable in all respects. The two doses of letrozole caused similar prompt and profound suppression of plasma and urinary estrogens.[55] Letrozole 2.5 mg yielded an overall response rate (complete and partial tumor regression and disease stabilization for greater than 6 months) of 35% compared with 27% for letrozole 0.5 mg and 32% for megestrol acetate. However, the median duration of response for letrozole 2.5 mg was 33 months, compared with 18 months for both megestrol acetate and the lower dose of letrozole. There was a non-significant trend in time to tumor progression and survival that favors the letrozole 2.5 mg dose.

In a second and similar study involving 555 postmenopausal patients with advanced breast cancer progressing after tamoxifen therapy,[53] letrozole was compared with amino-glutethimide 250 mg twice a day and hydrocortisone (Table 6.3). Letrozole 0.5 mg daily produced a non-significant difference in objec-

tive response rate of 17% versus 12% for aminoglutethimide.[53] The median response duration was 23 months for letrozole, compared with 15 months for aminoglutethimide, and there was a statistically significant improvement in overall survival for the patients receiving letrozole. Moreover, letrozole produced less somnolence and skin rash. The results of these large, well-done, randomized trials suggest that the side-effect profile and the dosing schedules of both anastrozole and letrozole are superior to those of megestrol acetate and aminoglutethimide.

Recently a third multicenter randomized study (US02) of letrozole in patients with advanced breast cancer progressing on tamoxifen has been published.[58] This study had a similar design to that of the first study noted above,[52] in that patients were randomized to a standard dosage of megestrol acetate, letrozole 2.5 mg daily, or letrozole 0.5 mg daily. While the designs of the studies are similar, the results are somewhat different. In the US02 study, there was no difference in the objective response rates between megestrol acetate, letrozole 0.5 mg, and letrozole 2.5 mg. The time to progression (TTP) and time to treatment failure (TTF) were significantly better in the patients treated with letrozole 0.5 mg compared with those treated with megestrol acetate ($p = 0.044$ and $p = 0.018$, respectively), while the time to death (TTD) was of borderline significance ($p = 0.053$). There was no difference between letrozole 2.5 mg and megestrol acetate in terms of TTP, TTF, or TTD. There was a non-significant trend ($p = 0.073$ and $p = 0.076$) in favor of letrozole 0.5 mg versus 2.5 mg in terms of TTP and TTF, respectively. There was no difference between the two doses in terms of TTD.

The findings of this latest study are of interest in that letrozole 2.5 mg is the currently recommended and commercially available dose. These results also suggest that letrozole is in fact similar to other aromatase inhibitors in terms of the lack of unequivocal evidence of a dose response in large randomized clinical trials.

Table 6.2 Dose–response studies with third-generation aromatase inhibitors

Response parameters	Anastrozole[51]			Letrozole[52,53]		
	1 mg	10 mg	p	0.5 mg	2.5 mg	p
Overall survival	26.7 months	NR	NS	21.5 months[52] 21 months[53]	25.3 months 28 months	0.04
Objective response rate (CR + PR)	10.3%	8.9%	NS	12.8% 16.7%	23.6% 19.5%	0.004 NS
Clinical benefit (CR + PR + stable > 6 months)	35%	32%	NS	27% 32.8%	35% 36.3%	NS NS
Time to progression	5 months	5 months	NS	5.1 months 3.3 months	5.6 months 3.4 months	0.02 NS
Number in study		764			551 555	

NR, not reported; NS, not significant; CR, complete response; PR, partial response.

Vorozole

This agent is another third-generation non-steroidal oral aromatase inhibitor that is highly potent and specific for aromatase.[59] Its clinical efficacy appears to be similar to that of anastrozole and letrozole (Tables 6.1 and 6.2). Vorozole appears to be superior to aminoglutethimide/ hydrocortisone with respect to clinical benefit (i.e. complete and partial objective regression plus stabilization of disease for greater than 6 months) (Table 6.3). Its efficacy did not differ significantly from that of megestrol acetate, although it was associated with fewer side-effects. Because of the proven efficacy and prior approval of anastrozole and letrozole, further

clinical development of vorozole has been abandoned.

Exemestane

Exemestane is an irreversible (type I, mechanism-based) aromatase inactivator.[60–62] Its K_i for competitive inhibition is 4.3 nM and its K_{inact} for irreversible inactivation is 26 nM. Single-dose administration reveals a major reduction of plasma estrogens with this compound.[60] A dose of 25 mg daily inhibited aromatase activity as documented by the isotope kinetic technique by 97.9%. Thurlimann et al[61] reported an objective response – complete (CR)

Table 6.3 Comparison of first- with third-generation aromatase inhibitors

Response parameters	AG/HC vs vorozole[59]			AG/HC vs letrozole[53]		
	AG/HC	Vorozole	p	AG/HC	Letrozole	p
Overall survival	21.7 months	25.7 months	NS	20 months	28 months	0.002
Objective response rate (CR + PR)	18%	23%	0.085	12%	17%	0.06
Clinical benefit (CR + PR + stable > 6 months)	37%	47%	0.017	29.3%	32.8%	NR
Time to progression	6.0 months	6.7 months	NS	3.2 months	3.4 months	0.008
Number in study		556			555	

AG, aminoglutethimide; HC, hydrocortisone; NS, not significant; CR, complete response; PR, partial response; NR, not reported.

plus partial (PR) – in 12% and 33% of patients expressing primary or secondary resistance to aminoglutethimide.

Two phase II open-label trials examined the effects of 25 mg of exemestane daily by mouth in patients with progressive disease after initial treatment with tamoxifen.[63,64] In the US trial,[63] entry criteria included postmenopausal status and relapse while receiving tamoxifen for metastatic disease or within 12 months of discontinuing adjuvant tamoxifen. Additional criteria included ER and PgR positivity and absence of rapidly progressing or inflammatory disease. Of the 128 women entered, 28% experienced an objective response rate and 47% clini-cal benefit as defined as CR, PR, or stable disease for greater than 24 weeks. In the European trial of 137 patients, 31% experienced objective responses (i.e. CR or PR) and 59% clinical bene-fit.[64] Estrogen production fell by 90% as assessed by measurement of estrone sulfate levels, and the drug was well tolerated.

Phase III studies compared 25 mg of exemes-tane daily in 366 patients with megestrol acetate 40 mg four times daily in 403 women progress-ing after initial tamoxifen therapy.[65,66] Only two-thirds of patients were known to be ER-positive. Objective responses occurred in 15% of women on exemestane and 12% on megestrol acetate, and the clinical benefit was

37% and 35%, respectively (p = NS for both). Both TTP (p = 0.037) and overall survival (p = 0.039) were significantly better for exemestane than for megestrol acetate.

Exemestane has also been studied as a third-line agent to be used after tamoxifen and non-steroidal aromatase inhibitors.[67-69] A large trial evaluated a total of 241 patients who had been treated both with tamoxifen and with a non-steroidal aromatase inhibitor (anastrozole, fadrozole, or vorozole). The objective response rate was 7% and the clinical benefit 24%, with a median duration of response of 58 weeks. This study demonstrated the lack of complete cross-resistance between aromatase inhibitors.[67]

COMPARISON OF POTENCY OF AROMATASE INHIBITORS

The relative potencies of aromatase inhibitors can be determined in vitro as characterized as the inhibitory constant K_i or as the concentration that inhibits aromatase by 50%. However, these measurements do not provide information that can be extrapolated to patients, since the drug half-life and the amount of drug that can be given safely also contribute substantially to the degree of inhibition achievable in vivo. Consequently, the most useful comparator of potency among agents is measurement of the degree of aromatase inhibition in women with breast cancer. This requires highly sensitive and specific means of measuring aromatase inhibition. Plasma radioimmunoassay techniques are not sufficiently sensitive to precisely quantitate degree of suppression and the ultrasensitive estradiol bioassay has not been used to compare inhibitors.

The isotopic kinetic technique for quantitating total body aromatase activity serves then as the best method to compare the potency of various inhibitors in patients.[19-22] Jones et al[21] have compared a number of these agents and reviewed published studies of others. With this methodology, formestane inhibits aromatase by 92%, fadrozole by 93%, exemestane by 97.9%, anastrozole by 93%, vorozole by 98%, and letro-

zole by 99% (Figure 6.3). It is not clear whether the aromatase activity remaining during therapy is biologically important. Most biologic systems operate on a logarithmic dose–response basis. Since residual aromatase activity is 8% with formestane and only 1% with letrozole, these differences could have biologic relevance.

SUMMARY OF CONCLUSIONS FROM LARGE CLINICAL TRIALS WITH THIRD-GENERATION AROMATASE INHIBITORS AS SECOND-LINE THERAPY

These studies allow answers to four important questions:

1. Do higher doses of third-generation aromatase inhibitors produce greater clinical effects than lower doses?
2. Do third-generation inhibitors produce greater clinical benefit than the first-generation aromatase inhibitor amino-glutethimide?
3. Do the third-generation inhibitors produce greater clinical benefit than megestrol acetate?
4. Are aromatase inhibitors similar or superior in efficacy to tamoxifen?

A fifth question, 'Which is the most effective third-generation aromatase inhibitor?' cannot be answered until head-to-head comparisons between agents are made. Relative efficacy based upon results among very large but non-randomized trials cannot be validly interpreted, but provide trends to be tested in future studies.

With respect to the dose–response question (question 1), the two initial large studies suggested that 2.5 mg of letrozole was clinically more effective than the 0.5 mg dose. However, a second study[53] of similar design published recently failed to confirm this – indeed, if anything, there was a non-significant trend in favor of the 0.5 mg dose for TTP and TTF. No differences were demonstrated when comparing 1 mg with 10 mg daily of anastrozole (Table 6.2). With respect to the superiority of third-over first-generation inhibitors (question 2), letrozole at the 2.5 mg dosage produced significantly better responses than did aminoglutethimide with respect to duration of response, TTP, and TTF (Table 6.3). The objective response rates were also greater with letrozole than with aminoglutethimide, and the rate of side-effects was less than with the first-generation aromatase inhibitor. However, it should be noted that 9% of patients in the aminoglutethimide arm discontinued the drug because of side-effects. While there is no doubt that letrozole was a clinically more effective treatment than aminoglutethimide, it remains to be established how much of this benefit was due to better drug tolerability (and therefore to more patients remaining in the active treatment) or whether it was a more potent aromatase inhibitor. Finally, with respect to the superiority of third-generation inhibitors to other agents (question 3), exemestane and anastrozole were clearly superior to megestrol acetate with respect to overall patient survival (Table 6.1). Letrozole 0.5 mg was statistically superior in terms of TTP and TTF in one study, while letrozole 2.5 mg showed more objective responses in the study of similar design. The overall duration of survival was not significantly different, but there was a non-significant trend in favor of letrozole 0.5 mg ($p = 0.053$) in the US02 study. With greater maturity of these studies, differences in overall survival could emerge. It should be noted that earlier studies (as cited above) suggested equal efficacy of anastrozole and megestrol acetate but updated data demonstrate a clear enhancement of overall survival imparted by anastrozole when compared with megestrol. Vorozole, on the other hand, did not differ from megestrol acetate with respect to any parameter reflecting efficacy.

Each of these trials demonstrated that the third-generation aromatase inhibitors were better tolerated than megestrol acetate. Side-effects reported for letrozole and anastrozole were of low grade in severity, including mild headache, nausea, diarrhea, and hot flashes, and were infrequent. Significantly, letrozole and anastro-

zole were associated with less weight gain, dyspnea, thromboembolic events, and vaginal bleeding when compared with megestrol acetate.[45,52,58]

All three of these aromatase inhibitors – exemestane, anastrozole, and letrozole – are highly potent, specific, and well tolerated. Based upon the studies reviewed, these agents have now replaced megestrol acetate as second-line therapy after tamoxifen in postmenopausal women with metastatic breast carcinoma.

AROMATASE INHIBITORS VERSUS TAMOXIFEN AS FIRST-LINE THERAPY

The fourth clinical question asks where aromatase inhibitors are superior to tamoxifen. There are now data available that allow us to address this question.

Anastrozole

Two large randomized trials of similar design have been published, comparing 1 mg of anastrozole daily with 20 mg of tamoxifen as first-line therapy for metastatic breast cancer. A European trial with entry of 668 patients reported objective response rates of 32.9% with anastrozole and 32.6% with tamoxifen[70] and clinical benefit (i.e. CR, PR, or stable disease for more than 24 weeks) in 56.2% of patients receiving anastrozole and 56.5% on tamoxifen. No statistically significant differences emerged with respect to percentage disease progression or median TTP. Survival data are not yet available. The second trial[71] entered 171 patients into the anastrozole arm and 182 into the tamoxifen arm. Objective responses occurred in 21.1% of patients receiving anastrozole and 17.0% on tamoxifen. Clinical benefit was observed in 59.1% of women on anastrozole and 45.6% on tamoxifen (2-sided $p = 0.005$). TTP was significantly longer with anastrozole (11.1 months) than with tamoxifen (5.6 months), and this result was statistically significant ($p = 0.005$). These two large trials when combined[72] have been reported to show at least equivalent efficacy of aromatase inhibitors and tamoxifen overall, with a superiority for anastrozole in hormone-receptor-positive tumors. A longer period of observation is necessary to determine if survival differences will be observed in this study.

More recently, another European study has been reported comparing anastrozole with tamoxifen as initial endocrine therapy in patients with advanced breast cancer.[73] Patients entering this study had receptor-positive tumors. Anastrozole-treated patients showed a higher objective response and clinical benefit rate than patients who received tamoxifen. Anastrozole was associated with a significantly longer TTP than tamoxifen (10.6 months versus 5.3 months, respectively; $p < 0.05$). This study also reported that there was a survival advantage for the patients treated with anastrozole compared with tamoxifen ($p < 0.05$). This is the first study to report a survival advantage of a third-generation aromatase inhibitor over tamoxifen as first-line endocrine therapy for advanced breast cancer.

A potential advantage of the aromatase inhibitors is the lack of estrogenic effects associated with their use. Recent data suggest that estrogen-replacement therapy causes an increase in the rate of thromboembolic events in postmenopausal women. It is of interest then to examine the rate of these events in women receiving tamoxifen versus anastrozole. This is clearly of interest in terms of patients with advanced breast cancer, but it might be particularly significant in terms of adjuvant therapies, where patients tend to continue on endocrine agents for longer periods of time. In the two advanced breast cancer trials of similar design referred to above,[70,71] thromboembolic events were associated with the use of anastrozole in 4.8% and 4.1% of cases and with tamoxifen in 7.3% and 8.2%. These data suggest that the aromatase inhibitors might be preferable for patients with a history of prior thromboembolic events.

Letrozole

A large phase III randomized trial comparing letrozole versus tamoxifen as first-line endocrine therapy in patients with advanced breast cancer has also been reported.[74] This trial was initiated as a three-arm study comparing initial tamoxifen 20 mg daily (with subsequent crossover to letrozole on disease progression), initial letrozole 2.5 mg daily (with subsequent crossover to tamoxifen on disease progression), and the two agents given initially in combination. The third arm was discontinued owing to interactions between the two agents that affected the serum concentration of letrozole. The study was therefore continued as a two-arm crossover study. The reported results of this study relate to the therapeutic efficacy of the two agents given as first time therapy. Data on the crossover are not yet available.

Letrozole 2.5 mg was superior to tamoxifen 20 mg daily in terms of objective response rate (30% versus 20%, respectively) and clinical benefit (49% versus 38%, respectively). Letrozole was also statistically superior to tamoxifen in terms of TTP (9.4 versus 6.0 months, respectively; $p = 0.0001$) and TTF (9.1 versus 5.7 months, respectively; $p = 0.0001$). With longer follow-up, a more recent report of this study has shown no difference in overall survival between patients randomized to these two treatment sequences. There was no significant difference in overall survival between the two treatment arms, either by log-rank test ($p = 0.53$) or Wilcoxon test ($p = 0.08$).[75] Therefore, while letrozole provided an early advantage in TTP, it did not result in a long-term survival advantage when patients were crossed-over to tamoxifen. While this is an important finding, it does not negate the superior initial control achieved with an aromatase inhibitor over tamoxifen, which has now been recorded for both letrozole and anastrozole in advanced breast cancer.

Exemestane

Exemestane has also been compared with tamoxifen as first-line endocrine therapy in a small randomized phase II study. It should be noted that while the study was randomized, it was not blinded to either the patient or the clinician – i.e. it was an 'open' study. Data reported thus far suggested that patients treated with exemestane had better outcome in terms of objective response, clinical benefit, and TTP than those treated with tamoxifen.[76]

RELATIVE EFFICACY OF THIRD-GENERATION INHIBITORS

Table 6.4 compares several parameters observed with the various third-generation inhibitors when compared with megestrol acetate. Overall survival is quite similar with each agent, ranging from 25.3 months to 28

months. Objective response rates, on the other hand, appeared somewhat higher with letrozole (19.5% and 23.6%) than with vorozole (10.5%) and anastrozole (10.3%). The percentage of patients experiencing clinical benefit (i.e. objective response plus stabilization of disease for greater than 6 months) appeared similar for each therapeutic modality, and ranged from 47% with vorozole, to 35% with anastrozole, to 36.3 and 35% with letrozole. TTP appeared to be the shortest with vorozole (2.7 months) and somewhat longer but similar with anastrozole (5 months) and letrozole (3.4–5.6 months).

There is no direct comparison of any of these three aromatase inhibitors as first-line therapy. Any comparison, therefore, must be by indirect assessment of how they have each compared

Table 6.4 Comparison of third-generation aromatase inhibitors versus megestrol acetate

Response parameters	Vorozole[59]	Anastrozole[51]	Letrozole[52,53]
Overall survival	26 months	26.7 months	25.3 months[52] 28 months[53]
Objective response rate (CR + PR)	10.5%	10.3%	23.6% 19.5%
Clinical benefit (CR + PR + stable > 6 months)	47%	35%	35% 36.3%
Time to progression	2.7 months	5 months	5.6 months 3.4 months
Number in study	452	764	551 555

CR, complete response; PR, partial response.

versus tamoxifen in the studies detailed above. Such interstudy comparisons are fraught with difficulties (e.g. different entry criteria and different patient populations) and should be interpreted with much caution. In a recent review, Buzdar[77] summarized the main clinical outcomes. The similarities in outcome are interesting, and the table in Buzdar's article is reproduced here (Table 6.5). The percentage of patients with hormone-receptor-positive tumors is different in each study, and therefore of particular interest is the comparison of the three aromatase inhibitors in the subgroup of patients with receptor-positive tumors. This showed that for the primary objective of the studies (i.e. TTP), the benefit of each aromatase inhibitor over tamoxifen was remarkably similar (i.e. approximately 10 months versus 6 months) (Table 6.5).

Head-to-head comparisons are now required to determine if one aromatase inhibitor is significantly better than another. However, given the similar differences that have been seen with each of these aromatase inhibitors when compared with tamoxifen, one can estimate that it will require much larger studies (of over 1000 patients) to ensure adequate power to avoid a type 2 error when comparing between these aromatase inhibitors.

AROMATASE INHIBITORS VERSUS A PURE ANTIESTROGEN IN ADVANCED BREAST CANCER

Two randomized studies of similar trial design comparing anastrozole versus the pure antiestrogen fulvestrant (ICI 182,780, Faslodex) have been reported.[77–79] These were both second-line endocrine therapy trials in patients with advanced breast cancer who had failed prior tamoxifen treatment. They showed no significant difference in terms of objective response and clinical benefit rates nor in TTP. The two agents also had similar side-effect profiles.

COMPARISON OF ANTIESTROGENS WITH THIRD-GENERATION AROMATASE INHIBITORS IN THE ADJUVANT SETTING

Trials are ongoing to determine the efficacy of aromatase inhibitors versus tamoxifen versus the combination of antiestrogen and aromatase inhibitor. The largest trial is termed the ATAC trial – 'anastrozole alone versus tamoxifen alone and in combination' (i.e. anastrozole plus tamoxifen) for 5 years – and enrolled a total of 9366 patients. The ATAC trial recently reported the first efficacy data from trials of third-generation aromatase inhibitors as adjuvant therapy.

The mean age and mean weight of the patients and the hormone-receptor status of the primary tumors were well balanced between the three treatment arms (Table 6.6), as were primary treatment (i.e. surgery, radiotherapy, and chemotherapy), tumor size and grade, and nodal status.[80] The primary endpoints were disease-free survival and tolerability. With a median follow-up for 33.3 months, disease-free survival was significantly longer in the patients randomized to anastrozole compared with tamoxifen ($p = 0.0129$). The hazard ratio was 0.83 (95.2% confidence interval, CI = 0.71–0.96) in favor of anastrozole.[81,82] There was no significant difference between the combination of anastrozole and tamoxifen versus tamoxifen alone ($p = 0.77$). The findings were even more striking when patients with hormone-receptor-positive tumors were analyzed. The hazard ratio in favor of anastrozole versus tamoxifen was 0.78 (95.2% CI = 0.65–0.93) ($p = 0.0054$).[82]

The reduction in disease events was seen at all sites of disease – i.e. locoregional, distant, and contralateral – further confirming that the results do represent an overall improvement in efficacy of anastrozole over tamoxifen. The reduction was most marked in the reduction of contralateral breast cancers, where the hazard ratio was 0.42 (95.2% CI = 0.22–0.79) ($p = 0.007$) in favor of anastrozole compared with tamoxifen. There was no difference in the incidence of contralateral breast cancers between the combination and tamoxifen

Table 6.5 Comparison of third-generation aromatase inhibitors versus tamoxifen: analysis by hormone-receptor status

	Anastrozole combined analysis		Letrozole		Exemestane phase II trial	
	Anastrozole	Tamoxifen	Letrozole	Tamoxifen	Exemestane	Tamoxifen
Total no. of patients	511	510	453	454	57	50
CR + PR (%)	29	27	30	20	42	16
CR + PR + stable > 24 wks (%)	57	52	49	38	58	31
Median TTP (months)	8.5	7.0	9.5	6.0	8.9	5.2
% of patients dead	ND	ND	ND	ND	ND	ND
% of hormone-receptor-positive patients	60	60	66	67	89	86

	Anastrozole combined analysis: subgroup of ER$^+$ and/or PgR$^+$		Letrozole: subgroup of ER$^+$ and/or PgR$^+$		Anastrozole independent Spanish study: all ER$^+$ patients	
	Anastrozole	Tamoxifen	Letrozole	Tamoxifen	Anastrozole	Tamoxifen
Total no. of patients	305	306	294	305	121	117
CR + PR (%)	ND	ND	31	21	34	27
CR + PR + stable > 24 wks (%)	ND	ND	ND	ND	72	55
Median TTP (months)	10.7	6.4	9.7	6.0	12.6	5.3
% of patients dead	ND	ND	ND	ND	61	92
% of hormone receptor-positive patients	100	100	100	100	100	100

Reproduced by permission of *Breast Cancer On-line*.
CR, complete response; PR, partial response; TTP, time to progression; ND, no data; ER, estrogen receptor; PgR, progesterone receptor.

Table 6.6 Pretreatment patient and hormone-receptor details in the ATAC study

	Anastrozole	Tamoxifen	Combination
No. of patients	3125	3116	3125
Mean age (years)	64.1	64.1	64.3
Mean weight (kg)	70.8	71.1	71.3
Receptor status:			
% positive	83.7	83.3	84.0
% negative	7.4	8.0	6.9
% other	8.9	8.7	9.1

(hazard ratio = 0.84, 92.5% CI = 0.51–1.40) ($p = 0.5$).[82] These results are summarized in Figure 6.6.

Tolerability was the other primary endpoint of the study. Anastrozole appeared to be significantly better tolerated than tamoxifen in terms of endometrial cancer, vaginal bleeding/dis-charge, ischemic cerebrovascular events, thromboembolic events, hot flashes, and weight gain) ($p < 0.03$ for all). Tamoxifen was significantly better tolerated than anastrozole in terms of musculoskeletal disorders and fractures ($p < 0.03$ for both). The tolerability results are summarized in Figure 6.7.

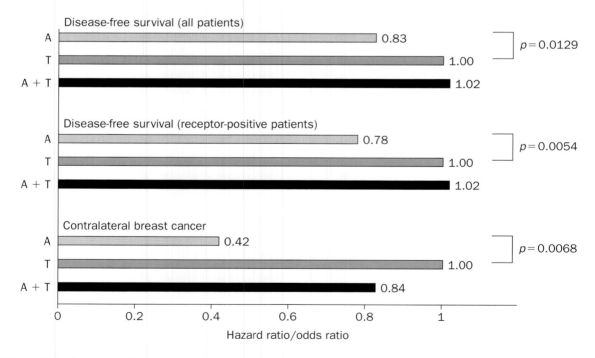

Figure 6.6 Summary of results from the ATAC trial. A, anastrozole; T, tamoxifen; (Reproduced from Fisher MD, O'Shaughnessy J. Anastrozole may be superior to tamoxifen as adjuvant treatment for postmenopausal patients with breast cancer. *Clin Breast Cancer* 2002; **2**: 269–71.)[80]

The initial findings of the ATAC study are therefore very encouraging, showing superior efficacy of anastrozole over tamoxifen for both disease-free survival and contralateral breast cancer. Nevertheless, longer follow-up and long-term data on bone mineral density and cognitive function are required. The differential actions of the anti-estrogens and aromatase inhibitors on non-breast tissues are likely to show up in the long-term side-effect profile as well as in differences in efficacy. Tamoxifen acts as an estrogen agonist on the uterus and increases the incidence of uterine cancer, whereas the aromatase inhibitors would be expected to reduce estrogenic stimulation on the uterus. The beneficial effects of tamoxifen on bone and potentially on the cardiovascular system differ from the potential of the aromatase inhibitors to accelerate the process of bone resorption and the incidence of cardiovascular disease. Subprojects within the ATAC trial are examining these issues in detail.

The results of ATAC and other adjuvant therapy trials involving third-generation aromatase inhibitors (i.e. anastrozole, letrozole, and examestane) should establish the relative efficacies of these two therapeutic strategies (i.e. tamoxifen or third-generation aromatase inhibitors) alone, in combination, or in sequence. However, just as important will be comparisons between different aromatase inhibitors – not only in terms of relative efficacy but also in terms of side-effect profiles. The level of inhibition of the aromatase enzyme

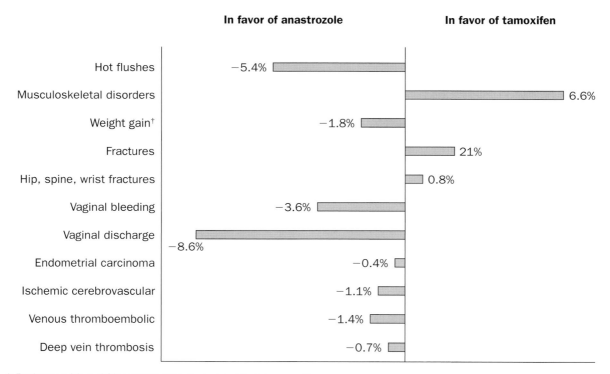

† Patients with >10% weight gain from baseline to year 2

Figure 6.7 Summary of the tolerability results from the ATAC trial showing the percentage differences between adverse events observed on anastrozole versus tamoxifen. (Reproduced from Fisher MD, O'Shaughnessy J. Anastrozole may be superior to tamoxifen as adjuvant treatment for postmenopausal patients with breast cancer. *Clin Breast Cancer* 2002; **2:** 269–71.)[80]

achieved by all third-generation aromatase inhibitors currently in development is over 95%. It is uncertain at this point whether relatively small differences in the percentage inhibition of the aromatase enzyme by these drugs may have marked differences on normal tissues (and therefore tolerability) or efficacy.

AROMATASE INHIBITORS AS NEOADJUVANT ENDOCRINE THERAPY

Endocrine therapy administered prior to surgery in an attempt to shrink the primary tumor is called neoadjuvant therapy. Dixon et al[83] conducted a trial comparing the use of letrozole, anatrozole, and tamoxifen in women with ER-positive (>20 fmol/mg cystosol protein) primary tumors. The tumors were T2 (>3 cm), T3, T4b, N0–1, and M0. Patients were treated for a period of 3 months before surgical excision. Ultrasound was used to precisely determine tumor size on therapy. With letrozole, either 2.5 or 10 mg daily (no dose–response differences were seen), the median reduction in tumor size was 81% (CI = 69–86%). With anastrozole, either 1 or 10 mg daily (again no dose–response differences were observed), the median reduction was 64% (CI = 52–76%). Tamoxifen produced a median reduction of 48% (CI = 27–48%). The authors suggested from this study that the aromatase inhibitors might be superior to tamoxifen in this setting. Further studies will be required to document this possibility.

MECHANISMS FOR LACK OF CROSS-RESISTANCE OF AROMATASE INHIBITORS AND ANTIESTROGENS

Logic would suggest that inhibitors of estrogen action, such as tamoxifen, would be completely cross-resistant with agents designed to block estrogen synthesis. However, early studies demonstrated that sequential responses to inhibitors of estrogen biosynthesis commonly occurred in patients initially responding to and then relapsing after treatment with the antiestrogen tamoxifen. For example, 25–50% of patients initially responding to tamoxifen and then relapsing experienced secondary tumor regressions in response to the aromatase inhibitor aminoglutethimide in combination with hydrocortisone.

POTENTIAL EXPLANATIONS FOR LACK OF CROSS-RESISTANCE AMONG HORMONAL THERAPIES

One potential explanation for the lack of cross-resistance between antiestrogens and aromatase inhibitors was raised by observations made during further study of the actions of the antiestrogens. A variety of data examining the effects of antiestrogens on various organs and in various species demonstrated that ER antagonists exert both hormone-agonistic and -antagonistic actions, depending upon the tissue studied.[84] For example, tamoxifen acts as a potent estrogen on bone, liver, pituitary, and uterus, while exerting antiestrogenic effects on breast. The various responses to antiestrogens could be modulated by adaptive mechanisms, such as, increased production of cyclic AMP or activation of the protein kinase A and C pathways.[84] Observations in xenograft models of human breast cancer were particularly striking with respect to this adaptive process. Initial exposure to tamoxifen caused tumor regression, but prolonged exposure allowed the tumor to adapt such that tamoxifen shifted from exerting estrogen-antagonistic to estrogen-agonistic effects. Re-transplant of the xenografts into additional animals allowed demonstration that tamoxifen stimulated these tumors to grow and that the pure antiestrogen fulvestrant could antagonize this estrogenic effect.[85]

These observations led to the hypothesis that in patients, breast tumors initially responding to tamoxifen but then regrowing had also undergone adaptation. Such tumors might then respond secondarily to agents such as the aromatase inhibitors that would lower estrogen levels but not be expected to exert estrogen-agonistic actions. The hypothesis of adaptation has also been used to explain why women appear to benefit to a greater extent from 5 than from 10 years of tamoxifen in the adjuvant setting. Adaptation to tamoxifen, occurring between 5 and 10 years of exposure to this agent, might allow tamoxifen to ultimately become a stimulator of growth of the remaining micrometastases.[85]

ADAPTIVE HYPERSENSITIVITY HYPOTHESIS

Another possible explanation for secondary responses to aromatase inhibitors following exposure to tamoxifen is the development of adaptive hypersensitivity to estradiol. This phenomenon was initially suggested by clinical observations demonstrating sequential tumor regressions in women undergoing oophorectomy followed by exposure to an aromatase inhibitor. Oophorectomy reduces estradiol levels from approximately 200 pg/ml (premenopausal levels) to 5–10 pg/ml (post-oophorectomy concentrations), resulting in tumor regression. The cancer then begins to regrow in the presence of these low estradiol levels but undergoes further regression when aromatase inhibitors lower levels further to 0.05–0.07 pg/ml. These observations are best explained by the hypothesis that long-term deprivation of estradiol can induce an adaptive sensitization of the tumor to estradiol. One could consider this to be analogous to Cannon's law of denervation hypersensitivity whereby estradiol deprivation causes hypersensitivity to estradiol.

We tested the estradiol hypersensitivity hypothesis directly in an in vitro cell culture system.[86] Breast cancer cells were deprived of estradiol over several months in culture by growing them in media stripped of estradiol by treatment with charcoal. This period of estrogen deprivation induced a four-log enhancement in sensitivity to the cell-proliferative effects of estradiol. The hypersensitivity phenomenon could be reversed by re-exposure of cells to estradiol, suggesting adaptive mecha-

nisms rather than selection of hypersensitive clones of cells.

Hypersensitivity to estradiol was also confirmed in an in vivo study using a nude mouse model.[87] Ovariectomized animals were inoculated with wild-type MCF-7 cells on one flank of the body and long-term estrogen-deprived (LTED) cells on the other flank. Plasma estradiol levels of the animals were clamped to 1.25, 2.5, 5, 10, and 20 pg/ml by Silastic implants containing different doses of estradiol. Tumor growth was monitored for a period of 2 months. Growth of LTED cells was stimulated by very low doses of estradiol that did not affect the growth rate of wild-type MCF-7 xenografts. At higher doses of estradiol, however, the growth rate of wild-type cells exceeded that of LTED cells (Figure 6.8). This observation was consistent with our in vitro data that long-term estrogen deprivation enhanced the sensitivity of MCF-7 cells to both stimulatory and inhibitory effect of estrogen.

Long-term exposure to tamoxifen might also result in the development of hypersensitivity to estradiol. Under these circumstances, a marked reduction of estradiol synthesis with an aromatase inhibitor would result in tumor regression. Taken together, these observations suggest that breast cancer cells adapt to the conditions of ambient hormonal exposure – either to tamoxifen or to estrogen deprivation. This adaptive process provides a plausible explanation for the sequential responses to various hormonal therapies observed clinically in women with breast cancer.

Development of adaptive hypersensitivity has practical implications for the use of aromatase inhibitors. If cells in culture can respond to 10 fm concentration of estradiol, then nearly complete inhibition of aromatase may be necessary to produce the most effective antitumor therapy. Even the most potent inhibitors available now allow 1% residual aromatase activity. It is not clear whether the inhibitors block aromatase in breast tumor tissue itself to the same degree. These concepts are of interest when considering the dose–response differences between 0.5 and 2.5 mg daily of letrozole.

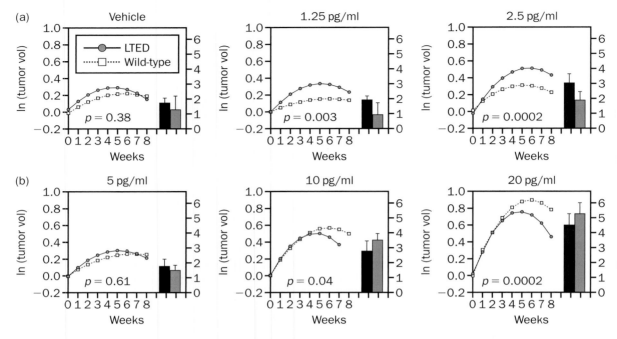

Figure 6.8 (a) Growth curves in wild-type and long-term estrogen-deprived (LTED) tumors in oophorectomized nude mice receiving only cholesterol-containing Silastic implants (vehicle control) and implants maintaining plasma estradiol levels at 1.25 and 2.5 pg/ml. The statistical significance of the differences between the wild-type and LTED tumors is indicated on each panel. The accompanying bars ± standard error of the mean represent mean area under the curve for each group, and are shown to illustrate variance among groups. The black bars are representative of volumes of LTED tumors and the crosshatched bars of wild-type tumors. The statistical significances indicated represent paired comparisons between integrated tumor volumes and not between mean areas under the various curves. Integrated tumor volumes were significantly higher in the LTED than the wild-type tumors in response to 1.25 and 2.5 pg/ml, but not in oophorectomized animals. (b) Growth curves in wild-type and LTED tumors with plasma estradiol clamped at 5, 10, and 20 pg/ml.

Perhaps even more potent aromatase inhibitors could produce even greater clinical effects. This possibility is not supported by the lack of dose–response differences detected between 1 and 10 mg of anastrozole per day, but it does perhaps deserve further exploration.

FUTURE PERSPECTIVES

As discussed above, several new potent and highly specific aromatase inhibitors are now available for the treatment of breast cancer. They offer several distinct advantages over some older forms of endocrine therapy, including a well-understood mechanism of action, good toxicity profile, convenient dosing schedules, and the absence of estrogen effects on the endometrium. On the other hand, their long-term effects on bone mineral density and serum lipids are unknown.[88]

New clinical trials with these promising agents are either underway or are planned in order to address several questions, including their role in the treatment of premenopausal women as discussed above. Although presently approved only as second-line therapies after tamoxifen failure, aromatase inhibitors are now being tested as first-line endocrine treatment for metastatic breast cancer in direct comparison with antiestrogens. Moreover, non-steroidal aromatase inhibitors would not be expected to induce endometrial carcinoma in women, and so could be investigated both as adjuvant hormonal therapy as well as in the chemoprevention of human breast cancer. A few clinical studies have attempted to combine different classes of endocrine agents, but there are few clinical data to support this approach as being superior to using these agents in sequence to treat metastatic breast cancer, for example tamoxifen followed by an aromatase inhibitor, followed by a progestin. In clinical practice, the sequential use of hormonal agents can produce long-term palliation of hormone-dependent breast cancer. Eventually, however, the problem of hormone resistance is encountered. The mechanisms by which tumors become resistant to hormones in general are only partially understood. Refractoriness to therapy with aromatase inhibitors is related not to the failure of these agents to suppress estradiol levels, as might be seen if there were upregulation of aromatase, but rather is likely due to some other mechanism of hormone resistance.

The paracrine production of aromatase-specific growth factors and cytokines within the microenvironment of a breast tumor require further study. Greater understanding of the biologic interaction of these factors could lead, for example, to the development of new therapeutic strategies.

USE OF AROMATASE INHIBITORS FOR BREAST CANCER PREVENTION

Estrogens are considered carcinogenic for the breast through their ability to increase the rate of cellular proliferation and consequently to increase the number of genetic mutations, which is proportional to the number of cell divisions.[2] In addition, the increased rate of cell proliferation could reduce the time required for DNA repair. This is the commonly accepted mechanism of estradiol-induced carcinogenesis.

An additional mechanism has been proposed that involves the metabolism of estradiol to 4-hydroxyestradiol and then to the estradiol-3,4-quinone. This compound can bind covalently to guanine or adenine and result in depurination of that segment of DNA. Upon replication, these depurinated sites preferentially undergo point mutations. This process could act in an additive or synergistic fashion with the effect of estrogen to increase cell proliferation.

It has been postulated that antiestrogens might prevent breast cancer by blocking the cell-proliferative effects of estrogens. The aromatase inhibitors might prevent breast cancer by two mechanisms: reduction of cell proliferation by inhibition of estrogen levels and prevention of genotoxic metabolite formation by lowering tissue levels of estrogen. Coombes et al[89] have reported that formestane prevents NMU-induced rat mammary carcinoma, and Steele and colleagues[90] have shown that fadrozole completely inhibits the development of spontaneous breast tumors in aging Sprague–Dawley rats.

The aromatase inhibitors block both cell proliferation and the formation of genotoxic metabolites.[91–93] Breast tissue levels of estradiol are substantially suppressed with aromatase inhibitors. Consequently, formation of the genotoxic metabolites in tissue would also be substantially reduced with these agents. In comparison, antiestrogens would not alter the formation of genotoxic metabolites of estrogen, while still blocking the proliferative effects of estradiol. If the genotoxic hypothesis were correct, one would postulate that the aromatase inhibitors would be much more effective for prevention of breast cancer than tamoxifen. The aromatase inhibitors would block two pathways (cell proliferation and genotoxic estrogen formation), whereas tamoxifen would block only one (cell proliferation). In this regard, the ATAC trial showed a substantially greater reduction of new contralateral breast cancers (14) than observed in patients receiving tamoxifen (33) ($p < 0.05$). These data are consistent with predictions from the genotoxicity hypothesis. These considerations highlight the urgent need to explore in greater detail the precise mechanisms whereby estrogens cause breast cancer. If the genotoxicity hypothesis is correct, then new therapies could be directed toward more direct inhibition of the formation of 4-hydroxyestradiol and its quinone, potentially with use of inhibitors of cytochrome P450 1B1. This is the enzyme that blocks the conversion of estradiol to 4-hydroxyestradiol. At the present time, these concepts are relatively speculative, but potentially of great importance.

To assess whether aromatase inhibitors are superior to antiestrogens in the prevention of breast cancer, the optimal study would include patients at high risk of developing breast cancer. Women with a single breast cancer are at high risk of developing a contralateral second cancer, estimates of rates range from 0.5% to 1.0% of women per year for development of a contralateral breast cancer. For a 60-year-old woman, this rate is 1.5- to 3-fold higher than the average incidence of 1 in 243 women per year who develop their first primary tumor. Thus the ATAC trial with assessment of diagnosis of second primary tumors provides a powerful means of determining whether the aromatase inhibitors will prevent breast cancer. It is known that tamoxifen reduces the incidence of second primaries by 45% under these circumstances. While trials of primary prevention of breast cancer with aromatase inhibitors are being planned, one would expect results from the adjuvant trials to be forthcoming sooner.

In summary, recently reported clinical studies of highly potent aromatase inhibitors have shown that it is possible to develop specific, non-toxic compounds that reduce serum estradiol concentrations to undetectable levels in postmenopausal patients with advanced breast cancer. Some of these compounds may also in fact, effectively target intratumoral synthesis of estrogen by aromatase. These compounds are emerging as a valuable approach to the treatment of hormone-dependent breast cancer.

REFERENCES

1. Frantz AG, Wilson JD. Endocrine disorders of the breast. In: *Williams Textbook of Endocrinology*, 9th edn (Wilson JD, Foster DW, Kronenberg HM, Larsen PR, eds). Philadelphia: WB Saunders, 1998: 877–900.

2. Santen RJ, Yue W, Naftolin F et al. The potential of aromatase inhibitors in breast cancer prevention. *Endocr Rel Cancer* 1999; **6:** 235–43.

3. Santen RJ, Manni A, Harvey H, Redmond C. Endocrine treatment of breast cancer in women. *Endocr Rev* 1990; **11:** 221–65.

4. Dickson RB, Lippman ME. Growth factors in breast cancer. *Endocr Rev* 1995; **16:** 559–89.

5. Simpson ER, Zhao Y, Agarwal VR et al. Aromatase expression in health and disease. *Rec Prog Hormone Res* 1997; **52:** 185–213.

6. Simpson ER, Merrill JC, Hollub AJ et al. Regulation of estrogen biosynthesis by human adipose cells. *Endocr Rev* 1989; **10:** 136–48.

7. Simpson ER, Mahendroo MS, Means G et al. Tissue specific promoters regulate aromatase cytochrome P450 expression. *Clin Chem* 1993; **39:** 317–24.

8. Sasano H, Harada N. Intratumoral aromatase in human breast, endometrial and other malignancies. *Endocr Rev* 1998; **19:** 593–607.

9. Fishman J, Hahn EF. The nature of the final oxidative step in the aromatization sequence. *Steroids* 1987; **50:** 339–45.

10. Abul-Hajj YJ, Iverson R, Kiang DT. Aromatization of androgens by human breast cancer. *Steroids* 1979; **33:** 205–22.

11. Santen RJ, Martel J, Hoagland M et al. Stromal spindle cells contain aromatase in human breast tumors. *J Clin Endocrinol Metab* 1994; **79:** 627–32.

12. Miller WR, O'Neil JS. The importance of local synthesis of estrogen within the breast. *Steroids* 1998; **50:** 537–48.

13. Mor G, Yue W, Santen RJ et al. Macrophages, estrogen and the microenvironment of breast cancer. *J Steroid Biochem Mol Biol* 1998; **67:** 403–14.

14. Brodie A, Long B, Liu Y, Lu Q. Aromatase inhibitors and their anti-tumor effects in model systems. *Endocr Rel Cancer* 1999; **6:** 205–10.

15. Yue W, Wang J-P, Hamilton CJ et al. In situ aromatization enhances breast tumor estradiol levels and cellular proliferation. *Cancer Res* 1998; **58:** 927–32.

16. Harada N, Honda S, Hatano O. Aromatase

inhibitors and enzyme stability. *Endocr Rel Cancer* 1999; **6**: 211–18.

17. Brodie AM. Aromatase, its inhibitors and their use in breast cancer treatment, *Pharmacol Ther* 1993; **60**: 501–15.

18. Lipton A, Demers LM, Harvey HA et al. Letrozole (CGS 20267) – phase I study of a new potent aromatase inhibitor in breast cancer. *Cancer* 1995; **75**: 2132–8.

19. Grodin JM, Siiteri PK, MacDonald PC. Source of estrogen production in postmenopausal women. *J Clin Endocrinol Metab* 1973; **36**: 207–14.

20. Dowsett M, Jeffcoate SL, Santner S et al. Low dose aminoglutethimide and aromatase inhibition. *Lancet* 1985; **i**: 175–6.

21. Jones AL, MacNeil F, Jacobs S et al. The influence of intramuscular 4-hydroxyandrostenedione on peripheral aromatisation in breast cancer patients. *Eur J Cancer* 1992; **28A**: 1712–16.

22. Santen RJ, Santner S, Davis B et al. Aminoglutethimide inhibits extraglandular estrogen production in postmenopausal women with breast cancer. *J Clin Endocrinol Metab* 1978; **47**: 1257–65.

23. Samojlik E, Santen RJ, Worgul TJ. Plasma estrone-sulfate: assessment of reduced estrogen production during treatment of metastatic breast carcinoma. *Steroids* 1982; **39**: 497–507.

24. Lonning PE, Geisler J, Johannessen DC, Ekse D. Plasma estrogen suppression with aromatase inhibitors evaluated by a novel, sensitive assay for estrone sulphate. *J Steroid Biochem Mol Biol* 1997; **61**: 255–60.

25. Oerter-Klein K, Demers LM, Santner SJ et al. Use of ultrasensitive recombinant cell bioassay to measure estrogen levels in women with breast cancer receiving the aromatase inhibitor, letrozole. *J Clin Endocrinol Metab* 1995; **80**: 2658–60.

26. Santen RJ, Worgul TJ, Lipton A et al. Aminoglutethimide as treatment of postmenopausal women with advanced breast carcinoma: correlation of clinical and hormonal responses. *Ann Intern Med* 1982; **96**: 94–101.

27. Geisler J, Lien EA, Ekse D, Lonning PE. Influence of aminoglutethimide on plasma levels of estrone sulphate and dehydroepiandrostenedione sulphate in postmenopausal breast cancer patients. *J Steroid Biochem Mol Biol* 1997; **63**: 53–8.

28. Cocconi G. First generation aromatase inhibitors-aminoglutethimide and testololactone. *Breast Cancer Res Treat* 1994; **30**: 57–80.

29. Gale KE, Anderson JW, Tormey DC et al.

Hormonal treatment for metastatic breast cancer. An Eastern Cooperative Oncology Group phase III trial comparing aminoglutethimide to tamoxifen. *Cancer* 1994; **73**: 354–31.

30. Lipton A, Harvey HA, Santen RJ et al. A randomized trial of aminoglutethimide versus tamoxifen in metastatic breast cancer. *Cancer* 1982; **50**: 2265–8.

31. Smith IE, Harris AL, Morgan M et al. Tamoxifen versus aminoglutethimide in advanced breast carcinoma: a randomized cross-over trial. *BMJ* 1981; **283**: 1432–4.

32. Alonso-Munoz MC, Ojeda-Gonzalez MB, Beltran-Fabregat M et al. Randomized trial of tamoxifen versus aminoglutethimide and versus combined tamoxifen and aminoglutethimide in advanced breast cancer. *Oncology* 1988; **45**: 350–3.

33. Harvey HA, Lipton A, Santen RI et al. Phase I and phase II clinical trials of fadrozole hydrochloride in postmenopausal women with metastatic breast cancer. *Adv Clin Oncol* 1994; **2**: 155–8.

34. Santen RJ, Demers LM, Lynch J et al. Specificity of low dose fadrozole hydrochloride (CGS 16949A) as an aromatase inhibitor. *J Clin Endocrinol Metab* 1991; **73**: 99–106.

35. Buzdar AU, Smith R, Vogel C et al. Fadrozole HCL (CGS-16949A) versus megestrol acetate treatment of postmenopausal patients with metastatic breast carcinoma: results of two randomized double blind controlled multi-institutional trials. *Cancer* 1996; **71**: 2503–13.

36. Trunet PF, Vreeland F, Royce C et al. Clinical use of aromatase inhibitors in the treatment of advanced breast cancer. *J Steroid Biochem Mol Biol* 1997; **61**: 241–5.

37. Thurlimann B, Beretta K, Bacchi M et al. First line fadrozole HCL (CGS 16949A) versus tamoxifen in postmenopausal patients with advanced breast cancer. *Ann Oncol* 1996; **7**: 471–96.

38. Falkson CI, Falkson HC. A randomized study of CGS 16949A (fadrozole) versus tamoxifen in previously untreated postmenopausal patients with metastatic breast cancer. *Ann Oncol* 1996; **7**: 465–9.

39. Santen RJ, Worgul TJ, Samojlik E et al. A randomized trial comparing surgical adrenalectomy with aminoglutethimide plus hydrocortisone in women with advanced breast cancer. *N Engl J Med* 1981; **305**: 545–51.

40. Swain SM, Steinberg SM, Bagley C, Lippman ME. Tamoxifen and fluoxymesterone versus

tamoxifen and danazol in metastatic breast cancer – a randomized study. *Breast Cancer Res Treat* 1988; **12**: 51–7.

41. Brodie AM, Wing LY. In vitro and in vivo studies with aromatase inhibitor 4-hydroxyandrostenedione. *Steroids* 1987; **50**: 89–103.

42. Brodie AMH, Romanoff ID, Williams KIH. Metabolism of the aromatase inhibitor 4-hydroxy-4-androstenedione-3,17-dione by male rhesus monkeys. *J Steroid Biochem* 1981; **14**: 693–6.

43. Goss PE, Powles TJ, Dowsett M et al. Treatment of advanced postmenopausal breast cancer with an aromatase inhibitor, 4-hydroxyandrostenedione: phase II report. *Cancer Res* 1986; **46**: 4823–6.

44. Hoffken K, Jonat W, Possinger K et al. Aromatase inhibition with 4-hydroxyandrostenedione in the treatment of postmenopausal patients with advanced breast cancer. A phase II study. *J Clin Oncol* 1990; **8**: 875–80.

45. Buzdar AU, Jonat W, Howell A et al. Anastrozole, a potent and selective aromatase inhibitor, versus megestrol acetate in postmenopausal women with advanced breast cancer: results of overview of two phase III trials. *J Clin Oncol* 1996; **14**: 2000–11.

46. Buzdar AU. Anastrozole: a new addition to the armamentarium against advanced breast cancer. *Am J Clin Oncol* 1998; **21**: 161–6.

47. Kleeberg UR, Dowsett M, Carrion RP et al. A randomized comparison of oestrogen suppression with anastrozole and formestane in postmenopausal patients with advanced breast cancer. *Oncology* 1997; **54**(Suppl 2): 19–21.

48. Howell A, Mackintosh J, Jones M et al. The definition of the 'no change' category in patients treated with endocrine therapy and chemotherapy for advanced carcinoma of the breast. *Eur J Cancer Clin Oncol* 1998; **24**: 1567–72.

49. Robertson JFR, Willsher PC, Cheung KL, Blamey RW. The clinical relevance of static disease (no change) category for 6 months on endocrine therapy in patients with breast cancer. *Eur J Cancer* 1997; **33**: 1774–9.

50. Robertson JFR, Howell A, Buzder A et al. Static disease on anastrozole provides similar benefit as objective response in patients with advanced breast cancer. *Breast Cancer Res Treat* 1999; **58**: 157–62.

51. Buzdar AU, Jonat W, Howell A et al.

Anastrozole versus megestrol acetate in the treatment of postmenopausal women with advanced breast carcinoma: Results of a survival update based on a combined analysis of data from two mature phase III trials. *Cancer* 1998; **83**: 1142–52.

52. Dombernowsky P, Smith I, Falkson G et al. Letrozole, a new oral aromatase inhibitor for advanced breast cancer: double-blind randomized trial showing a dose effect and improved efficacy and tolerability compared with megestrol acetate. *J Clin Oncol* 1998; **16**: 453–61.

53. Gershanovich M, Chaudri H, Campos D et al. Letrozole, a new oral aromatase inhibitor: randomised trial comparing 2.5 mg daily, 0.5 mg daily and aminoglutethimide in postmenopausal women with advanced breast cancer. *Ann Oncol* 1998; **9**: 639–45.

54. Schiweck K, Bhatnagar AS, Batzl CH, Lang M. Anti-tumor and endocrine effects of non-steroidal aromatase inhibitors on estrogen-dependent rat mammary tumors. *J Steroid Biochem Mol Biol* 1993; **44**: 633–6.

55. Demers LM, Lipton A, Harvey HA et al. The efficacy of CGS 20267 in suppressing estrogen biosynthesis in patients with advanced stage breast cancer. *J Steroid Biochem Mol Biol* 1993; **44**: 647–9.

56. Dowsett M, Jones A, Johnston SRD. In vivo measurement of aromatase inhibition by letrozole (CGS 20267) in postmenopausal patients with breast cancer. *Clin Cancer Res* 1995; **1**: 1511–15.

57. Iveson TJ, Smith IE, Ahern J et al. Phase I study of the oral non-steroidal aromatase inhibitor CGS 20267 in postmenopausal patients with breast cancer. *Cancer Res* 1993; **53**: 266–70.

58. Buzdar A, Douma J, Davidson N et al. Phase III multicenter, double-blind, randomised study of letrozole, an aromatase inhibitor for advanced breast cancer, versus megestrol acetate. *J Clin Oncol* 2001; **19**: 3357–66.

59. Goss P. Pre-clinical and clinical review of vorozole, a new third generation aromatase inhibitor. *Breast Cancer Res Treat* 1998; **49**: S59–65.

60. Lonning E. Pharmacological profiles of exemestane and formestane, steroidal aromatase inhibitors used for treatment of postmenopausal breast cancer. *Breast Cancer Res Treat* 1998; **49**: S45–52.

61. Thurlimann B, Paridaens R, Seroin D et al. Third-line hormonal treatment with exemestane in post-menopausal patients with advanced

breast cancer progressing on aminoglutethimide: a phase II multicentre multinational study. Exemestane Study Group. *Eur J Cancer* 1997; **33**: 1767–73.

62. Evans TRJ, Salle ED, Ornati G et al. Phase I and endocrine study of exemestane (FCE 24304), a new aromatase inhibitor, in postmenopausal women. *Cancer Res* 1992; **52**: 5933–9.

63. Jones S, Belt R, Cooper B et al. A phase II study of antitumor efficacy and safety of exemestane as second-line hormonal treatment of post-menopausal patients with metastatic breast cancer refractory to tamoxifen. *Breast Cancer Res Treat* 1998; **50**: 304 (Abst 436).

64. Kvinnsland S, Anker G, Dirix LY et al. Activity of exemestane, an irreversible, oral, aromatase inhibitor in metastatic postmenopausal breast cancer patients failing tamoxifen. *Eur J Cancer* 1998; **34**(Suppl 5): S91 (Abst 408).

65. Kaufmann M, Bajetta E, Dirix LY et al. Survival advantage of exemestane over megestrol acetate in postmenopausal women with advanced breast cancer refractory to tamoxifen: results of a phase III randomized double blind study. *Proc Am Soc Clin Oncol* 1999; **18**: 109a (Abst 412).

66. Kaufmann M, Bajetta E, Dirix LY et al. Exemestane is superior to megestrol acetate after tamoxifen failure in postmenopausal women with advanced breast cancer: results of a phase III randomised double-blind trial. The Exemestane Study Group. *J Clin Oncol* 2000; **18**: 1399–411.

67. Lonning PE, Bajetta E, Murray R et al. A phase II study of exemestane in metastatic breast cancer patients failing non-steroidal aromatase inhibitors. *Breast Cancer Res Treat* 1998; **50**: 304 (Abst 435).

68. Jones S, Chang A, Lusch C et al. A phase II confirmatory study of antitumor efficacy and safety of exemestane as third line hormonal treatment of postmenopausal patients with metastatic breast cancer refractory to tamoxifen. *Breast Cancer Res Treat* 1998; **50**: 305 (Abst 437).

69. Jones S, Vogel C, Arkhipov A et al. Multicenter, phase II trial of exemestane as third-line hormonal therapy of postmenopausal women with metastatic breast cancer. *J Clin Oncol* 1999; **17**: 3418–25.

70. Bonneterre J, Thurlimann B, Robertson JFR et al. Anastrozole versus tamoxifen as first-line therapy for advanced breast cancer in 668 post-menopausal women: results of the Tamoxifen or Arimidex Randomised Group Efficacy and Tolerability Study. *J Clin Oncol* 2000; **18**: 3748–57.

71. Nabholtz J, Buzdar A, Pollak M et al. Anastrozole is superior to tamoxifen as first-line therapy for advanced breast cancer in post-menopausal women: results of a North American multicenter randomised trial. *J Clin Oncol* 2000; **18**: 3758–67.

72. Nabholtz JM, Bonneterre J, Buzdar AU et al. Preliminary results of two multi-center trials comparing the efficacy and tolerability of Arimidex (anastrozole) and tamoxifen in post-menopausal women with advanced breast cancer. *Breast Cancer Res Treat* 1999; **57**: 31 (Abst 27).

73. Milla-Santos A, Milla L, Rallo L et al. Anastrozole versus tamoxifen in hormone dependent advanced breast cancer. A phase II randomised trial. *Breast Cancer Res Treat* 2000; **64**: 54 (Abst 173).

74. Mouridsen H, Gershanovich M, Sun Y et al. Superior efficacy of letrozole versus tamoxifen as first-line therapy for postmenopausal women with advanced breast cancer. Results of a phase III study of the International Letrozole Breast Cancer Group. *J Clin Oncol* 2001; **19**: 2596–606.

75. Mouridsen H, Sun Y, Gershanovich M et al. Final survival analysis of the double-blind, ran-domized multinational phase III trial of letrozole (Femara) compared to tamoxifen as first-line hormonal therapy for advanced breast cancer. *Breast Cancer Res Treat* 2001; **69**: 211 (Abst 9).

76. Paridaens R, Dirix LY, Beex L et al. Exemestane is active and well tolerated as first-line hormonal therapy of metastatic breast cancer patients: results of a randomised phase II trial. *Proc Am Soc Clin Oncol* 2000; **19**: 38A (Abst 316).

77. Buzdar AU. Aromatase inhibitors in breast cancer. *Breast Cancer On-line* 2001; 4.

78. Howell A, Robertson JFR, Quaresma AJ et al. Comparison of efficacy and tolerability of Faslodex™ (anastrozole) in postmenopausal (PM) women with advanced breast cancer (ABC) – preliminary results. *Breast Cancer Res Treat* 2000; **64**: 27 (Abst 6).

79. Osborne CK, Pippen J, Jones SE et al. 'Faslodex' (ICI 182,780) shows longer duration of response compared to 'Arimidex' (anastrozole) in post-menopausal (PM) women with advanced breast cancer (ABC). *Breast Cancer Res Treat* 2000; **64**: 27 (Abst 7).

80. Fisher MD, O'Shaughnessy J Anastrozole may

be superior to tamoxifen as adjuvant treatment for postmenopausal patients with breast cancer. *Clin Breast Cancer* 2002; **2:** 269–71.

81. Baum M. The ATAC (Arimidex, Tamoxifen, Alone or in Combination) adjuvant breast cancer trial in post-menopausal women. *Breast Cancer Res Treat* 2001; **69:** 210 (Abst 8).

82. Tobias J. Anastrozole (A) is superior to tamoxifen (T) in treatment of postmenopausal (PM) women with early breast cancer (EBC) – first results of the ATAC ('Arimidex', Tamoxifen, Alone or in Combination) trial. *Eur J Cancer* 2002; in press.

83. Dixon JM, Love CDB, Renshaw L et al. Lessons from the use of aromatase inhibitors in the neoadjuvant setting. *Endocr Rel Cancer* 1999; **6:** 227–30.

84. Santen RJ. Long term tamoxifen therapy: Can an antagonist become an agonist? *J Clin Endocrinol Metab* 1997; **81:** 2027–9.

85. Gottardis MM, Jordan VC. Development of tamoxifen-stimulated growth of MCF-7 tumors in athymic mice after long-term antiestrogen administration. *Cancer Res* 1988; **48:** 5183–7.

86. Masamura S, Santner SJ, Heitjan DF, Santen RJ. Estrogen deprivation causes estradiol hypersensitivity in human cancer cells. *J Clin Endocrinol Metab* 1995; **80:** 2918–25.

87. Shim W-S, Conaway M, Masamura S et al. Estradiol hypersensitivity and MAP kinase expression in long term estrogen deprived human breast cancer cells in vivo. *Endocrinology* 2000; **141:** 396–405.

88. Harvey HA. Aromatase inhibitors in clinical practice; current status and a look to the future. *Semin Oncol* 1996; **23:** 33–8.

89. Coombes RC, Wilkinson JR, Bliss JM et al. 4-Hydroxyandrostenedione in the prophylaxis of N-methyl-N-nitrosourea induced mammary tumourigenesis. *Br J Cancer* 1991; **64:** 247–50.

90. Gunson DE, Steele RE, Chau RY. Prevention of spontaneous tumors in female rats by fadrozole hydrochloride, an aromatase inhibitor. *Br J Cancer* 1995; **72:** 72–5.

91. Jefcoate CR, Liehr JG, Santen RJ et al. Tissue-specific synthesis and oxidative metabolism of estrogens. *J Natl Cancer Inst Monogr* 2000; **27:** 95–112.

92. Santen RJ. Symposium overview. *J Natl Cancer Inst Monogr* 2000; **27:** 15–16.

93. Estrogens as endogenous carcinogens in the breast and the prostate. *J Natl Cancer Inst Monogr* 2000; **27:** 1–159.

7

Progestational agents

Julie J Olin, Hyman B Muss

CONTENTS • Introduction • Clinical efficacy • Comparisons with other agents • Other effects and toxicity • Current role of progestins in hormonal therapy

INTRODUCTION

Progestational agents have been used in the treatment of metastatic breast cancer for over 40 years. The development of orally administered synthetic progestins was led by the seminal work of Stoll, who reported the results of a non-randomized comparative study of six progestins in women with advanced breast cancer in the mid 1960s.[1] Use of the two best known progesterone agents, medroxyprogesterone acetate (MPA) and megestrol acetate (MA), was described in 23 patients. Even at low doses of MPA 200–400 mg/day and MA 30 mg/day, an 18% response rate was noted by Stoll.[2]

The cellular mechanisms by which progestins inhibit tumor growth and induce tumor regression are unclear. Progestins can bind to progesterone, androgen, and glucocorticoid receptors,[3] in addition to lowering estradiol, estrone, testosterone, androstenedione,[4] adrenocorticotropic hormone, and cortisol levels.[5] Progestins have also been shown to have a direct cytotoxic effect on several cell lines, and can decrease the production of mitogenic cytokines. In spite of these effects, the major mechanism of action of progestins remains elusive.

CLINICAL EFFICACY

Metastatic disease

Over the past four decades, multiple clinical trials utilizing MPA and MA have been performed. While both synthetic progestins are usually given orally, MPA may also be administered intramuscularly. Given its two routes of administration, coupled with a broad range of potential doses, trials using MPA are particularly diverse. Doses ranging from 500 mg intramuscularly twice a week to 4000 mg/day orally have produced response rates ranging from 15% to 67% in previously treated and untreated patients.[6] To further evaluate the possible treatment outcome differences associated with the oral versus intramuscular administration routes of high-dose MPA, two randomized trials[7,8] involving 213 patients with advanced breast cancer were performed in Europe in the early 1980s. These studies found similar response rates of approximately 17–23%, with a median duration of remissions of about 1 year. While the toxicity profile associated with high-dose MPA consisted mainly of weight gain and tremors, intramuscular therapy was also associated with pain and/or infection at the injection site in approximately 12–15% of patients. See Table 7.1.

Multiple trials utilizing MA have been performed. In 16 studies[9] involving 1342 evaluable

Table 7.1 Medroxyprogesterone acetate in advanced breast cancer[a]

Study[b]	Dose/schedule	No. of patients	CR + PR rate (%)	Previous hormone therapy
Hortobagyi	400 mg/day p.o.	10	67	
	800 mg/day p.o.	29	37	
	(Total)	(39)	(44)	30/39
Hedley	600 mg/day p.o.	105	20	78/105
Haller	400 mg/day p.o.	32	47	13/32
Cavalli	500 mg i.m. biw × 4 weeks → 500 mg i.m. qw	93	15	76/93
	versus			
	1000 mg i.m. qd × 4 weeks → 500 mg i.v. qw	91	33	75/91
Falkson	1440 mg/m^2/day p.o. × 6 months → 500 mg/m^2 qd	23	22	23/23
Guarnieri	4000 mg p.o. qd × 30 days → 1000 mg p.o. qd	26	27	8/26

Abbreviations: CR, complete response; PR, partial response; biw, twice per week; qw, once per week; qd, every day; p.o., orally; i.m., intramuscularly; i.v., intravenously.
[a] Permission granted courtesy of WB Saunders in *Seminars in Oncology*.[6]
[b] The studies quoted are located in reference 6.

patients, the overall response rate was 26%, with a range of 14–44%. See Table 7.2. Fifty complete responses (3.7%) were observed, along with 306 partial responses (22.7%). The majority of studies used MA at 160 mg/day administered either once a day or in four divided doses. Fifty complete responses (3.7%) were observed along with 306 partial responses (22.7%). The median duration of remission ranged from 2.2 to 22 months in the 11 trials that included such data. In analyzing multiple separate variables such as response rates of metastatic foci and the effects of menopausal status, hormone receptor status, and prior therapy received for advanced breast cancer, several observations were noted. The response rates of measurable skin and soft tissue disease (41%) exceeded those of bony and visceral involvement (27% and 26%, respectively).

Virtually all of the patients were postmenopausal women, although a small subset of 19 premenopausal patients were identified from three of the trials and demonstrated a response rate of 42%. The duration of menopause correlated with the potential response to MA therapy. In two of the large trials[6] comprising over 300 patients, markedly higher response rates were seen in patients who had a well-established postmenopausal status of over 5–10 years duration. Data with regard to estrogen receptor (ER) and progesterone receptor (PgR) status were available in five trials. Response rates were highest (43%) in patients whose tumors contained both ER and PgR and lowest in tumors devoid of either receptor. While all of the patients accrued in the 16 trials[9] had previously treated advanced breast cancer, precise data regarding the effect of prior thera-

Table 7.2 Summary of trials evaluating megestrol acetate for the treatment of breast cancer[a]

Study[b]	No. of evaluable patients	No. of males	Total daily dose (mg)	Dosing frequency	No. of CRs	No. of PRs	Response rate (%)	Median response duration (months)
Robertson et al	221	0	320	Twice a day	2	34	16	14.0
Ansfield et al	161	1	160	Four times a day	0	48	30	6.5
Alexieva-Figusch et al	160	0	60–180	?	0	48	30	—
	136	0	180	?	8	23	23	12.0
Gregory et al	124	1	160	Four times a day	5	24	24	22.0
Allegra et al	91	0	160	Four times a day	10	22	35	9.6
Lundgren et al	74	0	160	Every day	5	18	31	13.0
Muss et al	61	0	160	Four times a day	5	12	25	7.7
Benghiat et al	49	0	160	Every day	1	14	31	⩾10
Ross et al	48	0	160	Four times a day	0	15	31	7.0
Morgan	46	0	160	Four times a day	5	9	30	—
Wander et al	43	0	160	Every day	2	9	26	—
Johnson et al	43	2	160	Four times a day	5	14	44	—
Blackledge et al	37	0	160	Four times a day	1	8	24	5.0
Ingle et al	28	0	$150/m^2$	Three times a day	1	3	14	2.2
Carpenter and Peterson	20	1	160	Every day	0	5	25	—
Total	1342	5			50	306	26	

Abbreviations: CR, complete response; PR, partial response.
[a]Permission granted courtesy of WB Saunders in *Seminars in Oncology*.[9]
[b]The studies quoted are located in reference 9.

pies on response to MA were deemed insufficient to allow proper analysis.

As summarized by Schacter et al,[9] a study by Wander and colleagues compared MA 160 mg/day with MPA 1000 mg/day orally in a randomized trial of 87 postmenopausal patients with advanced breast cancer.[9] Virtually identical response rates of 26% and 30% and response durations of 8–9 months were seen.

A number of studies have suggested a possible dose–response relationship for the progestins in advanced breast cancer therapy. In a randomized phase III trial of high-dose MPA in 184 postmenopausal patients, Cavalli et al[10] compared MPA 1000 mg/day intramuscularly for 1 month with MPA 500 mg intramuscularly twice weekly for 1 month. Following the high-dose versus low-dose MPA induction, MPA was further administered at 500 mg intramuscularly on a weekly basis. A 33% response rate was seen in the high-dose MPA arm, compared with a 15% response to low-dose therapy. While toxicity was similar in both treatment arms, the two different schedules of MPA did not influence the time to disease progression or overall survival. This trial sparked a flurry of interest in the concept of dose intensification of hormonal therapy utilizing either MPA orally or MA.

Several trials using high-dose versus low-dose oral MPA have been performed. Rose et al[11] randomly assigned 201 patients with advanced breast cancer to receive 300 mg/day versus 900 mg/day of oral MPA. The overall response rates were 16% and 23%, respectively. The time to progression was significantly longer in patients treated with high-dose MPA, whereas response duration and survival were not. Hortobagyi et al[12] treated 39 post-menopausal patients with MPA at 400 mg/day versus 800 mg/day. An overall response rate of 67% was seen in the 10 patients given low-dose MPA, versus a 37% response rate seen in the 29 patients treated with high-dose MPA. In a larger randomized trial of 124 patients with advanced breast cancer that contained both pre- and postmenopausal women, Gallagher et al[13] tested MPA at doses of 300 mg/day versus 1000 mg/day. Response rates were 24% for both treatment arms. Both treatments were associated with a high incidence of bone pain relief but a low objective response rate in bony metastatic foci. Both response duration (10 months versus 11 months) and survival (13 months versus 11 months) were not significantly different for the two treatments. Further evaluation of high-dose MPA has most recently been studied in Japan. A randomized trial of oral MPA 1200 mg and 600 mg was conducted in 80 patients with advanced breast cancer.[14] There were no significant differences between the two treatment arms in terms of response rate, duration of response, overall survival, or toxicity.

The superior oral availability of MA compared with MPA led to three large trials of high-dose MA. Muss et al[15] randomly assigned 172 patients with advanced breast cancer (virtually all of whom had been previously treated with tamoxifen) to receive standard-dose MA 160 mg/day or high-dose MA 800 mg/day. High-dose MA resulted in a superior complete plus partial response rate (27% versus 10%), time to treatment failure (median 8.0 months versus 3.2 months), and survival (median 22.4 months versus 16.5 months) when compared with standard-dose therapy. Weight gain was the most distressing side-effect, with 13% of standard-dose and 43% of high-dose patients gaining more than 8 kg. Four major cardiovascular events, including two deep venous thromboses, one thrombotic stroke, and one fatal myocardial infarction, occurred in patients receiving high-dose therapy. Only one deep venous thrombotic event was noted in the standard-dose arm. Thirty-four patients who failed to respond to standard-dose MA were crossed-over to receive high-dose MA, and none responded.

The second dose-intensified MA trial was a phase I/II trial of 57 patients using doses of MA ranging from 480 to 1600 mg/day.[16] Three patients were entered at each of these escalating dose levels of 480, 800, and 1280 mg/day. Forty-eight patients were then treated at 1600 mg/day. While responses were noted at each dose level, the overall response rate was 32% in patients with measurable disease. The most promising results occurred in a subset of 27 patients who displayed progressive disease after being treated with standard doses of MA. After crossover, a 15% response rate, including one complete response and three partial responses, was noted with high-dose MA. Ten crossover patients (37%) had stable disease lasting a median of 5.4 months. In addition, 2 of 14 patients with primary resistance to initial therapy with tamoxifen had objective responses, including one complete response and one partial response, to high-dose MA. Although classic chemotherapy-defined dose-limiting toxicity was not reached, substantial weight gain (median 5 kg) occurred in 71% of patients at the 1600 mg dose level.

Results from both Muss and Abrams provided rationale for the Cancer and Leukemia Group B (CALGB) to develop a randomized phase III trial of 368 women with metastatic breast cancer treated with either standard-dose MA at 160 mg/day, 5 times the standard dose at 800 mg/day, or 10 times the standard dose at 1600 mg/day.[17] The response rates were 23%, 27%, and 27% for the 160, 800, and 1600 mg/day arms, respectively. Median durations of response were 17, 14, and 8 months for the 160, 800, and 1600 mg/day arms, respectively. No significant differences in the treatment arms were noted for time to disease progression or for survival. The median survival was 28 months in the standard-dose MA arm, 24 months in the mid-dose arm, and 29 months in the high-dose arm. The most frequently reported side-effect, weight gain, was clearly dose-related. Approximately 20% of patients on the two higher-dose arms reported weight gain of more than 20% of their prestudy weight, compared with only 2% in the 160 mg/day dose arm. Five patients died of thromboembolic causes that were felt to be treatment-related, with one death on the 800 mg/day dose arm and four deaths on the 1600 mg/day dose arm. With a median follow-up of 8 years, this large multi-institutional trial failed to demonstrate any advantage for dose escalation of MA in the therapy of advanced breast cancer.

Adjuvant therapy

Most clinical trials of progestins have been performed in women with metastatic breast cancer. In the adjuvant setting, Pannuti et al[18] treated 151 premenopausal patients with six cycles of CMF (cyclophosphamide, methotrexate, and 5-fluorouracil (5-FU)) versus CMF and concurrent high-dose (HD) MPA. One hundred and thirty-eight postmenopausal patients were also randomly assigned to receive HD-MPA versus no adjuvant therapy. The majority of patients had primary breast tumors 2–5 cm in size coupled with node-positive disease, although node-negative cases were also included. HD-MPA included MPA 1000 mg twice daily orally for 1 month followed by 500 mg twice daily orally for 5 months. With a median follow-up of 3 years, no significant differences in disease-free or overall survival were found in the postmenopausal patients. In the postmenopausal portion of the study, a statistically significant lower number of recurrences was observed in the progestin-treated patients with three or less positive lymph nodes, although no

overall survival benefit was detected. Both ER-positive and ER-negative patients were eligible, and receptor status was unknown in over half the cases enrolled.

Focan et al[19] compared adjuvant HD-MPA with observation in 240 pre- and postmenopausal patients with node-negative breast cancer. MPA was administered intramuscularly at 500 mg/day for 1 induction month, followed by 500 mg intramuscularly twice weekly for 5 maintenance months. With a median follow-up of 3 years, significant increases in relapse-free and overall survival were found in the progestin-treated group. The relapse-free and overall survival rates were 94% and 99% respectively in the HD-MPA arm, versus 73% and 89% in the control arm. Side-effects for HD-MPA included a mean weight gain of 7.4 kg and tremor, cramps, headaches, and vaginal spotting in 10–15% of patients. Approximately 20% of patients were ER-negative in this trial, although overall the ER status was unknown in about half the cases enrolled.

Hupperets et al[20] randomly assigned 408 pre- and postmenopausal women with node-positive breast cancer to CAF (cyclophosphamide, doxorubicin, and 5-FU) for six cycles versus CAF coupled with concurrent HD-MPA for 6 months. Progestin therapy included MPA 500 mg intramuscularly daily for 28 days followed by 500 mg intramuscularly twice a week for 5 months. While the 5-year disease-free survival rate was 59% in the chemohormonally treated group, compared with 49% in the chemotherapy-only group, no difference in overall survival was found. In subgroup analysis, a slight survival advantage for CAF plus MPA over CAF alone was found in elderly patients between 55 and 70 years of age with small breast primaries. The chemotherapy- and progestin-treated group experienced a mean weight gain of 5.5 kg, whereas weight gain in the CAF group did not exceed 1.8 kg. Approximately two-thirds of patients were ER-positive in this trial.

These data suggest that progestins may be beneficial in the adjuvant setting. Although further research in this area may be of interest, it is unlikely that progestins would prove to be superior to other hormonal agents in standard use for adjuvant therapy. Moreover, weight gain associated with chronic progestins would likely be a highly undesirable side-effect for women treated in the adjuvant setting.

COMPARISONS WITH OTHER AGENTS

Progestins have been tested in multiple trials against other hormonal therapies, including tamoxifen and several aromatase inhibitors. The comparison of MA and tamoxifen in post-menopausal women with advanced breast cancer has been extensively documented in four randomized trials. See Table 7.3. In each trial, MA 40 mg four times a day was compared with tamoxifen 10 mg twice a day. The cumulative response rate was 28% for MA and 32% for tamoxifen.[1] In a study by Muss et al[21] of 136 eligible patients, the estimated 1-year survival rate was 77% for the MA-treated group and 85% for the tamoxifen-treated group. The 2-year survival rates were 57% and 69%, respectively. After adjustment for multiple pretreatment variables, the difference in survival between the

two regimens was significant ($p = 0.04$) in favor of tamoxifen.

The MA versus tamoxifen trials also had crossover components.[1] Treatment with MA after tamoxifen failure was compared with treatment with tamoxifen after MA failure. The rate of response to MA after tamoxifen failure (16%) was similar to the response rate to tamoxifen after MA failure (12%). The results of these crossover studies seem to indicate that MA and tamoxifen are non-cross-resistant therapies.

Like MA, MPA has been compared with tamoxifen in randomized trials. In the study by van Veelen et al,[22] 129 previously untreated postmenopausal women with advanced breast cancer were randomly assigned to receive MPA 900 mg/day orally or tamoxifen 40 mg/day. No significant differences were found in the overall response rate (44% versus 35%), median duration of remission (17 months versus 23 months), or median survival (20 months versus 26 months). Interesting findings of this study included marked improvement in the response rate of MPA-treated patients with osseous metastases as well as in patients over 70 years of age. After crossover from tamoxifen to MPA, 8 of 31 patients responded, while no responses

Table 7.3 Megestrol acetate versus tamoxifen in advanced breast cancer[a]

Study[b]	Megestrol acetate		Tamoxifen	
	No. of responses/patients	Response rate (%)	No. of responses/patients	Response rate (%)
Ingle et al	4/28	14	7/27	26
Johnson et al	20/49	40	14/49	28
Alexieva-Figusch et al	31/136	23	17/80	21
Morgan	14/46	30	17/48	35
Ettinger et al	32/91	35	42/99	42
Muss et al	17/69	25	20/65	31
Total	118/419	28	117/368	32

[a]Permission granted courtesy of WB Saunders in *Seminars in Oncology*.[1]
[b]The studies quoted are located in reference 1.

were seen in the 27 patients who were crossed-over from MPA to tamoxifen.

In a follow-up trial by Muss et al,[23] 182 endocrine-naive postmenopausal patients were randomly assigned to receive MPA 1000 mg/day orally or tamoxifen 20 mg/day. While the overall response rate in the MPA-treated group was significantly higher than that seen with tamoxifen (34% versus 17%, respectively), this failed to translate into improved time to treatment failure or survival. As in the van Veelen et al study, patients with bony metastases had a significantly higher partial response rate with MPA compared with tamoxifen (33% versus 13%, respectively). Similar responses to crossover from one agent to the other were noted. While both agents were associated with minimal toxicity, weight gain was markedly more apparent with progestin therapy. Thirty-five percent of the MPA-treated patients gained more than 9 kg, as opposed to only 2% on tamoxifen.

Several generations of aromatase inhibitors now exist. While both MPA and MA have been compared with aminoglutethimide (AG), more recent trials of second- and third-generation aromatase inhibitors have compared these agents only with MA. In the study of 85 postmenopausal women by Samonis et al,[24] patients were randomly assigned to receive AG 1000 mg/day plus replacement hydrocortisone, MPA 500 mg intramuscularly for 1 month and twice weekly thereafter, or combined therapy of AG and MPA without replacement hydrocortisone. All three treatment arms displayed similar response rates and durations of response.

In a similarly designed three-arm trial by the Southwest Oncology Group (SWOG),[25] 288 postmenopausal women were randomly assigned to receive MA 160 mg/day, AG 1000 mg/day with replacement hydrocortisone, or combination MA and AG. This study failed to show a difference in any of the three arms with regard to response rates, time to treatment failure, or survival. Toxicity was greater in the two AG arms with respect to fatigue, nausea and vomiting, and rash.

Several large randomized trials have compared the newer aromatase inhibitors with MA.[26–29] See Table 7.4. Complete and partial response rates of 10–25% coupled with similar rates of stable disease were found in both the aromatase inhibitor- and MA-treated patients. The only mature study that showed an improvement in survival with AI therapy over megestrol was the large multinational trial of anastrozole by Buzdar et al.[30] Use of anastrozole 1 mg daily compared with MA 40 mg four times daily led to a prolongation of survival of slightly over 4 months. When compared with MA, aromatase inhibitor therapy was associated with markedly fewer side-effects. While mild antiestrogenic side-effects of hot flashes and nausea were occasionally associated with aromatase inhibitor therapy, troublesome weight gain and potentially life-threatening thromboembolic disease was dramatically less. Given the similar response rates yet improved side-effect profiles compared with MA, the second- and third-generation aromatase inhibitors[31] have become the therapy of choice in postmenopausal receptor-positive patients who have developed metastases while on adjuvant tamoxifen or have shown progression of metastatic disease while on tamoxifen. Aromatase inhibitors are not very effective in premenopausal women because of the high level of estradiol synthesis in the ovaries.

OTHER EFFECTS AND TOXICITY

Several trials have investigated the addition of progestins to chemotherapy. As with other chemoendocrine combinations, there is no convincing evidence that combining progestins with chemotherapy in the metastatic setting improves survival. Progestins may protect against leukopenia, allowing for higher doses of chemotherapy.[32] Progestins have also been suggested as palliative agents for bone pain in patients with extensive skeletal metastases.[33]

The major complication of progestin therapy is the potential for substantial weight gain, which has led to the use of progestins for

Table 7.4 Aromatase inhibitors versus megestrol acetate (MA)

Formestane versus MA[20]	Formestane (250 mg i.m. biw)	MA (40 mg qid)
No. of patients	91	86
Median TTP (months)	4	3.7
CR + PR rate (%)	17	17
Stable disease ⩾ 24 weeks (%)	25	22
Median survival (months)	NA	NA

Exemestane versus MA[21]	Exemestane (25 mg daily)	MA (40 mg qid)
No. of patients	366	403
Median TTP (months)	4.7	3.8
CR + PR rate (%)	15	12
Stable disease ⩾ 24 weeks (%)	22	23
Median survival (months)	NR	28.4

Vorozole versus MA[22]	Vorozole (2.5 mg daily)	MA (40 mg qid)
No. of patients	225	227
Median TTP (months)	2.6	3.3
CR + PR rate (%)	9.7	6.8
Stable disease ⩾ 24 weeks (%)	11.7	17.1
Median survival (months)	26.3	28.8

Letrozole versus MA[23]	Letrozole (2.5 mg daily)	MA (40 mg qid)
No. of patients	174	189
Median TTP (months)	5.6	5.5
CR + PR rate (%)	24[a]	16
Stable disease ⩾ 6 months (%)	11	15
Median survival (months)	25.3	21.5

Anastrozole versus MA[24]	Anastrozole (1 mg daily)	MA (40 mg qid)
No. of patients	263	253
Median TTP (months)	4.8	4.6
CR + PR rate (%)	13	12
Stable disease ⩾ 24 weeks (%)	30	28
Estimated 2-year survival rate (%)	56	46
Median survival (months)	27	23

Abbreviations: i.m., intramuscularly; biw, twice per week; qid, four times per day; TTP, time to progression; CR + PR, complete plus partial responses; NA, not addressed; NR, not reached.
[a]$p < 0.05$.

patients with HIV- and cancer-related cachexia.[34] Progestins are also associated with a higher than anticipated frequency of thromboembolic phenomena. Vaginal bleeding, especially withdrawal bleeding following discontinuation of MA, is common in postmenopausal women.

CURRENT ROLE OF PROGESTINS IN HORMONAL THERAPY

Progestins, like other endocrine agents, are most likely to be effective in patients with ER- and/or PgR-positive tumors. They should be considered for postmenopausal women with metastatic breast cancer who have responded or have had prolonged periods of stable disease after antiestrogens and oophorectomy. In postmenopausal women with metastatic breast cancer who have responded or have had prolonged periods of stable disease after antiestrogens and newer aromatase inhibitors, progestins are also worthy of consideration. For patients selected for progestin treatment, we recommended using standard doses of MA (160 mg daily) or MPA (500 mg daily) via the oral route. There is currently no defined role for progestins in the adjuvant setting.

REFERENCES

1. Sedlacek SM. An overview of megestrol acetate for the treatment of advanced breast cancer. *Semin Oncol* 1988; **15**: 3–13.
2. Stoll BA. Progestin therapy of breast cancer: comparison of agents. *BMJ* 1967; **3**: 338–41.
3. Teulings FA, Van Gilse HA, Henkelman MS et al. Estrogen, androgen, glucocorticoid, and progesterone receptors in progestin-induced regression of human breast cancer. *Cancer Res* 1980; **40**: 2557–61.
4. Dowsett M, Lal A, Smith IE et al. The effects of low and high-dose medroxyprogesterone acetate on sex steroids and sex hormone binding globulin in postmenopausal breast cancer patients. *Br J Cancer* 1987; **55**: 311–13.
5. Mahlke M, Grill HJ, Knapstein P et al. Oral high-dose medroxyprogesterone acetate (MPA) treatment: cortisol/MPA serum profiles in relation to breast cancer regression. *Oncology* 1985; **42**: 144–9.
6. Haller DG, Glick JH. Progestational agents in advanced breast cancer: an overview. *Semin Oncol* 1986; **13**: 2–8.
7. Paridaens R, Becquart D, Vanderlinden B et al. Oral versus intramuscular high-dose medroxyprogesterone acetate (HD-MPA) in advanced breast cancer. A randomized study of the Belgian Society of Medical Oncology. *Anticancer Res* 1986; **6**: 1089–94.
8. Beex L, Bourghouts J, van Turnhout J et al. Oral versus IM administration of high-dose medroxyprogesterone acetate in pretreated patients with advanced breast cancer. *Cancer Treat Rep* 1987; **71**: 1151–6.
9. Schacter LP, Rozeneweig M, Canetta R et al. Overview of hormonal therapy in advanced breast cancer. *Semin Oncol* 1990; **17**: 38–46.
10. Cavalli F, Goldhirsch A, Jungi F et al. Randomized trial of low- versus high-dose medroxyprogesterone acetate in the induction treatment of postmenopausal patients with advanced breast cancer. *J Clin Oncol* 1984; **2**: 414–19.
11. Rose C, Mauridsen HT, Engelsman E et al. Treatment of advanced breast cancer with medroxyprogesterone acetate. *Proc Am Soc Clin Oncol* 1985; **4**: 57.
12. Hortobagyi GN, Buzdar AU, Frye D et al. Oral medroxyprogesterone acetate in the treatment of metastatic breast cancer. *Breast Cancer Res Treat* 1985; **5**: 321–6.
13. Gallagher CJ, Cairnduff F, Smith IE. High-dose versus low-dose medroxyprogesterone acetate: a randomized trial in advanced breast cancer. *Eur J Cancer Clin Oncol* 1987; **23**: 1895–900.
14. Koyama H, Tominaga T, Asaishi K et al. A randomized controlled comparative study of oral medroxyprogesterone acetate 1,200 and 600 mg in patients with advanced or recurrent breast cancer. *Oncology* 1999; **56**: 283–90.
15. Muss HB, Case LD, Capizzi RL et al. High- versus standard-dose megestrol acetate in women with advanced breast cancer: a phase III trial of the Piedmont Oncology Association. *J Clin Oncol* 1990; **8**: 1797–805.
16. Abrams JS, Parnes H, Aisner J. Current status of

high-dose progestins in breast cancer. *Semin Oncol* 1990; **17:** 68–72.

17. Abrams J, Aisner J, Cirrincione C et al. Dose-response trial of megestrol acetate in advanced breast cancer: Cancer and Leukemia Group B phase III study 8741. *J Clin Oncol* 1999; **17:** 64–73.

18. Pannuti F, Martoni A, Cilenti G et al. Adjuvant therapy for operable breast cancer with medroxyprogesterone acetate alone in post-menopausal patients or in combination with CMF in premenopausal patients. *Eur J Cancer Clin Oncol* 1988; **24:** 423–9.

19. Focan C, Baudoux A, Beauduin M et al. Adjuvant treatment with high-dose medroxy-progesterone acetate in node-negative early breast cancer. A 3-year interim report on a ran-domized trial (I). *Acta Oncol* 1989; **28:** 237–40.

20. Hupperets PS, Wils J, Volovics L et al. Adjuvant chemohormonal therapy with cyclophos-phamide, doxorubin and 5-fluorouracil (CAF) with or without medroxyprogesterone acetate for node-positive breast cancer patients. *Ann Oncol* 1993; **4:** 295–301.

21. Muss HB, Wells HB, Paschold EH et al. Megestrol acetate versus tamoxifen in advanced breast cancer: 5-year analysis – a phase III trial of the Piedmont Oncology Association. *J Clin Oncol* 1988; **7:** 1098–106.

22. van Veelen H, Willemse PHB, Tjabbes T et al. Oral high-dose medroxyprogesterone acetate versus tamoxifen: a randomized crossover trial in postmenopausal patients with advanced breast cancer. *Cancer* 1986; **58:** 7–13.

23. Muss HB, Case LD, Atkins JN et al. Tamoxifen versus high-dose oral medroxyprogesterone acetate as initial endocrine therapy for patients with metastatic breast cancer: a Piedmont Oncology Association study. *J Clin Oncol* 1994; **12:** 1630–8.

24. Samonis G, Margioris AN, Bafaloukos D et al. Prospective randomized study of amino-glutethimide (AG) versus medroxyprogesterone acetate (MPA) versus AG + MPA in generalized breast cancer. *Oncology* 1994; **51:** 411–15.

25. Russell CA, Green SJ, O'Sullivan J et al. Megestrol acetate and aminoglutethimide/hydrocortisone in sequence or in combination as second-line endocrine therapy of estrogen recep-tor positive metastatic breast cancer: a Southwest Oncology Group phase III trial. *J Clin Oncol* 1997; **15:** 2494–501.

26. Thürlimann B, Catiglione M, Hsu-Schmitz SF et al. Formestane versus megestrol acetate in post-menopausal breast cancer patients after failure of tamoxifen: a phase III prospective randomised cross over trial of second-line hormonal treat-ment (SAKK 20/90). *Eur J Cancer* 1997; **33:** 1017–24.

27. Kaufman M, Bajetta E, Dirix LY et al. Survival advantage of exemestane (Aromasin) over mege-strol acetate in postmenopausal women with advanced breast cancer refractory to tamoxifen: results of a phase II randomized double-blind study. *Proc Am Soc Clin Oncol* 1999; **18:** 109a.

28. Goss PE, Winer EP, Tannock IF et al. Randomized phase III trial comparing the new potent and selective third-generation aromatase inhibitor vorozole with megestrol acetate in postmenopausal advanced breast cancer patients. *J Clin Oncol* 1999; **17:** 52–63.

29. Dombernowsky P, Smith I, Falkson G et al. Letrozole, a new oral aromatase inhibitor for advanced breast cancer: double-blind random-ized trial showing a dose effect and improved efficacy and tolerability compared with mege-strol acetate. *J Clin Oncol* 1998; **16:** 453–61.

30. Buzdar AU, Jonat W, Howell A et al. Anastrozole vs megestrol acetate in the treat-ment of postmenopausal women with advanced breast carcinoma: results of a survival update based on a combined analysis of data from two mature phase III trials: Arimidex Study Group. *Cancer* 1998; **82:** 1142–52.

31. Muss HB. New hormones for advanced breast cancer. *Cancer Control* 1999; **6:** 12–16.

32. Focan C, Baudoux A, Beauduin M et al. Improvement of hematological and general tol-erance to CMF by high-dose medroxyproges-terone acetate (HD-MPA) adjuvant treatment for primary node positive breast cancer (analysis of 100 patients). *Anticancer Res* 1986; **6:** 1095–9.

33. Martoni A, Longhi A, Canova N et al. High-dose medroxyprogesterone acetate versus oophorec-tomy as first-line therapy of advanced breast cancer in premenopausal patients. *Oncology* 1991; **48:** 1–6.

34. Cruz JM, Muss HB, Brockschmidt JK et al. Weight changes in women with metastatic breast cancer treated with megestrol acetate: a compari-son of standard versus high-dose therapy. *Semin Oncol* 1990; **17:** 63–7.

8

The clinical efficacy of progesterone antagonists in breast cancer

Walter Jonat, Marius Giurescu, John FR Robertson

CONTENTS • Introduction • Onapristone • Mifepristone • Summary

INTRODUCTION

The search for active and safe alternatives to current systemic therapies is one of the main objectives of current breast cancer research. Over the last three decades since the discovery of the estrogen receptor (ER), the development of new endocrine agents has in the main been aimed at either preventing the production of estrogens (e.g. ovarian ablation with gonadotropin-releasing hormone (GnRH) analogues, aromatase inhibition) or blocking their effect by competition for ER (e.g. selective ER modulators (SERMs) and pure antiestrogens). Such developments have focused, indirectly or directly, on the ER as a target for manipulation of tumour growth. This approach is supported by the finding that the response to such therapies is related to the expression of ER by breast tumours.[1–3] However, it is also known that response to 'antiestrogen therapies' (in the broadest sense) also correlates with the expression of another sex steroid receptor, the progesterone receptor (PgR).[1,3]

The importance of PgR in breast cancer is controversial. Since the promotor region of PgR contains an estrogen response element (ERE; see Chapter 9), PgR expression may serve as a marker of endocrine dependence, providing indication of a functional PgR.[4] As described in Chapter 14, substantial in vitro and in vivo evidence suggests that PgR serves as a biologically important molecule in breast cancer behaviour. Moreover, preclinical studies indicate that blockade of PgR function inhibits proliferation and induces apoptosis (see Chapter 14). Therefore, clinically practical PgR inhibitors have been developed. These are overtly active small molecules that appear to function by binding to PgR and inhibiting pathways downstream of PgR. Two agents, onapristone and mifepristone, have been evaluated in clinical trials, and, as described below, have activity in patients with metastatic disease. Although commercial support for these two agents has recently waned, the concept of PgR inhibition in breast cancer is sufficiently well founded to justify its inclusion in any textbook of endocrine therapy.

Mifepristone (RU38486) was the first progesterone antagonist reported to be useful in the treatment of patients with advanced breast cancer; these were tumours that had developed resistance to prior endocrine therapies.[5,6] Prior to these clinical reports, mifepristone had been reported to inhibit the growth of human breast cancer cell lines in vitro[7,8] and in vivo.[9,10] Indeed, in the latter studies,[10] antiprogestin and antiestrogenic treatment were reported to have additive antitumour effects. Treatment with mifepristone for 3 weeks resulted in decreased expression of ER, although this was slightly less than seen with tamoxifen. In contrast, mifepristone decreased the expression of PgR almost to zero, whereas tamoxifen caused an increase in PgR expression. In the in vivo experiments, mifepristone caused an increase in plasma serum estradiol and progesterone.[10] As noted below, these findings are different to those reported recently using onapristone in a phase II clinical study.[11]

The progesterone antagonist onapristone [11β-(4-dimethylaminophenyl)-17α-hydroxy-17-(3-hydroxypropyl)-13α-estra-4,9-dien-3-one], was also reported to exhibit tumour-inhibitory effects in several hormone-dependent mammary tumours in animal models. As described in detail in Chapter 14, the main mechanism of action of onapristone appears to be the induction of terminal differentiation, leading to cell death.[12,13] Its antitumour activity in mouse MXT mammary tumours and rat DMBA- or MNU-induced mammary tumours was as strong as that of tamoxifen or oophorectomy.[14] Toxicological studies carried out in two species (monkey and rat) over a 12-month period did not reveal any changes that could have precluded the use of onapristone in humans. In phase I studies, onapristone was given orally to healthy postmenopausal women in doses of up to 400 mg/day over a period of 14 days. The subjective tolerance of the drug was good. The laboratory parameters did not show any clinically relevant changes, and onapristone entered phase II studies in postmenopausal patients with advanced breast cancer that was tamoxifen-resistant (i.e. as second-line therapy) and a smaller study as first-line therapy in hormone-naive patients. Results of the latter study have been published,[15] but those of the former have not been, to date. This chapter continues the first publication of these data, which will therefore be described in more detail before being reviewed along with the previously published studies.

ONAPRISTONE

Onapristone in tamoxifen-resistant disease (phase II study)

A non-randomized, open, multicentre phase II study was conducted between December 1991 and May 1995 at 13 sites in Germany and the UK. The study was established to investigate the efficacy of onapristone when given in a dosage of 100 mg/day to postmenopausal patients with advanced breast cancer who had progressed on tamoxifen. The study was also designed to assess patient tolerability and to study the influence of onapristone on the levels of the relevant endocrine parameters (cortisol, androstenedione, estrone, and estradiol). The patient characteristics are described in Table 8.1.

Of the 101 evaluable patients, 1 had a complete remission, 9 had a partial remission, and 39 had stable disease for 3 months or more. This resulted in an overall clinical benefit of 49%. Table 8.2 shows the effect of onapristone on individual sites of disease. The most frequent metastatic site was bone (82 patients), followed by lymph nodes (29 patients), lung (25 patients), liver (22 patients), skin (20 patients), local recurrence (16 patients), and pleura (14 patients). A total of 42 patients out of 118 had visceral disease. A complete remission was observed at the site of a local recurrence. Partial remissions were observed in all other major localizations, except pleura.

Out of 10 remissions on onapristone, 8 were achieved in patients who had a benefit from palliative tamoxifen therapy in the form of either remission (3 patients) or stable disease (5 patients) (Table 8.3). Two remissions were registered in patients who had received tamoxifen as an adjuvant therapy. In 2 out of 12 primarily tamoxifen-resistant patients, disease stabilization was registered. No remission was observed in this group.

The response in the group of 33 evaluable patients with PgR-positive primary tumours was 4 patients with partial remission, 15 with stable disease, and 14 with progressive disease.

Table 8.1 Patient characteristics	
Sample size	**118**
Median age ($n = 118$)	62 years (range 40–86)
Menopausal status at diagnosis ($n = 118$):	
<2 years postmenopausal	16
⩾2 years postmenopausal	101
unknown	1
ER and/or PgR status at diagnosis ($n = 118$):	
ER^+/PgR^+	33
ER^+/PgR^-	13
ER^+/PgR unknown	7
ER^-/PgR^+	3
ER^-/PgR^-	6
ER^-/PgR unknown	2
ER unknown/PgR unknown	54
ER and/or PgR status at the start of study in patients with lesions accessible to biopsy ($n = 18$):	
ER^+/PgR^+	7
ER^+/PgR^-	4
ER^-/PgR^+	1
ER^-/PgR^-	5
ER^-/PgR unknown	1
Previous tamoxifen treatment ($n = 118$):	
palliative	90
adjuvant	28
Relapse-free interval in patients receiving initial palliative treatment ($n = 90$):	
<24 months	12
⩾24 months	55
unknown	23
Response to initial palliative treatment ($n = 90$):	
complete remission	5
partial remission	23
stable disease	38
progressive disease	12
unevaluable	8
unknown	4
Duration of previous adjuvant treatment ($n = 28$):	
<24 months	10
⩾24 months	12
unknown	6

Table 8.2 Response in individual sites of disease

Localization	Result						
	CR	PR	SD	PD	Not evaluable	Missing	Total
Bones		2	24	16	13	27	82
Lymph nodes		3	8	5	1	12	29
Lung		5	7	5	1	7	25
Liver		1	11	3	0	7	22
Skin		1	10	1	1	7	20
Local recurrence	1	1	5	0	0	9	16
Pleura		0	3	4	1	6	14
Other		0	5	0	4	5	14

CR, complete remission; PR, partial remission; SD, stable disease; PD, progressive disease.

Table 8.3 Response in relation to the results of previous antiestrogen therapy

Response to tamoxifen	Response to onapristone					
	CR/PR	SD	PD	Not evaluable	Missing	Total
CR/PR	3	15	6	2	2	28
SD	5	13	15	2	3	38
PD	0	2	9	0	1	12
Missing	0	2	2	0	0	4
Not evaluable	0	2	5	1	0	8

CR/PR, complete/partial remission; SD, stable disease; PD, progressive disease.

In 8 patients, the PgR status was established in biopsies taken prior to the start of onapristone treatment. The response in this group of patients was 2 patients with partial remission, 2 with stable disease, and 4 with progressive disease. In the group of patients whose tumours were PgR-negative, 2 partial remissions were observed.

The median time to progression was 4 months, and the median time to treatment failure was 3 months. The median time to progres-sion according to response was 11 months (complete or partial remission), 7 months (stable disease), and 3 months (progressive disease).

Onapristone was well tolerated, with the exception of liver function test (LFT) abnormalities. Other laboratory parameters were stable during treatment. Onapristone did not influence body weight or systolic and diastolic blood pressure (data not shown). No systematic changes in the serum concentrations of cortisol, androstenedione, estrone, and estradiol were observed during the study (data not shown). However, in 20 out of 32 patients with LFTs within normal range at baseline, elevations of one or more parameters – bilirubin, aspartate aminotransferase (AST), alanine aminotransferase (ALT), γ-glutamyl transpeptidase (GGT), lactate dehydrogenase (LDH), and alkaline phosphatase – were observed. LFTs started to increase after 0.5–1 month of treatment, and reached a maximum after 1 or 2 months. Subsequently, LFTs either stayed unchanged for the rest of the study or returned to normal.

In summary, a clinical benefit for onapristone of 49% compares favourably with results seen with other endocrine agents in patients who have progressed on tamoxifen, including megestrol acetate[16] and aromatase inhibitors.[17]

Onapristone in hormone-naive patients (phase II study)

As the above study of onapristone as second-line endocrine therapy was finishing, a small phase II study as first-line therapy was established.[15] In summary, this study set out to recruit 30 patients, but was stopped after 19 patients had been entered into the trial because the clinical development programme for onapristone was halted. Nonetheless, the agent appears to be active in this setting.

Of the 19 patients entered into the study, one was withdrawn after 4.5 months owing to marked elevation in the patient's LFTs. At this time, the patient had stable disease. In the remaining 18 patients, 10 achieved partial remission, 2 had durable stable disease (>24 weeks), and 6 had de novo progression. Thus, the overall clinical benefit was 66%. As previously reported, the majority of patients had hormone-receptor-positive tumours. Ten patients were ER-positive/PgR-positive, of whom 7 achieved partial remission, 1 had stable disease, and 2 had de novo progressive disease. Six patients had ER-positive/PgR-negative tumours, of whom 2 achieved partial remission, 2 had stable disease (1 of

whom was the patient withdrawn for LFT elevations after 4–5 months), and 2 had progressive disease. Two patients had ER-negative/PgR-negative tumours, both of whom showed de novo progression.

Overall, the clinical benefit rate of 66% (12 of 18 patients) is similar to the published remission rates for the antiestrogen tamoxifen,[18–20] the synthetic progestin megestrol acetate,[19–21] and aromatase inhibitors such as anastrozole.[22,23] There was no change in serum estradiol during the first 6 months (data not shown). LFT elevations were noted in the majority of patients. These were initially detected at 6 weeks, when the first on-treatment blood samples were taken. Later in the study, when LFT measurements were performed weekly, the elevations in LFTs were detected from weeks 1–2 onwards.

Onapristone (two doses) versus megestrol acetate (phase III study)

Given the favourable phase II results, a comparative trial of two doses of onapristone (50 mg/day and 100 mg/day) versus megestrol acetate was started. In view of the LFT results in the phase II studies, early review was carried out of the LFT results in this phase III study. Elevations of LFTs occurred with a higher incidence in the two onapristone arms, without clear signs of dose dependence. Subsequently, the development of onapristone was terminated by the sponsor. The mechanism of onapristone-associated liver toxicity is not fully understood. Taking into account (1) that LFT alterations were transient in a number of patients despite continued treatment, (2) that dose level, duration of treatment, and total exposure did not appear to play a role, and (3) onapristone's failure to elicit comparable effects in animals, the likely mechanism could be an idiosyncratic reaction to onapristone rather than a direct hepatoxic effect.

Since no comparative trials with onapristone were completed, the potential of this drug in relation to current endocrine therapies could not be conclusively evaluated. Nevertheless, the level of clinical activity demonstrated by onapristone in the phase II studies indicated that progesterone antagonists have therapeutic potential in the treatment of breast cancer and supported the earlier studies of mifepristone.

MIFEPRISTONE

Mifepristone in tamoxifen-resistant disease (phase II studies)

The first clinical report of a progesterone antagonist in patients with breast cancer was of mifepristone as second-line therapy in advanced disease.[5,6] In the study by Romieu and colleagues,[5] 3 out of 22 patients achieved partial remission, with a further 9 showing stable disease. Klijn and colleagues[6] reported that 1 patient out of 11 achieved partial remission, with a further 6 showing stable disease. Together, these phase II studies reported on 33 patients with advanced breast cancer who were treated with mifepristone. Overall, 4 out of 33 patients (12%) achieved partial remission, with a further 15 (46%) showing stable disease. These results for second- and/or third-line endocrine therapy are consistent with the literature, and are similar to the results obtained with onapristone that have been described above.

Mifepristone in hormone-naive breast cancer (phase II study)

One further study of mifepristone in advanced breast cancer was reported by Perrault and colleagues.[24] A 10.7% objective response rate (complete plus partial remissions) and a 39.3% stable disease rate was reported for what the authors described as patients with untreated metastatic breast cancer. However, it should be noted that 43% of the patients had received a prior endocrine agent as adjuvant therapy, while 32% had received adjuvant chemotherapy. These prior systemic therapies, albeit as adjuvant

treatment, would have influenced the response rates when the patients received mifepristone for metastatic disease. In reality, therefore, mifepristone in this study was, for many of the patients, being used as a second endocrine agent on failure of adjuvant endocrine therapy, and the results seem more reflective of response rates reported for second-line endocrine therapies.

It should also be noted that mifepristone has been reported to cause an increase in serum estradiol.[6] In contrast, onapristone caused no such increase.[15] While the significance of this remains to be established, it is known that a 50–90% *decrease* in serum estradiol by aromatase inhibitors is associated with objective remissions. Whether the increases in serum estradiol seen with mifepristone have any effect on tumour growth is an intriguing but as yet unanswered question.

SUMMARY

The progesterone antagonists onapristone and mifepristone have been used in clinical studies in advanced breast cancer. Onapristone entered phase II clinical trials as both second-line and first-line endocrine therapy. Only the smaller first-line study has thus far been published, and therefore this is the first report of the larger phase II study of onapristone as second-line therapy. In this trial, 118 postmenopausal patients with systemic progressive disease resistant to antiestrogens received 100 mg/day onapristone orally. One hundred and one patients were evaluated for response, with the following results: 1 complete remission, 9 partial remissions, 39 cases of stable disease, and 52 cases of progressive disease. The median time to progression was 4 months. These findings, along with published phase II studies using another progesterone antagonist, mifepristone, which reported similar clinical efficacy, indicates that progesterone antagonists may have therapeutic potential in the treatment of breast cancer.

Mifepristone is currently being investigated

in combination with tamoxifen rather than as a single agent. The clinical development of onapristone has been stopped by the sponsor. Although clinically onapristone seemed to be well tolerated, its administration was associated with elevation of liver function tests in a significant number of patients. Nevertheless, the studies of antiprogestins to date have confirmed that this class of endocrine agent has clinical activity, providing impetus to search for newer antiprogestins.

REFERENCES

1. Osborne CK, Yochmowitz MG, Knight WA, McGuire WL. The value of estrogen and progesterone receptors in the treatment of breast cancer. *Cancer* 1980; **46:** 2884–8.
2. Williams MR, Todd JH, Ellis IO et al. Oestrogen receptors in primary and advanced breast cancer. *Br J Cancer* 1987; **55:** 67–73.
3. Robertson JFR, Cannon P, Nicholson RI, Blamey RW. Oestrogen and progesterone receptors as prognostic variables in hormonally treated breast cancer. *Int J Biol Markers* 1996; **11:** 29–33.
4. Clarke CL, Feil PD, Satyaswaroop PG. Progesterone receptor regulation by 17 beta-estradiol in human endometrial carcinoma grown in nude mice. *Endocrinology* 1987; **121:** 1642–8.
5. Romieu G, Maudelonde T, Ulmann A et al. The antiprogestin RU 486 in advanced breast cancer: preliminary clinical trial. *Bull Cancer* 1987; **74:** 455–61.
6. Klijn JGM, de Jong FH, Bakker GH et al. Antiprogestins, a new form of endocrine therapy for human breast cancer. *Cancer Res* 1989; **49:** 2851–6.
7. Bardon S, Vignon F, Chalbos D, Rochefort H. RU486, a progestin and glycocorticoid antagonist, inhibits the growth of breast cancer cells via the progesterone receptor. *J Clin Endocrinol Metab* 1985; **60:** 692–7.
8. Gill P, Vignon F, Bardon S et al. Difference between R5070 and the antiprogestin 486 in antiproliferative effects on human breast cancer cells. *Breast Cancer Res Treat* 1987; **10:** 37–45.
9. Bakker GH, Setyono-Han B, Henkelmann MS et al. Comparison of the actions of the antiprogestin mifepristone (RU486), the progestin mege-strol acetate, the LNRH-analog buserelin and ovariectomy in treatment of rat mammary tumours. *Cancer Treat Rep* 1987; **71:** 1021–7.
10. Bakker GH, Setyono-Han B, Portengan H et al. Endocrine and anti-tumour effects of combined treatment with an anti-progestin and antioestrogen or luteinizing hormone-releasing hormone agonist in female rats bearing mammary tumours. *Endocrinology* 1989; **125:** 1593–8.
11. Crook SJ, Brook D, Robertson JFR. Biological and molecular mechanisms of the progesterone receptor antagonist, onapristone. *Proc Am Assoc Cancer Res* 2001; **42:** 893 (Abst 4789).
12. Michna H, Schneider MR, Nishino Y, El Etreby MF. The antitumour mechanism of progesterone antagonists is a receptor mediated antiproliferative effect by induction of terminal cell death. *J Steroid Biochem* 1989; **34:** 447–53.
13. Michna H, Nishino Y, Neef G et al. Progesterone antagonists: tumor-inhibiting potential and mechanism of action. *J Steroid Biochem Mol Biol* 1992; **41:** 339–48.
14. Schneider MR, Michna H, Nishino Y, El Etreby MF. Antitumor activity of the progesterone antagonists ZK 98.299 and RU 38.486 in the hormone-dependent MXT mammary tumor model of the mouse and the DMBA- and the MNU-induced mammary tumor models of the rat. *Eur J Cancer Clin Oncol* 1989; **25:** 691–701.
15. Robertson JFR, Willsher P, Winterbottom L et al. Onapristone, a progesterone receptor antagonist, as first-line therapy in primary breast cancer. *Eur J Cancer* 1999; **35:** 214–18.
16. Cheung KL, Willsher PC, Pinder SE et al. Predictors of response to second-line endocrine therapy for breast cancer. *Breast Cancer Res Treat* 1997; **45:** 219–24.
17. Buzdar AU, Jonat W, Howell A et al. Anastrozole, a potent and selective aromatase inhibitor, versus megestrol acetate in postmenopausal women with advanced breast cancer: results of overview analysis of two phase III trials. *J Clin Oncol* 1996; **14:** 2000–11.
18. Robertson JFR, Willsher P, Cheung KL, Blamey RW. The clinical relevance of static disease (no change) category for 6 months on endocrine therapy in patients with breast cancer. *Eur J Cancer* 1997; **33:** 1774–9.
19. Morgan LR. Megestrol acetate v tamoxifen in advanced breast cancer in postmenopausal patients. *Semin Oncol* 1985; **12:** 43–7.
20. Ingle JN, Creagan ET, Ahmann DL et al.

Randomised clinical trial of megestrol acetate versus tamoxifen in paramenopausal or castrated women with advanced breast cancer. *Am J Clin Oncol* 1982; **5:** 155–60.

21. Muss HB, Wells HB, Paschold EH et al. Megestrol acetate versus tamoxifen in advanced breast cancer: 5 year analysis – a phase III trial of the Piedmont Oncology Association. *J Clin Oncol* 1988; **6:** 1098–106.

22. Nabholtz JM, Buzdar A, Pollak M et al. Anastrozole is superior to tamoxifen as first-line therapy for advanced breast cancer in postmenopausal women: results of a North American multicenter randomised trial. *J Clin Oncol* 2000; **18:** 3758–67.

23. Bonneterre J, Thurlimann B, Robertson JFR et al. Anastrozole versus tamoxifen as first-line therapy for advanced breast cancer in 668 postmenopausal women: results of the Tamoxifen or Arimidex Randomised Group Efficacy and Tolerability study. *J Clin Oncol* 2000; **18:** 3748–57.

24. Perrault D, Eisenhauer EA, Pritchard KI et al. Phase II study of progesterone antagonist mifepristone in patients with untreated metastatic breast carcinoma: a National Cancer Institute of Canada Clinical Trials Group study. *J Clin Oncol* 1996; **14:** 2709–12.

Part II
Biological Aspects of Endocrine Therapies

9

Cellular and molecular actions of estrogens and antiestrogens in breast cancer

Robert I Nicholson, Tracie-Ann Madden, Sian Bryant, Julia MW Gee

CONTENTS • Introduction • Molecular biology of the target receptor for estrogens – ERα • ERα variants • ERβ subtype • ERα activation by estrogens • Crosstalk between estrogen and growth factor signalling pathways • Estrogen withdrawal • The ERα protein and antiestrogens • Summary

INTRODUCTION

Since the discovery of the target receptor for estrogen (ER) in 1958,[1] a massive literature has accumulated on the ER and endocrine response in breast cancer, where it has proved a useful, if imprecise, predictor of therapeutic benefit to multiple types of antihormonal therapy.[2] In biological terms, the ER acts as a ligand-dependent nuclear transcription factor that regulates the expression of genes containing estrogen response elements (EREs) within their promoters, and antihormone therapies act to either (i) limit the tissue availability of estrogens, and hence the formation of active ER complexes, or (ii) bind to the ER and attenuate/alter ER-mediated gene expression profiles.

In this context, this chapter outlines those molecular actions of estrogens and antiestrogens that allow a fuller appreciation of the mechanisms leading to endocrine-induced therapeutic remissions in breast cancer patients, and that help to define the processes whereby response is subverted to generate de novo and acquired endocrine resistance (see Chapters 10 and 12). In addition to the now well-described functional domain structure of the ER and its interactions with EREs, emphasis will also be placed on several more recently identified elements of ER signalling, including the contribution made to the tissue-selective actions of ER by the presence of ER subtypes and variants, co-activators/co-repressors, and crosstalk between ER and growth factor signalling elements.[3]

MOLECULAR BIOLOGY OF THE TARGET RECEPTOR FOR ESTROGENS – ERα

ERα gene structure and its regulation

The human *ER* gene (now termed *ERα*) was first cloned and sequenced from MCF-7 human breast cancer cells in 1986 by two separate groups working concurrently.[4,5] It is located on chromosome 6, extends over 140 kbp, and consists of eight exons[6] separated by seven large intronic regions,[7] and it is a member of the nuclear receptor superfamily, of which more than 150 different members are now known. It is expressed in the female accessory sex organs, in the skeletal and cardiovascular systems, and in those areas of the brain influencing sexual behaviour.[8] In each of these tissues, the *ERα* gene product is a phosphorylated protein[9] consisting of 595 amino acids[4,10] with a molecular weight of 67 kDa, although this can vary depending on the degree of receptor hyperphosphorylation.[11–14]

The transcriptional regulation of the *ERα* gene is extremely complicated; however, there have been several recent advances that contribute to the understanding of the mechanisms involved. The *ERα* gene possesses two promoters, P_0 and P_1, from which its transcription can be initiated.[15] The principal transcriptional start site is P_1,[4] although this appears to vary depending on tissue/cell type.[14] Additionally, a 75 bp region of the 5′ untranslated leader sequence of the *ERα* gene has been discovered that augments the expression from the *ERα* promoter.[16] This region contains two binding sites for estrogen receptor factor 1 (ERF-1) protein. ERF-1 is the AP-2γ member of the AP-2 transcription factor family. This protein is increased in ERα-positive breast cancers,[16,17] suggesting that a direct correlation exists between the expression of ERF-1 and the expression of ERα.[18] Further work undertaken

by McPherson and colleagues[19] has shown that ERF-1 activates *ERα* gene transcription by binding to the imperfect palindrome CCCT-GCGGGG within the promoter of the *ERα* gene.

Finally, Tang and colleagues[20] have recently identified an additional transcriptional enhancer (35 bp) in the human *ERα* gene upstream of the major human ERα mRNA start site, termed ER-EH0. ER-EH0 appears to be active in ERα-positive cells, but not ERα-negative cells. It is a 12-*O*-tetradecanoylphorbol-13-acetate-responsive element (TPA-RE)-containing region, although methylation interference assays suggest that binding of factors occurs both on the AP-1 site and its adjacent base pairs, both being required for enhancer activity.[20]

Mutational studies of both ERF-1 and ER-EH0 have confirmed the ER-EH0 enhancer element as the predominant *cis*-acting factor in the differential expression of ERα.[20]

ERα protein structure

Transfection studies characterizing the activity of various *ERα* deletion mutants have revealed that the ERα protein, like other family members, consists of six distinct functional domains labelled A–F (Figure 9.1).[14,21,22] These contain specific amino acid sequences that (i) facilitate

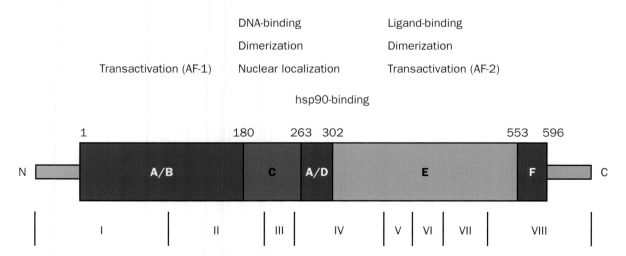

Figure 9.1 Structural and functional domains of the estrogen receptor ERα.

the localization of the receptor within the nucleus of the cell, (ii) allow it to bind steroid hormone, dimerize, and associate with specific DNA response elements, and (iii) finally promote transcriptional regulation of responsive genes. The culmination of these events in breast cancer is often tumour growth.

The A/B region

The A/B domain in *ERα*, encoded by exon 1 and part of exon 2, has an intrinsic transcriptional activation function known as AF-1,[23] the activity of which is independent of estrogen (and antiestrogen) binding. This is in contrast to the second transactivation function of *ERα*, located in the E region and requiring estrogen for activity (see below). Although in most instances both AF-1 and AF-2 appear to function together for optimal transcriptional activity, there is considerable experimental evidence to indicate that the contribution made by AF-1 to overall ER activity varies between cell types and gene promoters. Thus, while introduction of an *ERα* gene lacking AF-2 into chicken embryo fibroblasts has been shown to promote 60–70% of wild-type ER activity,[24] an identical construct introduced into HeLa and CV1 cells shows only 1–5% of the transcriptional activity of wild-type ER.[22] Conversely, while an *ERα* construct lacking AF-1 (but possessing AF-2), showed considerably reduced ER activity on the pS2-ERE-containing promoter in HeLa cells, no reduction in transcriptional activity from the vitellogenin-ERE-containing promoter was seen in these cells.[22]

Importantly, among the requirements for full activation of AF-1 in vitro is phosphorylation of the serine residue at position 118 of ERα, potentially through the Ras/MAPK (mitogen-activated protein kinase) cascade of growth factor signalling pathways.[25] Activation of this pathway, therefore, could potentially promote the expression of ER-regulated genes dependent upon AF-1, even in the absence of estrogens or the presence of antiestrogens. Such regulation is discussed more thoroughly late in this chapter.

The C region

The C region of ERα has been identified as the DNA-binding domain (DBD), consisting of a core sequence of 66 amino acids rich in cysteine residues.[7,26] It is the most highly conserved section of the ERα between species[27] and between other nuclear receptors.[28] The region is folded into two zinc-stabilized DNA-binding 'fingers' (CI and CII),[29,30] encoded by exons 2 and 3, with each exon encoding a single zinc finger.[7] Each zinc finger binds a zinc atom via cysteine residues, producing a stable 13-amino-acid loop.[27]

The zinc fingers are important for the recognition of specific ERE sequences located upstream of the promoters of genes regulated by estrogen.[31] These two zinc fingers are structurally and functionally distinct from each other. The N-terminal finger is involved in DNA sequence recognition by providing specific contacts with the nucleotides in the major groove of the ERE sequence. It is believed that the three amino acids at the base of this zinc finger are the most crucial for discrimination of ERE binding.[32–34] The C-terminal finger mediates high-affinity DNA binding by providing the phosphate backbone contacts and the dimerization interface between the two DBDs of the ERα homodimer bound at the response element.[35,36]

Although both zinc fingers are required for DNA binding, they are insufficient alone for high-affinity binding.[27] ER-deletion studies by Kumar and Chambon[37] have demonstrated that sequences located downstream of region C are required for stabilization of the ERα–ERE complex, although such sequences do not take part in the recognition of the ERE. Indeed, it now appears that there are several amino acid residues other than those found within the zinc fingers that are necessary for high-affinity DNA binding. These include regions employed for nuclear localization or targeting, receptor dimerization, and binding of heat-shock proteins.[27]

The D region

The D region is considered to be a 'hinge' segment that separates the DNA-binding domain (region C) and the ligand-binding domain (region E) of the receptor, encoded by part of exon 4.[38] Mutations of this region have been reported to induce no effects on estrogen binding or on the transcriptional capability of ERα in HeLa cells.[22] However, a nuclear localization motif consisting of 48 amino acids is C-terminal to the zinc fingers in region D, and is apparently required to tether unliganded receptor in the nucleus.[39–41] This section of the receptor consists of three stretches of basic amino acids at residues 256–260, 266–271, and 299–303 that are highly conserved between species. A second nuclear localization signal is also believed to exist in region E of the receptor.[42]

The E region

The E region of ERα is hydrophobic and is known as the hormone-binding domain (HBD); it consists of approximately 250 amino acids encoded by exons 4–8.[7,10] Affinity labelling experiments have determined that HBD integrity is necessary for the binding of the natural ligand estrogen to the ER.[43,44] The hormone-binding domain can only be obtained as a trypsin-resistant fragment in its occupied form, indicating that a ligand-induced change in its structure has occurred. This region also contains the principal dimerization activity of the receptor as well as the ligand-dependent transactivation function (AF-2).[38] In addition, region E is involved in the binding of hsp90 to the receptor.[27] Following the binding of estrogens, this region provides some interacting surfaces on the receptor to allow interconnections with other cellular proteins, including various cofactors (discussed in detail later in this chapter).

The E domain is believed to comprise a hydrophobic 'pocket' that facilitates the binding of ligand.[4,7,10,45] Eight or nine highly conserved heptad repeats associated with regions of hydrophobicity are thought to be involved in this hydrophobic pocket formation.[46] It has been shown that ERα mutants that contain these heptad repeats but not the remainder of the HDB and DBD undergo spontaneous dimerization.[47] It was concluded that because

the dimerization of normal ERα protein is usually dependent on the binding of ligand, sites important for receptor dimerization are masked in unliganded receptors and unmasked on binding of ligand.

The ERα principal dimerization domain resides within the C-terminus end of this region, in exon 7.[48–50] This region mediates most of the interaction between the two ERα molecules.[48] The phosphorylation of tyrosine 537 is also a necessary step for the formation of the hERα dimer,[11,12] and is phosphorylated by p60[c-Src] independently of estradiol treatment.[12] A second weaker dimerization site is located in the C region of the receptor, believed to be on the second zinc finger encoded by exon 3.[36]

The activity of AF-2 in region E depends on a number of dispersed elements that occur throughout the HBD and that are brought together on estrogen binding.[10,18,51,52] In essence, the elements of the entire HBD appear to be necessary for AF-2 activity,[10,27,53] with mutational studies showing that alterations in amino acids throughout the HBD can eliminate AF-2 activity without necessarily affecting the receptor's hormone-binding function.[54] Halachmi et al[55] have identified a 160 kDa protein known as ERAP 160, which interacts with the HBD/AF-2 domain of ERα. It has been suggested that this protein is involved in AF-2 estrogen transcriptional activity, because the ability of ERα to activate transcription in the presence of estrogen parallels its ability to bind ERAP 160. In addition to ERAP 160, Cavailles et al[56] have also identified several proteins that interact with the wild-type ERα HBD/AF-2 domain.

Reports have suggested the presence of a third transactivation domain, AF-2a, containing a hormone-independent transcriptional activation function, which has been localized to the N-terminal portion of AF-2 between amino acids 282 and 351.[57,58]

The binding of hsp90 to ERα also appears to include numerous sections of region E,[27] which seem to overlap the regions involved in both nuclear localization[40] and receptor dimerization.[49,59] hsp90 bound to the receptor seems to inhibit dimerization and therefore any subsequent DNA binding.[60] However, surprising results were achieved by Picard et al,[41] following experimentation using yeast mutants in which the expression of hsp90 was considerably reduced. It was found that unliganded steroid receptors remained transcriptionally inactive even though they were virtually free of all bound hsp90. In addition, it was shown that the introduction of ligand only slightly activated these receptors, thus suggesting that hsp90 could well be functioning not only by steric hindrance, but possibly also by facilitating the events subsequent to its dissociation from the receptor.[27] Region D may also be involved to a limited extent in the binding of hsp90 to the receptor protein.[27]

The F region

ERα contains a 42-amino-acid C-terminal region (not well conserved between species) known as the F region, encoded by the 3′ portion of exon 8.[21] Recent studies have revealed that the presence of the C-terminal F domain is important in the transcriptional activation and repression of estrogen-regulated genes by antiestrogens and that it affects the magnitude of ligand-bound ERα bioactivity in a cell-specific manner.[61]

ERα VARIANTS

Considerable interest has recently been directed towards the expression of structurally altered ERαs that may either contribute to or interfere with normal estrogen ERα signalling. Since there is currently no evidence for genomic deletion or significant mutations or amplications of the *ERα* gene, recent research has focused on the existence of alterations in the ERα mRNA, and several independent groups have reported the existence of altered ERα mRNA within both normal and malignant human breast tissue and human breast cancer cell lines. Such alterations in ERα frequently involve changes at the exon/intron boundaries, usually as a result of alternative splicing. Following transcription of the gene, the primary transcript (pre-mRNA)

has the same organization as the gene. Pre-mRNA is cleaved so that sequences corresponding to introns are excised and discarded. The remaining RNA segments corresponding to exons are spliced together to form mRNA. The location of these splice sites is dictated by the intron/exon boundaries. Although the majority of genes give rise to a single type of spliced mRNA, RNAs of some genes follow patterns of alternative splicing, when a single gene gives rise to more than one mRNA sequence. The structure and function of some of the variant ERα mRNAs found in human breast cancers are summarized in Table 9.1, and the exon 5 and 7 variants are briefly discussed below.

Exon 5 and 7 variants in ERα mRNA

Fuqua et al[62] were the first group to isolate an ERα variant lacking exon 5 of the HBD, from ERα-negative/progesterone receptor (PgR)-positive breast tumours in vivo. This variant has since been shown to exist in ERα-positive/PgR-positive breast cancers and several human breast cancer cell lines, including ERα-negative cell lines.[62-65] The precise deletion of this exon results in an interruption in translation after codon 370. While a major portion of the estrogen-binding domain (including AF-2) is missing from the variant, the AF-1 domain and DBD remain intact. It was initially demonstrated that the exon 5 ERα deletion variant was capable of stimulating the transcriptional activity of an ERE through the constitutive transactivation of AF-1, in the absence of estrogen. However, the activity of this variant was only about 10–15% of that of the wild-type ERα in a yeast reporter system. The potential relevance of the exon 5 ERα deletion variant has also been examined in ERα-negative MDA-MB-231 breast cancer cells. Tzukerman and colleagues[66] concluded that while estrogen was absolutely required for wild-type activity, the exon 5 deletion variant was active in the absence of exogenous hormone. From these results, it has been suggested that the exon 5 ERα deletion variant might be a potent dominantly acting receptor in estrogen-

Table 9.1 Examples of variant/mutated forms of ER mRNA reported in human breast cancers in vivo and their predicted activity

Region of ER	Type of mRNA error	Error	Predicted activity of alterations in these regions if translated	Ref
A/B	Base-pair substitution	Silent G → C substitution at nucleotide 261	Enhancement of elimination or AF-1 activity	240–242
C	Insertion	Insertion of 84 amino acids at the exon 3/intron boundary, resulting in a premature stop codon	Prevention or diminished ability of ER to recognize its response elements, as a result of reduced or absent DNA-binding domain (DBD)	243, 244
	Splice variant	Exon 2 deletion, predicted to code for a 17 kDa ER protein prematurely terminated after exon 1		14, 68, 244
	Splice variant	Exon 3 deletion only (predicted to code for an ER protein of 61 kDa)		68, 70, 245
D	Splice variant	Exon 4 deletion only	Effects on the nuclear localization of the receptor and hence functionality	246–249
E	Splice variant	Exon 4 deletion only	Detrimental effects (enhancement, reduction, or elimination) on hormone binding, activation of AF-2, dimerization, or nuclear localization	246–247
	Splice variant	Exon 5 deletion, resulting in an interruption in translation after codon 370		62–65, 67
	Splice variant	Exon 7 deletion, predicted to code for a truncated protein		68, 69, 250
	Substitution	42 bp replacement in exon 6, would generate a truncated ER if translated		251
	Deletion	1 bp deletion in exon 6, would generate a truncated ER if translated		251

sensitive tissues, including human breast cancer, where it may confer a cellular ability to survive in a reduced estrogenic environment.[67] Indeed, the exon 5 ERα deletion variant has been stably transfected into MCF-7 cells that express abundant wild-type ERα, and has been shown to induce estrogen-independent growth.[67]

The exon 7 deletion variant was first reported by Wang and Miksicek[68] in T47-D human breast cancer culture cells. Fuqua et al[69] subsequently reported the presence of this receptor variant in human breast tumours, and suggested it to be transcriptionally inactive; however, when co-expressed with wild-type ERα in a yeast expression vector system, it acted in a dominant-negative manner. Fuqua et al[69] proposed that as the variant was overexpressed in approximately one-half of the ERα-positive/PgR-negative tumours, it may be responsible for this discordant phenotype. In contrast to these results, Miksicek et al,[70] who identified the same variant in T47-D cells,[68] found it to be non-functional in HeLa cells.

ERβ SUBTYPE

In 1996, Kuiper et al,[71] isolated from a rat prostate cDNA library a new type of ER, designated ERβ. This previously unrecognized moiety was subsequently shown to be also present in many human and mouse tissues, where it shows important differences in tissue distribution to the classical ERα.[72,73] Thus, in contrast to ERα, ERβ is not highly expressed in the major female accessary sex organs (except the ovaries), rather it is more abundant in several male organs and in different parts of the central nervous system. Importantly, gene knockout experiments in mice have established that while the loss of ERα results in a severely impaired development of the uterus, ovary, and mammary gland after puberty and the animals were infertile,[74] mice devoid of ERβ were found to have relatively normal uteri and mammary glands and were fertile, although they showed reduced ovarian function.[75]

In the human form, ERβ shows an overall 47% homology to the translated portion of ERα and maps to chromosome 14q23–24.[76] The greatest homology is in the DNA- and hormone-binding domains, suggesting common estrogenic ligands and DNA response elements (Figure 9.2). Indeed, recent studies have shown that the α and β forms of the ER can heterodimerize and bind with high affinity to several EREs.[77] Estrogen-activated ERβ, however, unlike ERα, does not appear to efficiently promote growth-factor-induced AP-1 activity.[78] Although a number of variants of ERβ have also been reported, including one with a hormone-binding-domain deletion,[79] their contribution, if any, to ER signalling is unknown.

ERα ACTIVATION BY ESTROGENS

Normally, in the absence of ligand, ERα resides in a large molecular complex with multiple heat-shock proteins.[80] The most potent ligand for ERα is estradiol, with the weaker estrone and estriol activating ERα by similar mechanisms. Estrogens, owing to their fat-soluble nature, rapidly diffuse through the plasma membrane, move into the nucleus of the cell,[81] and bind to ERα via the HBD.[82] This binding of estrogens to ERα results in displacement of the heat-shock proteins and allows phosphorylation of ERα at several serine residues within its N-terminal portion.[18] Indeed, the basal level of ERα phosphorylation increases three- to fourfold on exposure to estradiol.[83] Although the cellular kinases that actually promote this phosphorylation have yet to be fully determined, following these events the receptor protein undergoes a conformational change allowing for a productive association and transcriptional synergism between AF-1 and AF-2.[84] These changes permit receptor homodimerization and subsequent binding to *cis*-acting elements within the enhancers of target genes,[14] resulting in the rapid formation of a relatively unstable ERα–ERE complex.[85] This, coupled with the recruitment of cofactors (see below), allows the activation of estrogen-responsive genes such as the progesterone receptor,[86] *pS2*,[87]

ERα sites of expression: uterus and mammary gland

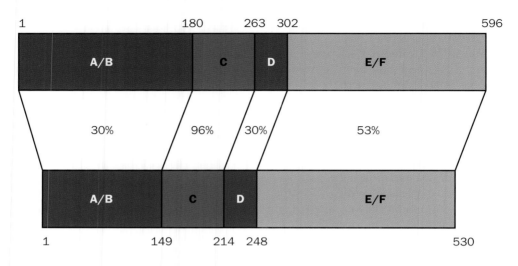

Figure 9.2 Structural comparison of ERα and ERβ.

LIV1,[88] and c-*myc*.[89] Such events may lead to cell cycle entry and progression, following the expression of cell cycle regulatory genes,[90,91] thus resulting in cell proliferation. Additionally, several genes associated with cell survival, such as *bcl-2*[92,93] and *TGF-α*,[94] are also upregulated in estradiol-treated cells in vitro and ERα-positive tissues in vivo, with increased estrogen-induced cell survival contributing significantly to breast cancer growth responses to this steroid.[95]

As stated above, the recruitment of cofactors

(termed co-activators) is now known to significantly enhance ERα-dependent transcription (Figure 9.3). SPT6, isolated from *Saccharomyces cerevisiae*, was shown to be capable of modulating ERα-mediated transcription in both yeast and mammalian cells. It is believed that this proposed co-activator interacts specifically with the C terminus of the ERα.[96] A second steroid receptor co-activator, SRC-1 (steroid receptor co-activator 1), characterized using a yeast two-hybrid system,[97] has been shown to enhance the transcriptional activity of ERα. Furthermore,

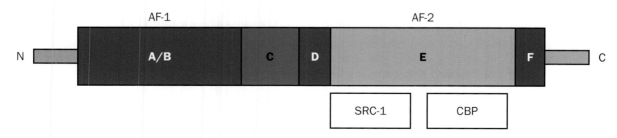

Figure 9.3 Cofactors associated with ERα signalling.

SRC-1 is also involved in enhancing the transcriptional activities of the progesterone receptor, the retinoic acid receptor, the thyroid hormone receptor, and the glucocorticoid receptor. As a result, SRC-1 may play a complex role in steroid receptor regulation. cAMP response-element binding protein (CREB)-binding protein (CBP)[98] can also interact with the members of the steroid hormone nuclear receptor family, and is able to enhance transcriptional activity.[99] Ectopic expression of CBP enhances estrogen-dependent ERα transcriptional activity tenfold compared with the ectopic expression of SRC-1.[98] When CBP and SRC-1 are co-expressed ectopically, ERα-mediated transcription is enhanced in a synergistic manner. Of further interest is the cell cycle regulatory protein cyclin D1, which also appears able to behave as an ERα cofactor to upregulate ERα-mediated transcription.[100] Rubino et al[101] reported a novel protein Brx, which binds specifically to ERα. Furthermore, they found that the overexpression of Brx in transfection experiments using an estrogen-responsive reporter revealed that Brx augmented gene activation by ERα in an element-specific and ligand-dependent manner. As well as co-activators, another class of proteins exists that repress the basal transcription of ERα (co-repressors). One putative co-repressor has recently been identified, known as SMRT (silencing mediator of retinoic acid and thyroid hormone receptors).[102]

In addition to transcriptional activation of ERE-containing genes by ERα, it can bind to and influence genes containing the thyroid hormone response element (TRE),[103–105] the TPA-RE[106,107] Sp1 sites,[108,109] and NF-κB sites.[110] Such events are enabled by protein–protein interactions,[111] and, as in the case of the TPA-RE, are markedly enhanced by the presence of estrogens[78] and the AP-1 complex components c-Fos/c-Jun.[107]

Although ER malfunction in tumours is chiefly manifest by the overexpression of ERα, it is currently unclear as to what degree ER subtypes and variants contribute to the overall cellular actions of estrogens on breast cancer cells, where they are certainly expressed in a proportion of breast tumours, albeit at lower levels than ERα.[112,113] Estrogens may thus induce a cocktail of active receptor forms, the balance of which, together with cofactor availability, determines the pattern of gene expression and thereby the biological responses experienced by breast cancer cells in response to these steroid hormones.

CROSSTALK BETWEEN ESTROGEN AND GROWTH FACTOR SIGNALLING PATHWAYS

As stated above, it is likely that ER signalling is central to mitogenesis in responsive breast cancers, with steroid hormone occupancy of the receptor efficiently driving cell growth and survival together with expression of target genes bearing either EREs or composite response elements that bind receptors in addition to other transcription factors. However, it is increasingly being proposed that such events proceed most efficiently in an appropriate growth factor environment, with steroid hormone and growth factor signalling pathways 'crosstalking' to reinforce each others' signalling.[3] While many of the relevant growth factors and their receptors are expressed by the breast cancer epithelial cells, thereby potentially working in an autocrine manner, additional paracrine factors may be liberated from the surrounding stroma. In each instance, several potential points of interaction between steroid hormone and growth factor signalling pathways have been identified.[3] A number of these are detailed below, and are illustrated in Figure 9.4.

The ER is a target for growth-factor-induced kinase activity (Figure 9.4: 1)

The activity of many transcription factors is regulated by phosphorylation and dephosphorylation, which involves various signal transduction pathways. Numerous studies have now shown that the ERα protein is subject to extensive phosphorylation and activation by several

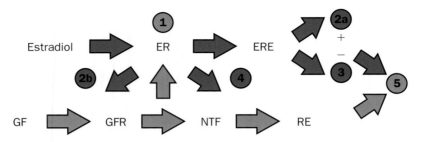

Figure 9.4 Points of crosstalk between ER and growth factor signalling pathways (ER, estrogen receptor; ERE, estrogen response element; GF, growth factor; GFR, growth factor receptor; NTF, nuclear transcription factor; RE, response element).

peptide growth factors – for example insulin-like growth factor I (IGF-I),[114] epidermal growth factor (EGF) and transforming growth factor α (TGF-α),[115] and heregulin[116] – events that can subsequently initiate ERE-mediated gene expression.[117,118] These events are believed to be effected by downstream signal transduction molecules such as mitogen-activated protein (MAP) kinase (MAPK), which, as stated previously, has been shown to activate ERα, possibly by a direct phosphorylation of serine 118 located in the A/B region of ERα (Figure 9.5).[25] Additional transduction molecules demonstrated to target the ERα to date include casein kinase II, pp90[rSk1], protein kinase Cδ (PKCδ), cyclin A/cdk2, Rho-pathway elements, and p60[c-Src].[83,100,119–123] Significantly, growth factors and downstream signal transduction pathways appear to differentially regulate the two transcriptional activator functions of ERα (i.e. AF-1 and AF-2), with the former being more responsive to EGF, TGF-α, and MAP kinase signalling.[115] While activation by these factors occurs most efficiently in the presence of estrogens, their promotion of AF-1 and AF-2 responses certainly appears adequate for initiating transcription in the absence of the steroid hormone. An increasing number of additional cell signalling pathways appear to also impact on the bioactivity of ERα, including the pineal hormone melatonin,[124] neurotransmitters such as dopamine,[125] and second messengers (includ-

ing cAMP).[126] An emerging concept for steroid hormone receptors is therefore that they not only function as direct transducers of steroid hormone effects but, as members of the cellular nuclear transcription factor pool, also serve as key points of convergence for multiple signal transduction pathways.[3]

Estrogens stimulate positive elements of growth factor signalling pathways (Figure 9.4: 2a, b)

Estrogen sensitivity and endocrine response have been extensively investigated in experimental models of human breast cancer both in vitro and in vivo. Based on these studies, it is becoming increasingly evident that estrogens can promote the autocrine expression of growth factor signalling pathway components (Figure 9.4: 2a), notably TGF-α,[94] IGF-II,[127] and growth factor receptors (e.g. the EGF receptor (EGFR)[128] and the insulin-like growth factor receptor (IGF-1R)[129] in estrogen-responsive (MCF-7 and T47-D) and estrogen-dependent (ZR-75-1) human breast cancer cell lines. In the latter instance, IGF-1R has also been shown to be activated by estrogen,[130,131] subsequently recruiting downstream signalling components, notably including insulin receptor substrate 1 (IRS-1),[130–132] which in turn may be estrogen-regulated.[133] Such actions, which are often

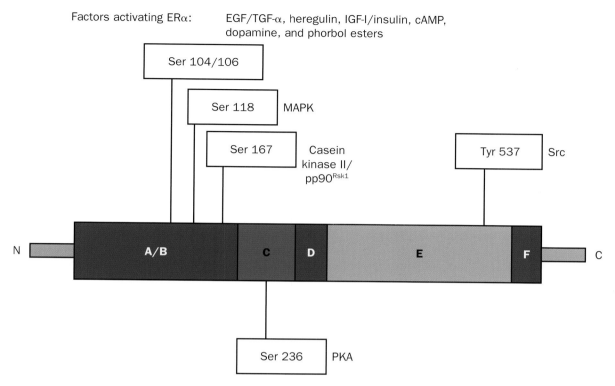

Figure 9.5 Phosphorylation sites on ERα (EGF, epidermal growth factor; TGF-α, transforming growth factor α; IGF-I, insulin-like growth factor I; MAPK, mitogen-activated protein kinase; PKA, protein kinase A).

antagonized by antiestrogens,[129,131] could significantly supplement the cellular growth responses directly primed by estrogens.[126] In addition, it appears that estrogens directly stimulate (while antiestrogens inhibit) the tyrosine kinase activities both of the EGFR-related protein c-ErbB2 (HER2/Neu)[134] and of c-Src,[135] the activation of which can provide important mitogenic signals to epithelial cells (Figure 9.4: 2b) through the recruitment of the p21[Ras]/Raf/MAP kinase pathway. Indeed, such estrogen-inducible functions, which occur through specific plasma membrane estrogen-binding proteins,[136] may provide an early mechanism for raising MAP kinase activity and hence ERα phosphorylation.

Commonly, the frequency with which a cell divides in vitro is dependent upon its adherence, increasing as cells spread out over the extracellular matrix. This may facilitate not only increased nutrient uptake, but also the ability of the cell to capture growth factors, this being particularly evident at focal adhesion contacts, which function as sites for priming of intracellular signals.[137] In this light, estrogens, in addition to stimulating growth factor signalling pathways directly, can promote cell/cell and cell/matrix adhesion,[138,139] thereby facilitating growth-factor-directed cell proliferation. Estrogens have thus been shown to induce the laminin receptor, together with various extracellular matrix components and cell membrane adhesion proteins[140] events that may be blocked by antiestrogens.[138] Indeed, the antiestrogen toremifene has been shown to inhibit the phorbol-ester-enhanced $\alpha_2\beta_1$-integrin-dependent adhesion of MCF-7 breast carcinoma cells.[141]

Estrogens inhibit negative elements of growth factor signalling pathways
(Figure 9.4: 3)

As well as the positive influences exerted by estrogens on growth factor signalling pathways detailed above, it is notable that in parallel they diminish (while antiestrogens induce) the expression of the growth-inhibitory factor TGF-β[142] in several estrogen-responsive human breast cancer cell lines. Estrogens thus serve to inhibit the expression of a factor that is implicated in the induction of programmed cell death[143] and that acts through the p38^{Jun} kinase (JNK) pathway.[144]

Additionally, however, it is of particular significance that estrogens have been reported to inhibit expression of tyrosine phosphatases in ERα-positive breast cancer cells to increase growth factor mitogenic activity, while both steroidal and non-steroidal antiestrogens increase phosphatase activity.[145,146] Tamoxifen, for example, inhibits the mitogenic activity of EGF by promoting significant dephosphorylation of EGFR, an effect believed to be ERα-mediated.[145,147] It appears that such EGFR dephosphorylation is accomplished via an increase in tyrosine phosphatase activity, as evidenced not only by an effective inhibition by sodium orthovanadate (a broad-spectrum phosphatase inhibitor), but also by a time- and dose-dependent increase in membrane phosphatase activity with the antiestrogen.[145] In this light, two tyrosine phosphatases have been identified that appear to be regulated by estrogens and antiestrogens: LAR and FAP-1 respectively.[146] Significantly, antisense inhibition of FAP-1 expression abolishes the antiestrogen-mediated inhibition of growth factor mitogenic activity, although the 'pure' antiestrogen fulvestrant (ICI 182,780, Faslodex) appears to retain inhibitory activity under these conditions, suggesting that the effects of this compound are FAP-1-independent.[146]

The ERα interacts with growth-factor-induced nuclear transcription factors
(Figure 9.4: 4)

An important feature of growth factor signalling is its potential to activate several profiles of nuclear transcription factors that subsequently serve to promote the expression of genes participating in a diversity of endpoints, including cell cycle progression. For example, in addition to its phosphorylation of the ERα protein, growth-factor-induced MAP kinase (Erk1/2) directly activates Elk-1/p62^{TCF}.[148] This latter transcription factor subsequently forms a ternary complex with p67^{SRF} (serum response factor) and primes c-Fos expression via the c-Fos serum response element.[148] Similarly, JNK (which is also a member of the MAP kinase family[149,150]) phosphorylates the c-Jun protein, which subsequently heterodimerizes with c-Fos.[151] The resultant complex, AP-1, is of central importance since it directly targets the TPA-RE, a sequence found in the promoters of many genes involved in a plethora of cellular endpoints, including proliferation and survival.[152]

In this light, it has been reported that estrogens can significantly enhance growth-factor-induced AP-1 activity in hormone-sensitive breast cancer cells.[153] This feature is believed to be a consequence of productive protein/protein interactions between the ER and the AP-1 complex[111] – a phenomenon also recently demonstrated to occur between ERα and the transcription factor Sp1.[108,154–156] Thus, ERα appears able to activate genes containing AP-1 sites in their promoters,[107] providing a mechanism whereby ERα signalling may be markedly diversified. In contrast to the above, ERα may repress the activity of the transcription factor NF-κB,[157] which regulates the expression of many cytokines (such as interleukin (IL)-6) and growth factors.[158] ERα-dependent inhibition of IL-6 again appears to be mediated via a direct protein–protein interaction with NF-κB.[110]

Finally, it should be remembered that ER/ERE-mediated gene transcription is also significantly enhanced by the recruitment of several co-activators and/or by overcoming the effects of co-repressor proteins[159] that may feasibly be regulated by growth factor signal transduction pathways.[98,160] Of particular interest is the co-activator CREB-binding protein (CBP)/p300, which is believed to be a component of multiple signalling pathways, including cAMP signal transduction.[98,160]

Steroid hormone and growth factor signalling pathways influence common growth-regulatory genes (Figure 9.4: 5)

In order for cells to proliferate, they initially need to be recruited into the cell cycle and then be induced to progress through it. These outcomes are orchestrated by at least two series of events that can be jointly influenced by steroid hormone and growth factor signalling pathways:[161,162] firstly, the induction of intermediate early response genes, such as c-Fos, c-Jun,[163,164] and c-Myc,[89] and, secondly, the regulation of G_1 cyclins (e.g. cyclin D1) and their partner kinases and inhibitors that are involved in restriction-point control.[161,165] Joint activation of these pathways by estrogens and growth factors would, at a minimum, reinforce mitogenic signals to responsive cells, and might even result in synergistic interactions between overlapping elements. Additionally, it is likely that steroid hormones[166] and many growth factors[167–169] influence the expression of cell survival factors in endocrine-responsive cells, such as the Bcl-2 protein.[169,170]

ESTROGEN WITHDRAWAL

Estrogen withdrawal from breast cancer cells in vivo relies either on the surgical or medical ablation of the bodily sources of estrogen (see Chapter 2) or on the inhibition of the enzymes that manufacture the steroid (see Chapters 6 and 13). As such, the procedures act to effectively lower the cellular levels of activated ERs and thereby block estrogen-induced tumour growth.[171–173] Thus, in simple terms, estrogen-induced displacement of heat-shock proteins from ERα, as well as ERα phosphorylation, dimerization, DNA-binding, and recruitment of cofactors, would be expected to be reduced in treated patients, as would synergistic interactions between the estrogen-occupied ER and growth factor signalling elements. Certainly, sequential therapies that progressively lower the tissue availability of estrogens, such as treatment of premenopausal women with the luteinizing hormone-releasing hormone (LHRH) agonist goserelin, followed by aromatase inhibitors, can promote sequential tumour remissions.[174]

Importantly, however, even the most effective estrogen-withdrawal procedures do not (i) fully obliterate all circulating estrogen levels, or in fact influence the tissue availablity of other estrogenic steroid hormones (e.g. androstenediol) or dietary or environmental estrogens, (ii) fully reduce the cellular levels of ERs, or (iii) fully block growth factor signalling. A degree of ER activity may therefore be maintained in treated patients, potentially leading to either residual tumour growth responses or the development of resistance to estrogen withdrawal (see Chapter 10). This appears to be achieved primarily through the A/B region of ERα and hence through the AF-1 transcription activator function. Indeed, several studies have suggested that the phosphorylation of serine 118 by growth-factor-induced MAP kinase activity plays a central role in ligand-independent activation of ERα,[115] where this can be achieved by multiple growth factors, including IGF-1, heregulin-β, and EGFR.[114–116] As stated previously, additional phosphorylation sites are also present on serines 104, 106, and 167, with the last of these being activated by EGF-induced pp90[Rsk1].[122] In resistant cells it appears that the EGFR, and possibly c-ErbB2, may be central to these events, since their expression is believed to be held under negative control in hormone sensitive tissues by estrogens and is then upregulated in the absence of the steroid.[175–177] Certainly, in model systems, resistant cells appear capable of producing several ligands for the EGFR and thus establishing an autocrine growth-regulatory loop to drive tumour cell growth.[178–180]

THE ERα PROTEIN AND ANTIESTROGENS

The most significant recent advance in the endocrine treatment of breast cancer has been the introduction of antiestrogens. An extensive range of antiestrogens have now been developed that selectively block the action of estrogens by competing for binding of the target receptor and hence can exert inhibitory effects on responsive breast cancers (see Chapters 3–5). Such compounds, which elicit an active inhibition of ERα AF-2 transactivation capacity, are thus mechanistically distinguishable from estrogen withdrawal, which, as stated above, leaves the native receptor intact within target cells.

In general terms, antiestrogens can be classified into two major groups: those that have mixed estrogenic/antiestrogenic actions (partial antiestrogens or selective ER modulators, SERMs), and those that have no estrogen-like properties (pure antiestrogens). Of this large number of compounds, only a few have been clinically tested, and only one, tamoxifen (ICI 46,474, Nolvadex), a partial antiestrogen, has achieved widespread therapeutic use, as a result of its relatively low toxicity and inhibitory properties.

SERMs (exemplified by tamoxifen)

Over two decades ago, it was demonstrated that tamoxifen could interact directly with the ER and prevent estradiol binding and hence any induced activity.[181–186] Following this discovery, it was proposed that tamoxifen might possess anti-tumour efficacy, and as such was shown to inhibit breast cancer growth by competitively blocking the ER and thereby inhibiting estrogen-induced tumour growth. Such studies have provided the foundation for a revolution in breast cancer therapy over the last twenty years. Thus, tamoxifen is the endocrine therapy of choice for all stages of breast cancer (see Chapter 3).

The early molecular effects of antiestrogens on the receptor are similar to those induced by estrogens (as discussed earlier in this chapter), including the binding to the HBD of the receptor in the nucleus, the dissociation of heat-shock proteins[187] and the induction of phosphorylation of ERα at serine residues in the A/B domain,[18] albeit inefficiently.[114,119] Indeed, tamoxifen seems to form a receptor complex that is converted into a fully active form,[66,188–194] although, as a result of anomalies in its tertiary structure, the tamoxifen–ERα complex is only partially active in initiating the program of events leading to gene activation.[23,195]

Tamoxifen effectively inhibits AF-2 activity.[196] However, since there is no parallel inhibition of AF-1 activity, this agent functions as a partial antagonist of ERα[24,52,197] since AF-1 has the potential to function in a constitutive manner once the receptor binds to the target response element.[52] Thus, in situations where AF-1 and AF-2 can function independently of one another, tamoxifen would be predicted to act as an antagonist on gene promoters where activity is reliant on AF-2, but as an agonist when AF-1 is the determining factor. Tamoxifen may also act as a mixed agonist/antagonist if both AF-1 and AF-2 contribute to transcriptional activity. Possible examples of this hypothesis have been demonstrated in MCF-7 cells, where May and Westley[198] have shown that the partial agonistic activity inherent in the drug can differentially stimulate transcription of the *pNR-2* and *pNR-1* genes to 10% and 80% of the estrogen-induced value respectively. Consequently, whilst some genes remain transcriptionally silent following the binding of the tamoxifen–ERα complex to the adjacent ERE, it would seem that the promoters of others are unable to discriminate between the estradiol–ERα complex and the dysfunctional tamoxifen–ERα complex. Presumably, the AF-1 activity alone is sufficient to generate a response in such cases. However, it is notable that different regions of AF-1 appear to be associated with antiestrogen activation of transcription compared with estrogens.[197] Further complexity is added by the observations that growth-factor-induced phosphorylation of ERα can amplify the agonistic activity of tamoxifen[199] and that the third activation domain within ERα may function when AF-1 and AF-2 are inactive.[58] Similarly, since ER-ERE interactions have been shown to be influenced by the presence of co-activators/co-repressors (as discussed earlier in this chapter), it is possible that the effectiveness of antiestrogens that retain partial agonist activity may also be under the control of the ratio of these factors (as discussed by Seery et al,[200] who also give additional references). Indeed, the agonistic activity of 4-hydroxytamoxifen in HepG2 cells is enhanced by the expression of the SRC-1 co-activator and inhibited by the overexpression of the SMRT co-processor protein,[102] with a similar pattern being observed in HeLa cells.

In contrast to its partial agonistic effects on ERα-mediated transactivation, tamoxifen fails to activate a basal promoter linked to EREs in Cos-1 cells in the presence of ERβ. This phenomenon is believed to be a result of ERα-like AF-1 function being absent in ERβ.[201] Antiestrogens, including tamoxifen, hence inhibit ERβ/estradiol-dependent transactivation efficiently.[201]

Since tamoxifen has the capability to act as a partial agonist, it is likely that the antitumour effects of this form of therapy are not currently maximized. Indeed, recently developed pure antagonists, such as fulvestrant that eliminate the activity of both AF-1 and AF-2 appear to exhibit a greater efficacy in controlling hormone-dependent breast cancer.

Pure antiestrogens (exemplified by fulvestrant)

Pure antiestrogens (see Chapter 5) have now been developed, including ICI 164,384[202,203] and the clinically applied fulvestrant.[204,205] These compounds have a greater inhibitory efficacy compared with tamoxifen, in that they do not induce any estrogen-like effects and also block completely all of the stimulatory actions of estrogens.[206] Such antiestrogens were structurally based on estradiol with a long lipophilic side-chain attached at the 7α position, following the identification by Burcourt and colleagues[207] that such side-chains in this position in estradiol retained high affinity for ERα. In vivo studies have since demonstrated the potential advantage of fulvestrant over tamoxifen in the treatment of breast cancer. Studies performed in vitro examining the growth characteristics of the estrogen-responsive human breast cancer cell line MCF-7 demonstrated that while pure antiestrogens and tamoxifen both arrest the cell cycle in early G_1 phase,[208,209] the pure antiestrogens ICI 164,384 and fulvestrant proved to be more effective in decreasing the proportion of actively growing cells in an asynchronous population.[171,209,210]

Additionally, several studies[211–214] have demonstrated that tamoxifen-resistant MCF-7 cells retain sensitivity to the growth-inhibitory action of the pure antiestrogens. The antitumour effect of pure antiestrogens has been studied extensively using parallel in vivo xenograft models of human breast cancer in athymic nude mice.[210,215–217] In all cases, treatment with ICI 164,384 or fulvestrant slowed the tumour growth rate and again proved to be effective in breast tumours with acquired resistance to tamoxifen, blocking any tamoxifen-stimulated tumour growth.[215,216] Preliminary clinical trials with fulvestrant seem to be consistent with the inhibitory effects predicted from the model studies, and therefore emphasize the potential of fulvestrant as a first-line treatment of breast cancer,[218–220] although clinical studies are ongoing (see Chapter 5).

Several earlier studies have indicated that some pure antiestrogens block dimerization of the receptor complexes, thereby preventing their binding to EREs,[202,221] as a direct consequence of steric hindrance of the 7α side-chain.[222] However, there have since been numerous reports[190,223,224] demonstrating that the anomalous pure antiestrogen–ERα complex can bind EREs, but the transcriptional unit remains inactive. Again, it is possible that co-activators or co-repressors may control the transcriptional activity of pure antiestrogen–ERα–ERE complexes. In this light, McDonnell and colleagues[159] have demonstrated that deletion of Ssn6 (a yeast ER co-repressor) confers agonist activity on ICI 164,384, suggesting that pure antiestrogenic activity is mediated at least in part by the interaction with co-repressor proteins.[225]

Pure antiestrogens, in common with tamoxifen, appear to effectively block AF-2-mediated activity,[192,193] and studies examining the effects of pure antiestrogens on transactivation, in cell-free systems, again indicate that they permit constitutive AF-1-mediated activity.[52] However, such an event is unlikely to occur both in vitro and in vivo, since these compounds are believed to induce a severely perturbed receptor conformation and furthermore enhance rapid receptor degradation.[52]

In this light, the cellular content of ERα protein is markedly reduced following treatment with fulvestrant – an event that is believed to occur via a marked reduction in the protein's half-life.[226] This effect has been observed in breast cancer cells in culture,[226–228] in mouse uterine tissue,[229] and in breast tumours in situ.[218] Indeed, it has been found that the half-life of the receptor protein is reduced from five hours in the presence of estrogen to around one hour in the presence of pure antiestrogens, resulting in a 90–95% decrease in ERα protein levels in the presence of such compounds.[224,226] In contrast, *ERα* mRNA levels appear to be unaltered by pure antiestrogens.[224,230,231] Pure antiestrogens appear to bind to newly formed ERα protein in the cytoplasm (where it is synthesized) and prevent its subsequent transportation to the nucleus.[232] This paralysed receptor is then destroyed rapidly, thus preventing any estrogen-regulated events occurring.[18] Additionally, such receptor downregulation would also serve to preclude growth-factor-induced activation of ERα signalling, and thus offers a potential therapeutic advantage over both estrogen withdrawal and tamoxifen therapy. Such an advantage, while readily evident in several experimental models of breast cancer,[227,228] is currently being tested in the clinical disease. This unique property of the pure antiestrogens in lowering ERα levels has resulted in fulvestrant being termed a selective ER downregulator (SERD).

Non-ER actions of antiestrogens

Although the molecular basis of the antiestrogenic action is primarily attributed to interaction with the ER, tamoxifen has shown direct inhibitory effects on other cellular components, which may influence their biological profile in both ER-positive and ER-negative cells. As yet, comparable studies have not been performed for other antiestrogens, and thus the generality of their significance cannot be assessed.

There are several possible mechanisms by which non-ER-mediated antagonistic and agonistic activities of tamoxifen could occur, depending upon the concentration used, duration of exposure and target cell/tissue type. For example, tamoxifen inhibits calmodulin activation of cAMP-dependent phosphodiesterase, a key element in the regulation of the cellular levels of cAMP;[233] it elevates levels of the immunosuppressive cytokine TGF-β1, a molecule that, although often inhibitory to the growth of epithelial cells, is protective against bone loss.[234,235] Tamoxifen furthermore binds to a type II antiestrogen binding site, potentially elevating the cellular concentrations of the drug and its metabolites.[236] Of further interest is its general inhibition of PKC activity,[237,238] although the PKCε isoform appears to be activated by the antiestrogen.[239] Effects on signalling molecules such as cAMP and PKC could certainly be envisaged as having wider implications within ER-positive cells, given their potential involvement in receptor phosphorylation.

SUMMARY

Cellular signalling originating from estrogens is far from simplistic, with an elaborate molecular and protein biology and a diverse regulation encompassing a network of phosphorylation cascades.[3] Estrogens do, however, appear to exert many of their known activities through the ER, which, within the appropriate cellular context, can promote both cell proliferation and survival. Reversal of these endpoints with anti-hormonal drugs appears sufficient in some tumours to bring about long-lasting tumour remissions.

From the increasing complexity of ER signalling there arise not only the possibility of additional targeting of ER-related pathways to promote better and longer-lasting therapeutic responses and hence survival benefits, but also explanations as to why there are certain patients who, although expressing ERs, appear unable to use these proteins in a dominant fashion for growth and in whom reversal of such events may regenerate endocrine response (see Chapters 10 and 12). Future strategies to exploit this information (see Chapter 15) will hopefully continue to reduce breast cancer mortality rates.

REFERENCES

1. Jensen EV, Jacobson HI. Fate of steroidal estrogens in target tissues. In: *Biological Activities of Steroids in Relation to Cancers* (Pincus G, Voilmer EP, eds). New York: Academic Press, 1960: 161–74.

2. Nicholson RI, McClelland RA, Gee JM. Steroid hormone receptors and their clinical significance in cancer. *J Clin Pathol* 1995; **48**: 890–5.

3. Nicholson RI, Gee JM. Oestrogen and growth factor cross-talk and endocrine insensitivity and acquired resistance in breast cancer. *Br J Cancer* 2000; **82**: 501–13.

4. Green S, Walter P, Kumar V et al. Human oestrogen receptor cDNA sequence, expression and homology to *v-erb*A. *Nature* 1986; **320**: 134–9.

5. Greene GL, Gilna P, Waterfield M et al. Sequence and expression of human estrogen receptor complementary DNA. *Science* 1986; **231**: 1150–4.

6. Gosden JR, Middleton PG, Rout D. Localization of the human oestrogen receptor gene to chromosome 6q24–q27 by in situ hybridisation. *Cytogenet Cell Genet* 1986; **43**: 218–20.

7. Ponglikitmongkol M, Green S, Chambon P. Genomic organisation for the human oestrogen receptor gene. *EMBO J* 1988; **7**: 3385–8.

8. Simerly RB, Chang C, Muramatsu M, Swanson LW. Distribution of androgen receptor mRNA-containing cells in the rat brain: an in situ hybridization study. *J Comp Neurol* 1990; **294**: 76–95.

9. Weigel NL. Steroid hormone receptors and their regulation by phosphorylation. *Biochem J* 1996; **319**: 657–67.

10. Diab SG, Castles CG, Fuqua SAW. Role of altered estrogen receptors in breast cancer. In: *Hormones and Cancer* (Vedeckis WV, ed). Boston: Birkhäuser, 1996: 261–81.

11. Arnold SF, Vorojeikina DP, Notides AC. Phosphorylation of tyrosine 537 on the human estrogen receptor is required for binding to an estrogen response element. *J Biol Chem* 1995; **270**: 30205–12.

12. Arnold SF, Obourn JD, Jaffe H, Notides AC. Phosphorylation of the human estrogen receptor on tyrosine 537 in vivo and by src family tyrosine kinases in vitro. *Mol Endocrinol* 1995; **9**: 24–33.

13. Arnold SF, Melamed M, Vorojeikina DP et al. Estradiol-binding mechanism and binding capacity of the human estrogen receptor is regulated by tyrosine phosphorylation. *Mol Endocrinol* 1997; **11**: 48–53.

14. Ferguson AT, Lapidus RG, Davidson NE. The regulation of estrogen receptor expression and function in human breast cancer. In: *Biological and Hormonal Therapies of Cancer* (Foon KA, Muss HB, eds). Boston: Kluwer, 1998: 255–85.

15. Keaveney M, Klug J, Dawson M et al. Evidence of a previously unidentified upstream exon in the human oestrogen receptor gene. *J Mol Endocrinol* 1991; **6**: 111–15.

16. deConinck EC, McPherson LA, Weigel RJ. Transcriptional regulation of estrogen-receptor in breast carcinomas. *Mol Cell Biol* 1995; **15**: 2191–6.

17. Gee JM, Robertson JF, Ellis IO et al. Immunocytochemical analysis reveals a tumour suppressor-like role for transcription factor AP-2 in invasive breast cancer. *J Pathol* 1999; **189**: 514–20.

18. MacGregor JI, Jordan VC. Basic guide to the

mechanisms of antiestrogen action. *Pharmacol Rev* 1998; **50**: 151–96.

19. McPherson LA, Baichwal VR, Weigel RJ. Identification of ERF-1 as a member of the AP2 transcription factor family. *Proc Natl Acad Sci USA* 1997; **94**: 4342–7.

20. Tang Z, Treilleux I, Brown M. A transcriptional enhancer required for the differential expression of the human estrogen receptor in breast cancers. *Mol Cell Biol* 1997; **17**: 1274–80.

21. Kumar V, Green S, Staub A, Chambon P. Localisation of the oestradiol-binding and putative DNA-binding domains of the human oestrogen receptor. *EMBO J* 1986; **5**: 2231–6.

22. Kumar V, Green S, Stack G et al. Functional domains of the human estrogen receptor. *Cell* 1987; **51**: 941–51.

23. Metzger D, White JH, Chambon P. The human oestrogen receptor functions in yeast. *Nature* 1988; **334**: 31–6.

24. Tora L, White J, Brou C et al. The human estrogen receptor has two independent nonacidic transcriptional activation functions. *Cell* 1989; **59**: 477–87.

25. Kato S, Endoh H, Masuhiro Y et al. Activation of the estrogen receptor through phosphorylation by mitogen-activated protein kinase. *Science* 1995; **270**: 1491–4.

26. Green S, Kumar V, Theulaz I et al. The N-terminal DNA-binding 'zinc finger' of the oestrogen and glucocorticoid receptors determines target gene specificity. *EMBO J* 1988; **7**: 3037–44.

27. Castles CG, Fuqua SAW. Alterations within the estrogen receptor in breast cancer. In: *Hormone Dependent Cancer* (Pasqualini JR, Katzenellenbogen BS, eds). New York: Marcel Dekker, 1996: 81–108.

28. Leng X, Tsai SY, Tsai M-J. The nuclear hormone receptor superfamily: structure and function. In: *Hormones and Cancer* (Vedeckis WV, ed). Boston: Birkhäuser, 1996: 91–126.

29. Jeltsch JM, Krozowski Z, Quirin-Stricker C et al. Cloning of the chicken progesterone receptor. *Proc Natl Acad Sci USA* 1986; **83**: 5424–8.

30. Freedman LP, Luisi BF, Korszun ZR et al. The function and structure of the metal co-ordination sites within the glucocorticoid receptor DNA binding domain. *Nature* 1988; **334**: 543–6.

31. Green S, Chambon P. Oestradiol induction of a glucocorticoid-responsive gene by a chimaeric receptor. *Nature* 1987; **325**: 75–8.

32. Danielsen M, Hinck L, Ringold GM. Two amino acids within the knuckle of the first zinc finger specify DNA response element activation by the glucocorticoid receptor. *Cell* 1989; **57**: 1131–8.

33. Mader S, Kumar V, deVerneuil H, Chambon P. Three amino acids of the oestrogen receptor are essential to its ability to distinguish an oestrogen from a glucocorticoid-responsive element. *Nature* 1989; **338**: 271–4.

34. Umesono K, Evans RM. Determinants of target gene specificity for steroid/thyroid hormone receptors. *Cell* 1989; **57**: 1139–46.

35. Schwabe JWR, Neuhaus D, Rhodes D. Solution structure of the DNA-binding domain of the oestrogen receptor. *Nature* 1990; **340**: 458–61.

36. Schwabe JWR, Chapman L, Finch JT, Rhodes D. The crystal structure of the complex between the oestrogen receptor DNA-binding domain and DNA at 24A: how receptors discriminate between their response elements. *Cell* 1993; **75**: 567–78.

37. Kumar V, Chambon P. The estrogen receptor binds tightly to its responsive element as a ligand-induced homodimer. *Cell* 1988; **55**: 145–56.

38. Auchus RJ, Fuqua S. The oestrogen receptor. *Baillière's Clin Endocrinol Metab* 1994; **8**: 433–49.

39. Picard D, Yamamoto KR. Two signals mediate hormone-dependent nuclear-localization of the glucocorticoid receptor. *EMBO J* 1987; **6**: 3333–40.

40. Guiochon-Mantel A, Loosfelt H, Lescop P et al. Mechanisms of nuclear localization of the progesterone receptor: evidence for interaction between monomers. *Cell* 1989; **57**: 1147–54.

41. Picard D, Kumar V, Chambon P, Yamamoto KR. Signal transduction by steroid hormones: nuclear localization is differentially regulated in estrogen and glucocorticoid receptors. *Cell Regul* 1990; **1**: 291–9.

42. Dingwall C, Laskey RA. Nuclear targeting sequences – a consensus? *Trends Biochem Sci* 1991; **6**: 478–81.

43. Harlow KW, Smith DN, Katzenellenbogen JA et al. Identification of cysteine 530 as the covalent attachment site of an affinity-labeling estrogen (ketononestrol aziridine) and antiestrogen (tamoxifen aziridine) in the human estrogen receptor. *J Biol Chem* 1989; **164**: 17476–85.

44. Ratajczak T, Wilkinson SP, Brockway MJ et al. The interaction site for tamoxifen aziridine with the bovine estrogen receptor. *J Biol Chem* 1989; **264**: 13453–9.

45. Katzenellenbogen BS, Elliston JF, Monsma FJ et al. Structural analysis of covalently labeled estrogen receptors by limited proteolysis and monoclonal antibody reactivity. *Biochemistry* 1987; **26:** 2364–73.

46. Landschulz WH, Johnson PF, McKnight SL. The leucine zipper: a hypothetical structure common to a new class of DNA binding proteins. *Science* 1988; **240:** 1759–64.

47. Salomonsson M, Haggblad J, O'Malley BW, Sitbon GM. The human estrogen receptor hormone binding domain dimerizes independently of ligand activation. *J Steroid Biochem* 1994; **48:** 447–52.

48. Lees JA, Fawell SE, White R, Parker MG. A 22-amino-acid peptide restores the DNA-binding activity to dimerization-defective mutants of the estrogen receptor. *Mol Cell Biol* 1990; **10:** 5529–31.

49. Fawell SE, Lees JA, White R, Parker MG. Characterization and colocalization of steroid binding and dimerization activities in the mouse estrogen receptor. *Cell* 1990; **60:** 956–62.

50. White R, Fawell SE, Parker MG. Analysis of oestrogen receptor dimerization using chimeric proteins. *J Steroid Biochem Mol Biol* 1991; **40:** 333–41.

51. Webster NJG, Green S, Jin JR, Chambon P. The hormone binding domains of the estrogen and glucocorticoid receptors contain an inducible transcription activation function. *Cell* 1988; **54:** 199–207.

52. Berry M, Metzger D, Chambon P. Role of the two activating domains of the oestrogen receptor in the cell-type and promoter-context dependent agonistic activity of the anti-oestrogen 4-hydroxytamoxifen. *EMBO J* 1990; **9:** 2811–18.

53. Webster NJG, Green S, Tasset D et al. The transcription activation function located in the hormone-binding domain of the human oestrogen receptor is not encoded by a single exon. *EMBO J* 1989; **8:** 1441–6.

54. Danielian PS, White R, Lees JA, Parker MG. Identification of a conserved region required for hormone dependent transcriptional activation by steroid hormone receptors. *EMBO J* 1992; **11:** 1025–33.

55. Halachmi S, Marden E, Martin G et al. Estrogen receptor-associated proteins: possible mediators of hormone-induced transcription. *Science* 1994; **264:** 1455–8.

56. Cavailles V, Dauvois S, Danielian PS, Parker MG. Interaction of proteins with transcriptionally active estrogen receptors. *Proc Natl Acad Sci USA* 1994; **91:** 10009–13.

57. Pierrat B, Heery DM, Chambon P, Losson R. A highly conserved region in the hormone binding domain of the human estrogen receptor functions as an efficient transactivation domain in yeast. *Gene* 1994; **143:** 193–200.

58. Norris JD, Fan D, Kerner SA, McDonnell DP. Identification of a third autonomous activation domain within the human estrogen receptor. *Mol Endocrinol* 1997; **11:** 747–54.

59. Chambraud B, Berry M, Redeuilh G et al. Several regions of human estrogen receptor are involved in the formation of receptor-heat shock protein 90 complexes. *J Biol Chem* 1990; **265:** 20686–91.

60. Baulieu E-E. Steroid hormone antagonists at the receptor level: a role for the heat shock protein MW 90 000 (hsp90). *J Cell Biochem* 1987; **35:** 161–74.

61. Montano MM, Muller V, Trobaugh A, Katzenellenbogen BS. The carboxy-terminal F domain of the human estrogen receptor: role in the transcriptional activity of the receptor and the effectiveness of antiestrogens as estrogen antagonists. *Mol Endocrinol* 1995; **9:** 814–25.

62. Fuqua SAW, Fitzgerald SD, Chamness GC et al. Variant human breast tumor estrogen receptor with constitutive transcriptional activity. *Cancer Res* 1991; **51:** 1105–9.

63. Castles CG, Fuqua SA, Klotz DM, Hill SM. Expression of a constitutively active estrogen receptor variant in the estrogen receptor-negative BT-20 human breast cancer cell line. *Cancer Res* 1993; **53:** 5934–9.

64. Klotz DM, Castles CG, Hill SM. Variant ER mRNAs are expressed in the MDA-MB-330 and other human breast tumor cell lines. In: *Proceedings of the 75th Annual Meeting of the Endocrine Society, Las Vegas, NV,* 1993: 515.

65. Zhang Q-X, Borg A, Fuqua SAW. An exon 5 deletion variant of the estrogen receptor frequently coexpressed with wild-type estrogen receptor in human breast cancer. *Cancer Res* 1993; **53:** 5882–4.

66. Tzukerman MT, Esty A, Santisomere D et al. Human estrogen receptor transactivational capacity is determined by both cellular and promoter context and mediated by two functionally distinct intramolecular regions. *Mol Endocrinol* 1994; **8:** 21–30.

67. Fuqua SAW, Wiltschke C, Castles C et al. A role for estrogen receptor variants in endocrine resistance. *Endocr Rel Cancer* 1995; **2:** 19–25.

68. Wang Y, Miksicek RJ. Identification of a dominant negative form of the human estrogen receptor. *Mol Endocrinol* 1991; **5:** 1707–15.

69. Fuqua SA, Fitzgerald SD, Allred DC et al. Inhibition of estrogen receptor action by naturally occurring variant in human breast tumors. *Cancer Res* 1992; **52:** 483–6.

70. Miksicek RJ, Lei Y, Wang Y. Exon skipping gives rise to alternatively spliced forms of the estrogen receptor in breast tumour cells. *Breast Cancer Res Treat* 1993; **26:** 163–74.

71. Kuiper GG, Enmark E, Pelto-Huikko M et al. Cloning of a novel estrogen receptor expressed in rat prostate and ovary. *Proc Natl Acad Sci USA* 1996; **93:** 5925–30.

72. Mosselman S, Polman J, Dijkema R. ERβ: identification and characterization of a novel human estrogen receptor. *FEBS Lett* 1996; **392:** 49–53.

73. Kuiper GG, Carlsson B, Grandien K et al. Comparison of the ligand binding specificity and transcript tissue distribution of estrogen receptors α and β. *Endocrinology* 1997; **138:** 863–70.

74. Lubahn DB, Moyer JS, Golding TS et al. Alteration of reproductive function but not prenatal sexual development after insertional disruption of the mouse estrogen receptor gene. *Proc Natl Acad Sci USA* 1993; **90:** 11162–6.

75. Krege JH, Hodgin JB, Couse JF et al. Generation and reproductive phenotypes of mice lacking estrogen receptor beta. *Proc Natl Acad Sci USA* 1998; **95:** 15677–82.

76. Enmark E, Pelto-Huikko M, Grandien K et al. Human estrogen receptor β-gene structure, chromosomal localization, and expression pattern. *J Clin Endocrinol Metab* 1997; **82:** 4258–65.

77. Pettersson K, Grandien K, Kuiper GG. Gustafsson JA. Mouse estrogen receptor beta forms estrogen response element-binding heterodimers with estrogen receptor alpha. *Mol Endocrinol* 1997; **11:** 1486–96.

78. Paech K, Webb P, Kuiper GG et al. Differential ligand activation of estrogen receptors ERα and ERβ at AP1 sites. *Science* 1997; **277:** 1508–10.

79. Vladusic EA, Hornby AE, Guerra-Vladusic FK, Lupu R. Expression of estrogen receptor β messenger RNA variant in breast cancer. *Science* 1997; **277:** 1508–10.

80. Segnitz B, Gehring U. Subunit structure of the nonactivated human estrogen receptor. *Proc Natl Acad Sci USA* 1995; **92:** 2179–83.

81. King WJ, Greene GL. Monoclonal antibodies localize oestrogen receptor in the nuclei of target cells. *Nature* 1984; **307:** 745–7.

82. Rao GS. Mode of entry of steroid and thyroid hormones into cell. *Mol Cell Endocrinol* 1981; **21:** 97–108.

83. Le Goff P, Montano MM, Scodin DJ, Katzenellenbogen BS. Phosphorylation of the human estrogen receptor. Identification of hormone-regulated sites and examination of their influence on transcriptional activity. *J Biol Chem* 1994; **269:** 4458–66.

84. Kraus WL, McInerney EM, Katzenellenbogen BS. Ligand-dependent, transcriptionally productive association of the amino- and carboxyl-terminal regions of a steroid hormone nuclear receptor. *Proc Natl Acad Sci USA* 1995; **92:** 12314–18.

85. Cheskis BJ, Karathanasis S, Lyttle CR. Estrogen receptor ligands modulate its interaction with DNA. *J Biol Chem* 1997; **272:** 11384–91.

86. Read LD, Snider CE, Miller JS et al. Ligand-modulated regulation of progesterone receptor messenger ribonucleic acid and protein in human breast cancer cell lines. *Mol Endocrinol* 1988; **2:** 263–71.

87. Jakowlev SB, Breathnach R, Jeltsch JM et al. Sequence of pS2 mRNA induced by estrogen in the human breast cancer cell line, MCF-7. *Nucleic Acids Res* **12:** 2861–78.

88. Manning DL, Robertson JF, Ellis IO et al. Oestrogen regulated genes in breast cancer: association of pLIV1 with lymph node involvement. *Eur J Cancer* 1994; **30A:** 675–8.

89. Dubik D, Shui RPC. Transcriptional regulation of c-myc oncogene expression by estrogen in hormone responsive human breast cancer cells. *J Biol Chem* 1988; **263:** 12705–8.

90. Musgrove EA, Sutherland RL. Cell cycle control by steroid hormones. *Semin Cancer Biol* 1994; **5:** 381–9.

91. Sutherland RL, Hamilton JA, Sweeney KJ et al. Steroidal regulation of cell cycle progression. *Ciba Found Symp* 1995; **191:** 218–34.

92. Gee JM, Robertson JF, Ellis IO et al. Immunocytochemical localization of BCL-2 protein in human breast cancers and its relationship to a series of prognostic markers and response to endocrine therapy. *Int J Cancer* 1994; **59:** 619–28.

93. Leung LK, Wang TT. Paradoxical regulation of Bcl-2 family proteins by 17β-oestradiol in human breast cancer cells MCF-7. *Br J Cancer* 1999; **81**: 387–92.

94. Bates SE, Davidson NE, Valverius EM et al. Expression of transforming growth factor α and its messenger ribonucleic acid in human breast cancer: its regulation by estrogen and its possible functional significance. *Mol Endocrinol* 1988; **2**: 543–55.

95. Swiatecka J, Dzieciol J, Anchim T et al. Influence of estrogen, antiestrogen and UV-light on the balance between proliferation and apoptosis in MCF-7 breast adenocarcinoma cells culture. *Neoplasma* 2000; **47**: 15–24.

96. Baniahmad C, Nawaz Z, Baniahmad A et al. Enhancement of human estrogen receptor activity by SPT6: a potential coactivator. *Mol Endocrinol* 1995; **9**: 34–43.

97. Onate SA, Tsai SY, Tsai M-J, O'Malley BW. Sequence and characterization of a coactivator for the steroid hormone receptor superfamily. *Science* 1995; **270**: 1354–7.

98. Smith CL, Onate SA, Tsai MJ, O'Malley BW. CREB binding acts synergistically with steroid receptor coactivator-1 to enhance steroid receptor-dependent transcription. *Proc Natl Acad Sci USA* 1996; **93**: 8884–8.

99. Kamei Y, Heinzel T, Torchia J et al. A CBP integrator complex mediates transcriptional activation and AP-1 inhibition by nuclear receptors. *Cell* 1996; **85**: 403–14.

100. Zwijsen RM, Buckle RS, Hijmans EM et al. Ligand-independent recruitment of steroid receptor coactivators to estrogen receptor by cyclin D1. *Genes Dev* 1998: 3488–98.

101. Rubino D, Driggers P, Arbit D et al. Characterisation of Brx, a novel Dbl family member that modulates estrogen receptor action. *Oncogene* 1998; **16**: 2513–26.

102. Smith CL, Nawaz Z, O'Malley BW. Coactivator and corepressor of the agonist/antagonist activity of the mixed antiestrogen, 4-hydroxytamoxifen. *Mol Endocrinol* 1997; **11**: 657–66.

103. Graupner G, Zhang XK, Tzukerman M et al. Thyroid hormone receptors repress estrogen receptor activation of a TRE. *Mol Endocrinol* 1991; **5**: 365-72.

104. Zhang XK, Wills KN, Graupner G et al. Ligand binding domain of thyroid hormone receptors modulates DNA binding and determines their bifunctional roles. *New Biol* 1991; **3**: 169–81.

105. Yarwood NJ, Gurr JA, Sheppard MC, Franklyn JA. Estradiol modulates thyroid hormone regulation of the human glycoprotein hormone alpha subunit gene. *J Biol Chem* 1993; **268**: 21984–9.

106. Schuermann M, Hennig G, Muller R. Transcriptional activation and transformation by chimaeric Fos–estrogen receptor protein: altered properties as a consequence of gene fusion. *Oncogene* 1993; **8**: 2781–90.

107. Webb P, Lopez GN, Uht RM, Kushner PJ. Tamoxifen activation of the estrogen receptor/AP-1 pathway: potential origin for the cell-specific estrogen-like effects of antiestrogens. *Mol Endocrinol* 1995; **9**: 443–56.

108. Porter W, Wang F, Wang W et al. Role of estrogen receptor/Sp1 complexes in estrogen-induced shock protein 27 gene expression. *Mol Endocrinol* 1996; **10**: 1371–8.

109. Scholz A, Truss M, Beato M. Hormone-induced recruitment of Sp1 mediates estrogen activation of the rabbit uteroglobin gene in endometrial epithelium. *J Biol Chem* 1998; **278**: 4360–6.

110. Ray P, Ghosh SK, Zhang DH, Ray A. Repression of interleukin-6 gene expression by 17β-estradiol: inhibition of the DNA-binding activity of the transcription factors NF-IL6 and NF-κB by the estrogen receptor. *FEBS Lett* 1997; **409**: 79–85.

111. Rochefort H. Oestrogen- and anti-oestrogen-regulated genes in human breast cancer. *Ciba Found Symp* 1995; **191**: 254–65.

112. Desai AJ, Luqmani YA, Walters JE et al. Presence of exon 5-deleted oestrogen receptor in human breast cancer: functional analysis and clinical significance. *Br J Cancer* 1997; **75**: 1173–84.

113. Balleine RL, Hunt SM, Clarke CL. Coexpression of alternatively spliced estrogen and progesterone receptor transcripts in human breast cancer. *J Clin Endocrinol Metab* 1999; **84**: 1370–7.

114. Aronica SM, Katzenellenbogen BS. Stimulation of estrogen receptor-mediated transcription and alteration in the phosphorylation state of the rat uterine estrogen receptor by estrogen, cyclic adenosine monophosphate, and insulin-like growth factor-I. *Mol Endocrinol* 1993; **7**: 743–52.

115. Bunone G, Briand PA, Miksicek RJ, Picard D. Activation of the unliganded estrogen receptor by EGF involves the MAP kinase pathway and direct phosphorylation. *EMBO J* 1996; **15**: 2174–83.

116. Pietras RJ, Arboleda J, Reese DM et al. HER-2 tyrosine kinase pathway targets estrogen receptor and promotes hormone-independent growth in human breast cancer cells. *Oncogene* 1995; **10:** 2435–46.

117. Ignar-Trowbridge DM, Pimentel M, Parker MG et al. Peptide growth factor cross-talk with the estrogen receptor requires the A/B domain and occurs independently of protein kinase C or estradiol. *Endocrinology* 1996; **137:** 1735–44.

118. Lee AV, Weng CN, Jackson JG, Yee D. Activation of estrogen receptor-mediated gene transcription by IGF-I in human breast cancer cells. *J Endocrinol* 1997; **152:** 39–47.

119. Ali S, Metzger D, Bornert JM, Chambon P. Modulation of transcriptional activation by lig- and-dependent phosphorylation of the human oestrogen receptor A/B region. *EMBO J* 1993; **12:** 1153–60.

120. Arnold SF, Obourn JD, Jaffe H, Notides AC. Serine 167 is the major estradiol-induced phosphorylation site on the human estrogen receptor. *Mol Endocrinol* 1994; **8:** 1208–14.

121. Trowbridge JM, Rogatsky I, Garabedian MJ. Regulation of estrogen receptor transcriptional enhancement by the cyclin A/Cdk2 complex. *Proc Natl Acad Sci USA* 1997; **94:** 10132–7.

122. Joel PB, Smith J, Sturgill TW et al. pp90rsk1 regulates estrogen receptor-mediated transcription through phosphorylation of Ser-167. *Mol Cell Biol* 1998; **18:** 1978–84.

123. Lahooti H, Thorsen T, Aakvaag A. Modulation of mouse estrogen receptor transcription activity by protein kinase Cδ. *J Mol Endocrinol* 1998; **20:** 245–59.

124. Ram PT, Kiefer T, Silverman M et al. Estrogen receptor transactivation in MCF-7 breast cancer cells by melatonin and growth factors. *Mol Cell Endocrinol* 1998; **141:** 53–64.

125. Gangolli EA, Conneely OM, O'Malley BW. Neurotransmitters activate the human estrogen receptor in a neuroblastoma cell line. *J Steroid Biochem Mol Biol* 1997; **61:** 1–9.

126. Cho H, Katzenellenbogen BS. Synergistic activation of estrogen receptor-mediated transcription by estradiol and protein kinase activators. *Mol Endocrinol* 1993; **7:** 441–52.

127. Brunner N, Yee D, Kern FG et al. Effect of endocrine therapy on growth of T61 human breast cancer xenografts is directly correlated to a specific down-regulation of insulin-like growth factor II (IGF-II). *Eur J Cancer* 1993; **29A:** 562–9.

128. Berthois Y, Dong XF, Martin PM. Regulation of epidermal growth factor receptor by oestrogen and antioestrogen in the human breast cancer cell line MCF-7. *Biochem Biophys Res Commun* 1989; **159:** 126–31.

129. Freiss G, Prebois C, Rochefort H, Vignon F. Anti-steroidal and anti-growth factor activities of anti-oestrogens. *J Steroid Biochem Mol Biol* 1990; **37:** 777–81.

130. Richards RG, DiAugustine RP, Petrusz P et al. Estradiol stimulates tyrosine phosphorylation of the insulin-like growth factor-1 receptor and insulin receptor substrate-1 in the uterus. *Proc Natl Acad Sci USA* 1996; **93:** 12002–7.

131. Guvakova MA, Surmacz E. Tamoxifen interferes with the insulin-like growth factor I receptor (IGF-IR) signaling pathway in breast cancer cells. *Cancer Res* 1997; **57:** 2606–10.

132. Molloy CA, May FE, Westley BR. Insulin receptor substrate-1 expression is regulated by estrogen in the MCF-7 human breast cancer cell line. *J Biol Chem* 2000; **275:** 12565–71.

133. Westley BR, Clayton SJ, Daws MR et al. Interactions between the oestrogen and insulin-like growth factor signalling pathways in the control of breast epithelial cell proliferation. *Biochem Soc Symp* 1998; **63:** 35–44.

134. Matsuda S, Kadowaki Y, Ichino M et al. 17β-Estradiol mimics ligand activity of the c-erbB2 protooncogene product. *Proc Natl Acad Sci USA* 1993; **90:** 10803–7.

135. Migliaccio A, Pagano M, Auricchio F. Immediate and transient stimulation of protein tyrosine phosphorylation by estradiol in MCF-7 cells. *Oncogene* 1993; **8:** 2183–91.

136. Russell KS, Haynes MP, Sinha D et al. Human vascular endothelial cells contain membrane binding sites for estradiol, which mediate rapid intracellular signaling. *Proc Natl Acad Sci USA* 2000; **97:** 5930–5.

137. Weisberg E, Sattler M, Ewaniuk DS, Salgia R. Role of focal adhesion proteins in signal transduction and oncogenesis. *Crit Rev Oncog* 1997; **8:** 343–58.

138. Millon R, Nicora F, Muller D et al. Modulation of human breast cancer cell adhesion by estrogens and antiestrogens. *Clin Exp Metastasis* 1989; **7:** 405–15.

139. DePasquale JA. Cell matrix adhesions and localization of the vitronectin receptor in MCF-7 human mammary carcinoma cells. *Histochem Cell Biol* 1998; **110:** 485–94.

140. Castronovo V, Taraboletti G, Liotta LA, Sobel ME. Modulation of laminin receptor expression by estrogen and progestins in human breast cancer cell lines. *J Natl Cancer Inst* 1989; **81**: 781–8.

141. Maemura M, Akiyama SK, Woods VL Jr, Dickson RB. Expression and ligand binding of $\alpha_2\beta_1$ integrin on breast carcinoma cells. *Clin Exp Metastasis* 1995; **13**: 223–35.

142. Knabbe C, Lippman ME, Wakefield LM et al. Evidence that transforming growth factor-β is a hormonally regulated negative growth factor in human breast cancer cells. *Cell* 1987; **48**: 417–28.

143. Perry RR, Kang Y, Greaves BR. Relationship between tamoxifen-induced transforming growth factor β1 expression, cytostasis and apoptosis in human breast cancer cells. *Br J Cancer* 1995; **72**: 1441–6.

144. Hill CS. Signalling to the nucleus by members of the transforming growth factor-β (TGF-β) superfamily. *Cell Signal* 1996; **8**: 533–44.

145. Freiss G, Vignon F. Antiestrogens increase protein tyrosine phosphatase activity in human breast cancer cells. *Mol Endocrinol* 1994; **8**: 1389–96.

146. Freiss G, Puech C, Vignon F. Extinction of insulin-like growth factor-I mitogenic signaling by antiestrogen-stimulated Fas-associated protein tyrosine phosphatase-1 in human breast cancer cells. *Mol Endocrinol* 1998; **12**: 568–79.

147. Freiss G, Rochefort H, Vignon F. Mechanisms of 4-hydroxytamoxifen anti-growth factor activity in breast cancer cells: alterations of growth factor receptor binding sites and tyrosine kinase activity. *Biochem Biophys Res Commun* 1990; **173**: 919–26.

148. Gille H, Kortenjann M, Thomae O et al. ERK phosphorylation potentiates Elk-1-mediated ternary complex formation and transactivation. *EMBO J* 1995; **14**: 951–62.

149. Paul A, Wilson S, Belham CM et al. Stress-activated protein kinases: activation, regulation and function. *Cell Signal* 1997; **9**: 403–10.

150. Lewis TS, Shapiro PS, Ahn NG. Signal transduction through MAP kinase cascades. *Adv Cancer Res* 1998; **74**: 49–139.

151. Minden A, Lin A, Smeal T et al. c-Jun N-terminal phosphorylation correlates with activation of the JNK subgroup but not the ERK subgroup of mitogen-activated protein kinases. *Mol Cell Biol* 1994; **14**: 6683–8.

152. Pfahl M. Nuclear receptor/AP-1 interaction. *Endocr Rev* 1993; **14**: 651–8.

153. Philips A, Chalbos D, Rochefort H. Estradiol increases and anti-estrogens antagonize the growth factor-induced activator protein-1 activity in MCF7 breast cancer cells without affecting c-fos and c-jun synthesis. *J Biol Chem* 1993; **268**: 14103–8.

154. Duan R, Porter W, Safe S. Estrogen-induced c-fos protooncogene expression in MCF-7 human breast cancer cells: role of estrogen receptor Sp1 complex formation. *Endocrinology* 1998; **139**: 1981–90.

155. Sun G, Porter W, Safe S. Estrogen-induced retinoic acid receptor α1 gene expression: role of estrogen receptor–Sp1 complex. *Mol Endocrinol* 1998; **12**: 882–90.

156. Xie W, Duan R, Safe S. Estrogen induces adenosine deaminase gene expression in MCF-7 human breast cancer cells: role of estrogen receptor–Sp1 interactions. *Endocrinology* 1999; **140**: 219–27.

157. Nakshatri H, Bhat-Nakshatri P, Martin DA et al. Constitutive activation of NF-κB during progression of breast cancer to hormone-independent growth. *Mol Cell Biol* 1997; **17**: 3629–39.

158. Sharma HW, Narayanan R. The NF-κB transcription factor in oncogenesis. *Anticancer Res* 1996; **16**: 589–96.

159. McDonnell DP, Vegeto E, O'Malley BW. Identification of a negative regulatory function for steroid receptors. *Proc Natl Acad Sci USA* 1992; **89**: 10563–7.

160. Hanstein B, Eckner R, DiRenzo J et al. p300 is a component of an estrogen receptor coactivator complex. *Proc Natl Acad Sci USA* 1996; **93**: 11540–5.

161. Musgrove EA, Hamilton JA, Lee CS et al. Growth factor, steroid, and steroid antagonist regulation of cyclin gene expression associated with changes in T-47D human breast cancer cell cycle progression. *Mol Cell Biol* 1993; **13**: 3577–87.

162. Prall OW, Rogan EM, Sutherland RL. Estrogen regulation of cell cycle progression in breast cancer cells. *J Steroid Biochem Mol Biol* 1998; **65**: 169–74.

163. Morishita S, Niwa K, Ichigo S et al. Overexpressions of c-fos/jun mRNA and their oncoproteins (Fos/Jun) in the mouse uterus treated with three natural estrogens. *Cancer Lett* 1995; **97**: 225–31.

164. Mohamood AS, Gyles P, Balan KV et al. Estrogen receptor, growth factor receptor and

protooncogene protein activities and possible signal transduction crosstalk in estrogen dependent and independent breast cancer cell lines. *J Submicrosc Cytol Pathol* 1997; **29:** 1–17.

165. Lukas J, Bartkova J, Bartek J. Convergence of mitogenic signalling cascades from diverse classes of receptors at the cyclin D–cyclin-dependent kinase–pRb-controlled G1 checkpoint. *Mol Cell Biol* 1996; **16:** 6917–25.

166. Kyprianou N, English HF, Davidson NE, Isaacs JT. Programmed cell death during regression of the MCF-7 human breast cancer following estrogen ablation. *Cancer Res* 1991; **51:** 162–6.

167. Amundadottir LT, Nass SJ, Berchem GJ et al. Cooperation of TGFα and c-Myc in mouse mammary tumorigenesis: coordinated stimulation of growth and suppression of apoptosis. *Oncogene* 1996; **13:** 757–65.

168. Werner H, Le Roith D. The insulin-like growth factor-I receptor signaling pathways are important for tumorigenesis and inhibition of apoptosis. *Crit Rev Oncog* 1997; **8:** 71–92.

169. Wang Q, Maloof P, Wang H et al. Basic fibroblast growth factor downregulates Bcl-2 and promotes apoptosis in MCF-7 human breast cancer cells. *Exp Cell Res* 1998; **238:** 177–87.

170. Huang Y, Ray S, Reed JC et al. Estrogen increases intracellular p26Bcl-2 to p21Bax ratios and inhibits taxol-induced apoptosis of human breast cancer MCF-7 cells. *Breast Cancer Res Treat* 1997; **42:** 73–81.

171. Nicholson RI, Walker KJ, Bouzubar N et al. Estrogen deprivation in breast cancer. Clinical, experimental, and biological aspects. *Ann NY Acad Sci* 1990; **595:** 316–27.

172. Nicholson RI, Manning DL. Oestrogen deprivation. In: *Breast Cancer: Biological and Clinical Progress* (Doglotti L, Sapino A, Bassolati G, eds). Dordrecht: Kluwer, 1992: 279–89.

173. Nicholson RI. Recent advances in the antihormonal therapy of breast cancer. *Curr Opin Invest Drugs: Oncol Endocr Metab* 1993; **2:** 1259–68.

174. Dowsett M, Stein RC, Coombes RC. Aromatization inhibition alone or in combination with GnRH agonists for the treatment of premenopausal breast cancer patients. *J Steroid Biochem Mol Biol* 1992; **43:** 155–9.

175. Dati C, Antoniotti S, Taverna D et al. Inhibition of c-erbB-2 oncogene expression by estrogens in human breast cancer cells. *Oncogene* 1990; **5:** 1001–6.

176. Chrysogelos SA, Yardin RI, Lauber AH, Murphy JM. Mechanisms of EGF receptor regulation in breast cancer cells. *Breast Cancer Res Treat* 1994; **31:** 227–36.

177. deFazio A, Chiew YE, McEvoy M et al. Antisense estrogen receptor RNA expression increases epidermal growth factor receptor gene expression in breast cancer cells. *Cell Growth Diff* 1997; **8:** 903–11.

178. Vickers PJ, Dickson RB, Shoemaker R, Cowan KH. A multidrug-resistant MCF-7 human breast cancer cell line which exhibits cross-resistance to antiestrogens and hormone-independent tumor growth in vivo. *Mol Endocrinol* 1988; **2:** 886–92.

179. van Agthoven T, van Agthoven TL, Dekker A et al. Induction of estrogen independence of ZR-75-1 human breast cancer cells by epigenetic alterations. *Mol Endocrinol* 1994; **8:** 1474–83.

180. van den Berg HW, Claffie D, Boylan M et al. Expression of receptors for epidermal growth factor and insulin-like growth factor I by ZR-75-1 human breast cancer cell variants is inversely related: the effect of steroid hormones on insulin-like growth factor I receptor expression. *Br J Cancer* 1996; **73:** 477–81.

181. Hunter RE, Jordan VC. Detection of the 8s oestrogen binding component in human uterine endometrium during the menstrual cycle. *J Endocrinol* 1975; **65:** 457–8.

182. Jordan VC, Koerner S. Tamoxifen (ICI 46,474) and the human carcinoma 8s oestrogen receptor. *Eur J Cancer* 1975; **11:** 205–6.

183. Jordan VC, Koerner S. Inhibition of oestradiol binding to mouse uterine and vaginal oestrogen receptors by triphenylethylenes. *J Endocrinol* 1975; **64:** 193–4.

184. Nicholson RI, Golder MP. The effect of synthetic anti-oestrogens on the growth and biochemistry of rat mammary tumours. *Eur J Cancer* 1975; **11:** 571–9.

185. Jordan VC, Prestwich G. Binding of (^{3}H)tamoxifen in rat uterine cytosols: a comparison of swinging bucket and vertical tube rotor sucrose density gradient analysis. *Mol Cell Endocrinol* 1977; **8:** 179–80.

186. Jordan VC, Dix CJ. Effect of oestradiol benzoate, tamoxifen and mono-hydroxytamoxifen on immature rat uterine progesterone receptor synthesis and endometrial cell division. *J Steroid Biochem* 1979; **11:** 285–91.

187. Jordan VC, MacGregor JI, Tonetti DA. Tamoxifen: from breast cancer therapy to the

design of a postmenopausal hormone replacement therapy. *Osteoporosis Int* 1997; **1**: S52–7.

188. Tate AC, Greene GL, DeSombre ER et al. Differences between estrogen and antiestrogen : estrogen receptor complexes identified with an antibody raised against the estrogen receptor. *Cancer Res* 1984; **44**: 1012–18.

189. Martin PM, Berthois Y, Jensen EV. Binding of the antiestrogen exposes an occult antigenic determinant in the human estrogen receptor. *Proc Natl Acad Sci USA* 1988; **85**: 2533–7.

190. Pham TA, Elliston JF, Nawaz Z et al. Antiestrogens can establish nonproductive receptor complexes and alter chromatin structure at target enhancers. *Proc Natl Acad Sci USA* 1991; **88**: 3125–9.

191. Allan GF, Leng X, Tsai ST et al. Hormone and antihormone induce distinct conformational changes which are central to steroid receptor activation. *J Biol Chem* 1992; **267**: 19513–20.

192. McDonnell DP, Dana SL, Hoener PA et al. Cellular mechanisms which distinguish between hormone- and antihormone-activated estrogen receptor. *Ann NY Acad Sci* 1995; **761**: 121–37.

193. McDonnell DP, Clemm DL, Hermann T et al. Analysis of estrogen receptor function in vitro three distinct classes of antiestrogens. *Mol Endocrinol* 1995; **9**: 659–69.

194. Metzger D, Berry M, Ali S, Chambon P. Effect of antagonists on DNA binding properties of the human estrogen receptor in vitro and in vivo. *Mol Endocrinol* 1995; **9**: 579–91.

195. Jordan VC. Biochemical pharmacology of antiestrogen action. *Pharmacol Rev* 1984; **36**: 245–76.

196. Cai W, Hu L, Foulkes JG. Transcription-modulating drugs: mechanism and selectivity. *Curr Opin Biotechnol* 1996; **7**: 608–15.

197. McInerney EM, Katzenellenbogen BS. Different regions in activating function-1 of the human estrogen receptor required for antiestrogen- and estradiol-dependent transcription activation. *J Biol Chem* **271**: 24172–8.

198. May FEB, Westley B. Effects of tamoxifen and 4-hydroxytamoxifen on the pNR-1 and pNR-2 estrogen regulated RNAs in human breast cancer cells. *J Biol Chem* 1987; **262**: 15894–9.

199. Katzenellenbogen BS, Montano MM, Le Goff P et al. Antiestrogens: mechanisms and actions in target cells. *J Steroid Biochem Mol Biol* 1995; **53**: 387–93.

200. Seery LT, Gee JMW, Dewhurst OL, Nicholson RI. Molecular mechanisms of antioestrogen. In: *Pharmacological Handbook* (Oettel M, Schillinger E, eds). Berlin: Springer-Verlag, 1999: 201–20.

201. Tremblay GB, Tremblay A, Copeland NG et al. Cloning, chromosomal localization, and functional analysis of the murine estrogen receptor β. *Mol Endocrinol* 1997; **11**: 353–65.

202. Fawell SE, White R, Hoare S et al. Inhibition of estrogen receptor-DNA binding by the 'pure' antiestrogen ICI 164,384 appears to be mediated by impaired receptor dimerization. *Proc Natl Acad Sci USA* 1990; **87**: 6883–7.

203. Wakeling AW, Bowler J. ICI 182,780, a new antioestrogen with clinical potential. *J Steroid Mol Biol* 1992; **43**: 173–7.

204. Wakeling AE, Bowler J. Novel pure antioestrogens without partial agonist activity. *J Steroid Biochem* 1988; **31**: 645–53.

205. Nicholson RI, Gee JM, Bryant S et al. Pure antiestrogens. The most important advance in the endocrine therapy of breast cancer since 1896. *Ann NY Acad Sci* 1996; **784**: 325–35.

206. Wakeling AE. The future of new pure antiestrogens in clinical breast cancer. *Breast Cancer Res Treat* 1993; **25**: 1–9.

207. Burcourt R, Vignau M, Torelli V et al. New biospecific adsorbents for the purification of estradiol receptor. *J Biol Chem* 1978; **253**: 8221–8.

208. Musgrove EA, Wakeling AE, Sutherland RL. Points of action of estrogen antagonists and a calmodulin antagonist within the MCF7 human breast cancer cell cycle. *Cancer Res* 1989; **49**: 2398–404.

209. Wakeling AE, Newboult E, Peters SW. Effects of antioestrogens on the proliferation of MCF-7 human breast cancer cells. *J Mol Endocrinol* 1989; **2**: 225–34.

210. Wakeling AE, Dukes M, Bowler J. A potent specific pure antiestrogen with clinical potential. *Cancer Res* 1991; **51**: 3867–73.

211. Brunner N, Frandsen TL, Holst-Hansen C et al. MCF-7/LCC2: a 4-hydroxytamoxifen resistant human breast cancer variant that retains sensitivity to the steroidal antiestrogen ICI 182,780. *Cancer Res* 1997; **53**: 3229–32.

212. Hu XF, Veroni M, De Luise M et al. Circumvention of tamoxifen resistance by the pure anti-estrogen ICI 182780. *Int J Cancer* 1993; **55**: 873–6.

213. Wiseman LR, Johnson MD, Wakeling AE et al. Type I IGF receptor and acquired tamoxifen resistance in oestrogen-responsive human

breast cancer cells. *Eur J Cancer* 1993; **29A:** 2256–64.

214. Lykkesfeldt AE, Madsen MW, Briand P. Altered expression of estrogen regulated genes in a tamoxifen-resistant and ICI 164,384 and ICI 182,780 sensitive human breast cancer cell line, MCF-7/TAM^R-1. *Cancer Res* 1994; **54:** 1587–95.

215. Gottardis MM, Jiang S-Y, Jeng M-H, Jordan VC. Inhibition of tamoxifen-stimulated growth of an MCF-7 tumor variant in athymic mice by novel steroidal antiestrogens. *Cancer Res* 1989; **49:** 4090–3.

216. Osborne CK, Jarman M, McCague R et al. The importance of tamoxifen metabolism in tamoxifen-stimulated breast tumor growth. *Cancer Chem Pharmacol* 1994; **34:** 89–95.

217. Osborne CK, Coronado-Heinsohn EB, Hilsenbeck EB et al. *J Natl Cancer Inst* 1995; **87:** 746–50.

218. DeFriend DJ, Howell A, Nicholson RI et al. Investigation of a new pure antiestrogen (ICI 182780) in women with primary breast cancer. *Cancer Res* 1994; **54:** 408–14.

219. Dowsett M, Johnston SRD, Iveson TJ, Smith IE. Response to specific antioestrogen (ICI 182 780) in tamoxifen-resistant breast cancer. *Lancet* 1995; **345:** 525.

220. Howell A, DeFriend D, Robertson J et al. Response to a specific antioestrogen (ICI 182780) in tamoxifen-resistant breast cancer. *Lancet* 1995; **345:** 29–30.

221. Arbuckle ND, Dauvois S, Parker MG. Effects of antioestrogens on the DNA binding activity of oestrogen receptors in vitro. *Nucleic Acids Res* 1992; **20:** 3839–44.

222. Bowler M, Lilley TJ, Pittam JD, Wakeling AE. Novel steroidal pure antioestrogens. *Steroids* 1989; **54:** 71–99.

223. Sabbah M, Grouileux F, Sola B, Redeuil GR. Structural differences between the hormone and antihormone estrogen receptor complexes bound to the hormone response elements. *Proc Natl Acad Sci USA* 1991; **88:** 390–4.

224. Pink JJ, Jordan VC. Models of estrogen receptor regulation by estrogens and antiestrogens in breast cancer cell lines. *Cancer Res* 1996; **56:** 2321–330.

225. Horwitz KB, Jackson TA, Bain DL et al. Nuclear receptor coactivators and corepressors. *Mol Endocrinol* 1996; **10:** 1167–77.

226. Dauvois S, Danielian PS, White R, Parker MG. Antiestrogen ICI 164,384 reduces cellular receptor content by increasing its turnover. *Proc Natl Acad Sci USA* 1992; **89:** 4037–41.

227. Nicholson RI, Gee JM, Manning DL et al. Responses to pure antiestrogens (ICI 164384, ICI 182780) in estrogen-sensitive and -resistant experimental and clinical breast cancer. *Ann NY Acad Sci* 1995; **12:** 148–63.

228. Nicholson RI, Gee JM, Francis AB et al. Observations arising from the use of pure antioestrogens on oestrogen-responsive (MCF-7) and oestrogen growth-independent (K3) human breast cancer cells. *Endocr Rel Cancer* 1995; **2:** 115–21.

229. Gibson MK. Nemmers LA, Beckman WC Jr et al. The mechanism of ICI 164,384 antiestrogenicity involves rapid loss of estrogen receptor in uterine tissue. *Endocrinology* 1991; **129:** 2000–10.

230. McClelland RA, Gee JM, Francis AB et al. Short-term effects of the pure antioestrogen ICI 182780 treatment on oestrogen receptor, epidermal growth factor receptor, transforming growth factor-α protein expression in human breast cancer. *Eur J Cancer* 1996; **32A:** 413–16.

231. McClelland RA, Manning DL, Gee JM et al. Effects of short-term antiestrogen treatment of primary breast cancer on estrogen receptor mRNA and protein expression and on estrogen-regulated genes. *Breast Cancer Res Treat* **41:** 31–41.

232. Dauvois S, White R, Parker MG. The antiestrogen ICI 182780 disrupts estrogen receptor nucleocytoplasmic shuttling. *J Cell Sci* 1993; **106:** 1377–88.

233. Dewhurst LO, Gee JW, Rennie IG, MacNeil S. Tamoxifen, 17β-Oestradiol and the calmodulin antagonist J8 inhibit human melanoma cell invasion through fibronectin. *Br J Cancer* 1997; **75:** 860–8.

234. Noguchi S, Motomura K, Inaji H et al. Downregulation of transforming growth factor α by tamoxifen in human breast cancer. *Cancer* 1993; **72:** 131–6.

235. Butta A, MacLennan K, Flanders KC et al. Induction of transforming growth factor β1 in human breast cancer in vivo following tamoxifen treatment. *Cancer Res* 1992; **52:** 4261–4.

236. Piantelli M, Maggiano N, Ricci R et al. Tamoxifen and quercetin interact with type II oestrogen binding sites and inhibit the growth of human melanoma cells. *J Invest Dermatol* 1995; **105:** 248–53.

237. O'Brian CA, Liskamp RM, Solomon DH, Weinstein IB. Inhibition of protein kinase C by tamoxifen. *Cancer Res* 1985; **45:** 2462–5.

238. Gundimeda U, Chen Z-H, Gopalakrishna R. Tamoxifen modulates protein kinase C via oxidative stress in estrogen receptor-negative breast cancer cells. *J Biol Chem* 1996; **271:** 13504–14.

239. Cabot MC, Zhang Z-H, Cao H-T et al. Tamoxifen activates cellular phospholipase C and D and elicits protein kinase C translocation. *Int J Cancer* 1997; **7:** 567–74.

240. Garcia T, Lehrer S, Bloomer WD, Schachter B. A variant estrogen receptor messenger ribonucleic acid is associated with reduced levels of estrogen binding in human mammary tumors. *Mol Endocrinol* 1988; **2:** 785–91.

241. Taylor JA, Li Y, You M, Wilcox AJ, Liu E. B region variant of the estrogen receptor gene. *Nucleic Acids Res* 1992; **20:** 2895.

242. Marci P, Khoriaty G, Lehrer S et al. Corrigendum: Sequence of a human estrogen receptor variant allele. *Nucleic Acids Res* 1992; **20:** 2008.

243. Dotzlaw H, Murphy LC. Cloning and sequencing of a variant sized estrogen receptor (ER) mRNA detected in some human breast cancer biopsies: 13th Annual San Antonio Breast Cancer Symposium (abstract). *Breast Cancer Res Treat* 1990; **16:** 147.

244. Dotzlaw H, Alkhalaf M, Murphy LC. Characterisation of estrogen receptor variant mRNAs from human breast cancers. *Mol Endocrinol* 1992; **6:** 773–85.

245. Fuqua SAW, Chamness GC, McGuire WL. Estrogen receptor mutations in breast cancer. *J Cell Biochem* 1993; **51:** 135–9.

246. Koehorst SG, Jacobs HM, Thijssen JH, Blankenstein MA. Wild type and alternatively spliced estrogen receptor messenger RNA in human meningioma tissue and MCF-7 breast cancer cells. *J Steroid Biochem Mol Biol* 1993; **45:** 227–33.

247. Pfeffer U, Fecarotta E, Castagnetta L, Vidali G. Estrogen receptor variant messenger RNA lacking exon 4 in estrogen-responsive human breast cancer cell lines. *Cancer Res* 1993; **53:** 741–3.

248. Murphy LC, Dotzlaw H, Hamerton J, Schwarz J. Investigation of the origin of variant, truncated estrogen receptor-like mRNAs identified in some human breast cancer biopsy samples. *Breast Cancer Res Treat* 1993; **26:** 149–61.

249. Gotteland M, Desauty G, Delarue JC, Lui L, May E. Human estrogen receptor messenger RNA variants in both normal and tumor breast tissues. *Mol Cell Endocrinol* 1995; **112:** 1–13.

250. McGuire WL, Chamness GC, Fuqua SAW. Estrogen receptor variants in clinical breast cancer. *Mol Endocrinol* 1991; **5:** 1571.

251. Karnik PS, Kulkarni PS, Liu X-P, Budd GT, Bukowski RM. Estrogen receptor mutations in tamoxifen-resistant breat cancer. *Cancer Res* 1994; **54:** 349–53.

10

Clinical response and resistance to SERMs

Julia MW Gee, Tracie-Ann Madden, John FR Robertson, Robert I Nicholson

INTRODUCTION

Selective estrogen receptor modulators (SERMs) are compounds that (to put it simply) exert their actions by competing with estrogens for binding to the target steroid hormone receptor, the estrogen receptor (ERα). The nonsteroidal SERMs have a triphenylethylene or benzothiophene structure, and exhibit complex organ-, cell-, and gene-specific antagonistic and agonistic properties.[1] Thus, the triphenylethylene tamoxifen (ICI 46,474; Nolvadex) is antagonistic in breast cancer yet agonistic on bone, lipids, and the endometrium. Its derivatives droloxifene, toremifene, and idoxifene exhibit profiles reminiscent of that of tamoxifen. The benzothiophene raloxifene (previously known as keoxifene) is inhibitory in breast tumours, agonistic on bone and lipids, but interestingly fails to demonstrate the unwanted stimulation of the endometrium.

While these compounds all share an ability to inhibit estrogen-responsive breast cancer cells, the most widely used, well tolerated, and well studied SERM in clinical disease to date is tamoxifen. Tamoxifen treatment is associated with a patient response rate of about 50% in advanced disease[2] and a median response duration of about 19 months.[3] In the adjuvant setting, tamoxifen is currently the endocrine therapy of choice, irrespective of age or menopausal status. Benefits are particularly prominent following at least 5 years of treatment.[4] This chapter thus principally examines the breast tumour phenotype in relation to clinical response and resistance to this agent, with the key features of SERM-responsive and -resistant disease being summarized in Tables 10.1 and 10.2 respectively.

WHAT IS THE TUMOUR PHENOTYPIC PROFILE ASSOCIATED WITH DISEASE REMISSION ON TAMOXIFEN CHALLENGE?

About 30% of breast cancer patients enjoy tumour remissions of good quality (i.e. are complete and partial responders, CR/PR) and long duration on tamoxifen challenge, while excellent remissions can also be observed with other SERMs.[2,5] These cancers are often histologically of low grade and well differentiated, with minimal proliferative capacity (as assessed using Ki-67/MIB1 immunostaining)

Table 10.1 Features of SERM-responsive disease in the clinic

1. **Histological features**
   - Low-grade and well-differentiated
   - Lowly proliferative and hence retention of some features of normal growth regulation

2. **Importance for ERα signalling**
   - Enriched for ERα, ERα signalling elements (e.g. co-activators??), and estrogen-regulated genes (e.g. PR, pS2, LIV1)

3. **Preferred growth factor receptor and ligand profile**
   - Enriched for c-ErbB3/4, IGF1-R, IGFs (decreased EGFR, c-ErbB2, TGF-α)

4. **Intracellular signalling element profile**
   - Enriched for PKCδ
   - Detectable (but low) activation of Erk1/2 MAP kinases and AP-1 elements
   - Enriched for activated JNK and p38 MAP kinases
   - Enriched for PKA Riα

Table 10.2 Features of SERM-resistant disease in the clinic

1. **Histological features**
   - High-grade and poorly differentiated
   - Highly proliferative and hence growth deregulation (changes in cell cycle proteins??; loss of tumour suppressor function – e.g. *p53* mutation??)

2. **Aberrations in ERα signalling**
   - ERα loss, redundancy of ERα, retention of ERα
   - Loss or retention of estrogen-regulated genes
   - Change in co-activator : co-repressor ratio??
   - Role for ERβ??

3. **Changes in preferred growth factor receptor and ligand profile**
   - Enriched for EGFR, c-ErbB2, TGF-α (decreased c-ErbB3/4)
   - Changes in IGF signalling??
   - Role for TGF-β?

4. **Changes in intracellular signalling element profile**
   - Enriched for PKCα
   - Enriched for activation of Erk1/2 MAP kinases
   - Enriched for AP-1 elements

and limited nuclear pleomorphism on presentation.[3,5–11] The profound decrease in tumour cellularity that comprises a tamoxifen response as recorded at 6 months appears to result both from a reduction in proliferative capacity and from increased apoptotic events.[12–17] Increases in apoptosis and decreases in mitotic events have similarly been observed during cellular response to toremifene and idoxifene.[18,19] Since a relatively indolent growth profile is exhibited by the majority of tamoxifen-responsive tumours in the clinic, it is likely that any growth inputs are counterbalanced (as in the normal breast) by significant suppressive influences.[20–22] Certainly there is evidence of normal p53 signalling (i.e. minimal p53 expression), together with marked positivity for the tumour suppressor product p21$^{WAF1/Cip1}$ of the WAF1/cip1 gene[23–25] and expression of BRCA1 in such tumours.[26] Similarly, there may be a lack of aberrant expression of cell cycle components such as cyclin D1 within tamoxifen-responsive, good-prognosis cancers,[27] while the key inhibitor of apoptosis and cell cycle regulator, Bcl-2, is noted both in the normal breast and in responsive disease.[28,29] There is evidence for increased p21$^{WAF1/Cip1}$ and decreased cyclin D1 and Bcl-2 expression during tamoxifen therapy,[14,30–32] as well as increased normal p53 expression with droloxifene[33] – events that in total are likely to contribute towards the antiproliferative and pro-apoptotic effects of SERMs in responsive patients.

Recent molecular examination of the endocrine-responsive phenotype in clinical breast cancer using technologies such as immunocytochemistry and reverse transcriptase polymerase chain reaction (RT-PCR) has provided a wealth of important clues as to the identity of the various mitogenic/cell survival signal transduction pathways that underlie growth. These data will be presented in some detail below, but, in summary, examination of the tamoxifen-responsive breast cancer phenotype (and probably that responsive to additional SERMs) appears to confirm both a growth-promoting role for estrogen and a preferred profile of growth factor signalling pathways – a scenario in many ways comparable to that in the normal breast.[34,35] ERα appears to be an essential component of such growth. This protein is a member of the family of steroid-binding receptors that function as nuclear transcription factors[34–36] (see Chapter 9). ERα is regulated at many levels via hyperphosphorylation by ligand-dependent and ligand-independent factors, notably including certain peptide growth factors.[37] An increasing body of experimental data, supplemented by recent clinical studies examining the phenotypic profile during the tamoxifen-responsive phase of the disease, indicates that interactions between estrogen and growth factor signalling elements comprise the precise cellular targets for tamoxifen inhibition. However, definitive demonstration of the importance of the various pathway elements in SERM-responsive disease remains a goal for researchers that may be achieved from the future clinical application of pure anti-hormones such as fulvestrant (ICI 182,780, Faslodex)[38] as well as appropriate and selective signal transduction inhibitors.[35,39]

Estrogen receptor signalling elements in CR/PR disease

ERα and estrogen-regulated genes in tamoxifen response

Between 60% and 80% of all primary breast cancers on presentation demonstrate the principal target receptor for the steroid hormone estrogen, ERα (Figure 10.1a), and indeed many of these tumours overexpress this receptor in relation to normal breast.[40] ERα-positive patients are likely to enjoy a longer survival time,[40–42] with the principal site of metastasis being bone.[43] These tumours are often well differentiated (i.e. 90% grade I versus only 55% grade III).[44,45] Importantly, measurement of an ERα-positive status identifies an increased likelihood of remissions of good quality and duration following tamoxifen challenge, with 50–60% of ERα-positive patients exhibiting such responses.[5,9,40,42] Indeed, the presence of ERα in endocrine-responsive breast cancers is an

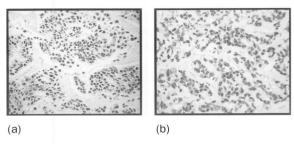

(a)   (b)

Figure 10.1 Immunocytochemical demonstration of steroid hormone receptors in SERM-responsive clinical breast cancer: (a) estrogen receptor (ERα); (b) progesterone receptor (PgR).

almost essential prerequisite (about 95%) for tamoxifen inhibition, with ERα expression also been associated with cellular responses to the additional SERMs idoxifene, toremifene, and droloxifene.[46–48] There is, moreover, some indication of an association between homogeneous, higher expression of ERα and increased likelihood of a tamoxifen response of long duration[9,49,50] – a feature that is also apparent with toremifene.[51] The excellent inhibitory responses that are elicited by SERMs in CR/PR disease mirror the substantial inhibitory effects of these agents consistently demonstrated in ERα-positive breast cancer in vitro. In total, the clinical and experimental SERM inhibitory data convincingly demonstrate the essential nature of ERα signalling with regard to the cell growth and survival of such tumours.[34,35,37,47,48]

SERM responses are likely to involve inhibition of key-growth regulatory genes bearing estrogen response element (ERE) sequences or additional response elements influenced by estrogen/ERα signalling (see Chapter 9). Such genes may include the estrogen-regulated nuclear transcription factors c-Fos and c-Myc and cell survival factors such as Bcl-2 and transforming growth factor α (TGF-α), since their expression often parallels proliferation and cellularity prior to and during clinical tamoxifen response.[15,31,32,52,53] In addition to such effects, however, estrogen/ERα signalling primes

expression of additional genes whose expression is perceived to again be dependent on functional estrogen/ERα signalling yet which fails to directly associate with proliferative capacity in clinical breast cancer material. These paradoxical data perhaps reflect important differences in the susceptibility of various estrogen-regulated genes to tamoxifen inhibition[52] – a feature that may be dependent on the promoter context, ERα activation functions 1 or 2 (AF-1/AF-2), the cellular complement of proteins interacting with the receptor, or the presence of additional response elements influenced by ERα signalling (see Chapter 9). Such genes notably include the progesterone receptor (*PgR*) (Figure 10.1b),[42] *pS2*, and *LIV1*.[54–57] These genes are frequently enriched in tumours that exhibit a good response to tamoxifen, with their expression being suppressed by long-term tamoxifen therapy.[58] Decreases in estrogen-regulated genes have similarly been noted during toremifene response.[18,59] PgR has been reported to be an independent predictive factor for response to tamoxifen,[60] and overall response rates of 77% have been reported for advanced tumours co-expressing ERα/PgR (versus only 27% of ERα-positive/PgR-negative).[44] Moreover, a 90% response rate has been achieved as a result of giving tamoxifen for a few days and then continuing therapy only where PgR levels increased (presumably reflecting the partial agonism exhibited on short-term challenge with tamoxifen acting via an intact ERα mechanism).[61]

ERα variants, mutations and ERβ in tamoxifen response

In contrast to the ERα data, preliminary studies indicate that there is unlikely to be a comparable relationship between expression of the additional recently identified estrogen receptor ERβ, and good response to tamoxifen.[62] This is certainly in agreement with our own findings at the mRNA level of no association with well-differentiated tumour types and indeed an inverse relationship between ERβ and ERα expression,[63] although examinations at the protein level remain somewhat at odds with these data.[64] Recent studies have also revealed that the ERα protein may be subject to very rare mutations, as well as the generation of several truncated or exon-deleted variant forms generated as a result of alternative splicing.[65] Some of these receptor forms, like ERβ, have been shown experimentally to maintain binding capabilities for tamoxifen, to form homo- and heterodimers with ERα, and hence to influence transactivation of EREs. However, there is no conclusive relationship between tamoxifen response and expression of variants and mutants,[66] although the mRNAs for several variants (e.g. δ2, 7, 4, and 5) are very commonly expressed at low levels in ERα-positive breast cancer with its inherently better prognosis, as well as within normal breast material.[67,68]

Transcription factors for ERα and ERa co-accessory proteins in tamoxifen response
Limited studies have demonstrated that molecules that enhance ERα gene expression,[69,70] such as the nuclear transcription factor AP-2/ERF-1, are enriched in lowly proliferative, low-grade tumours, which are often also tamoxifen responsive.[16] This expression profile may also be true for the co-activator proteins SRC-1 (steroid receptor co-activator)[71] and AIB1.[72] Such co-activators interact with ERα, acting as a bridge with the basal transcriptional machinery to enhance receptor transactivation of EREs and thus estrogen-regulated gene expression.

Positive growth factor signalling elements in CR/PR disease

Experimental studies have indicated that ERα activity is regulated at many levels by phosphorylation in a ligand-dependent or -independent manner.[37] Several peptide growth factors and their intracellular signalling pathways have been implicated in ligand-independent activation of ERα (see Chapter 9). However, as will be detailed below, examination of CR/PR disease for such signalling elements has revealed that there may be a preferred growth factor signalling pathway profile (i.e. c-ErbB3/4 and insulin-like growth factors) that sharply contrasts tamoxifen resistance. These transduction pathways are primed by ligands very often derived from stromal elements in close vicinity to the tumour epithelial cells comprising well-differentiated cancers. Moreover, there is increasing evidence that the preferred pathways interact closely with ERα, and that their key elements are targets for inhibition during tamoxifen response.

TGF-α, EGFR, and c-ErbB2 signalling elements
The type 1 ErbB family of plasma-membrane-spanning tyrosine kinase receptors currently has four distinct members: the epidermal growth factor (EGF) receptor (EGFR), c-ErbB2 (HER2/Neu), c-ErbB3 (HER3), and c-ErbB4 (HER4). Signal transduction by type 1 ErbB receptors is initiated via ligand-induced receptor homo- or heterodimerization and receptor tyrosine autophosphorylation (Figure 10.2).[39,73,74] There are prominent differences in structure and intrinsic catalytic activity between the ErbB receptors, as well as preferred ligands. For example, EGFR is activated by peptide growth factor ligands such as TGF-α or EGF, heregulins activate c-ErbB3, while c-ErbB2 appears to have no direct ligand (although activation of this receptor can still be elevated via heterodimerization). There is recruitment of specific Src homology 2 (SH2)-containing proteins, notably the adapter proteins Shc and Grb2. Shc and Grb2 in turn recruit other signalling proteins, including the guanine nucleotide exchange factor Sos1, which brings p21[Ras] into its active GTP-binding form, subsequently translocating Raf-1 kinase (mitogen-activated protein kinase kinase kinase, MAPKKK) and sequentially activating the MEK1/2 (MAPK/Erk kinase, MAPKK) and MAPK (e.g. Erk1/2, 'extracellular signal regulated kinase') phosphorylation cascade.[75-77] Such events culminate in activation and modulation of expression of a profile of nuclear transcription factors (e.g. AP-1 and Elk-1), thereby influencing a plethora of cellular endpoints such as proliferation, cell survival, and

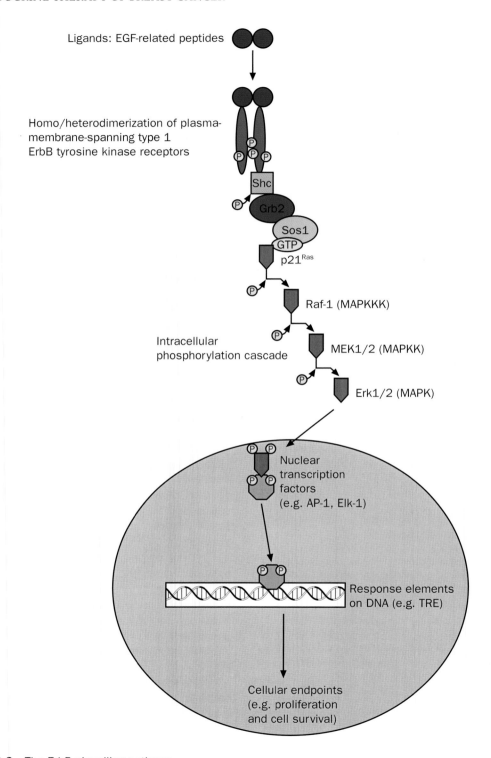

Figure 10.2 The ErbB signalling pathway.

differentiation. p21[Ras] signalling is not the only pathway to the nucleus employed by ErbB receptors, however, since the second messenger phosphoinositide-3'-kinase (PI3K) can also be recruited because c-ErbB3 bears a consensus for the SH2 domain of this enzyme. Furthermore, it has been postulated from experimental studies that crosstalk exists between the ErbB and ERα transduction pathways in breast cancer. Such crosstalk may involve ligand-independent ERα activation by ErbB signalling, for example, via phosphorylation of serine 118 in the activation function 1 (AF-1) region located within the A/B domain of ERα (see Chapter 9).[78,79]

Examination of the tamoxifen-responsive clinical breast cancer phenotype generally reveals only minimal expression of the EGFR and c-ErbB2 proteins in tumour epithelial cells. Indeed, in our own study, almost 80% of ERα-positive patients with minimal EGFR expression showed some degree of response, with 43% of patients obtaining CR/PR.[11,80,81] A similar (albeit weaker) association is seen with the c-ErbB2 protein.[11,80,81] Immunocytochemistry demonstrates any expression to be merely weakly cytoplasmic, with no positive correlations with proliferation.[80–82] In addition, only barely detectable levels of the tumour EGFR ligand TGF-α are generally expressed in the tumour epithelial cells comprising CR/PR disease, where there is again a lack of correlation with proliferation.[83,84] These data indicate that if there is any positive interaction with the ERα transduction pathway in clinical material, then this must occur in the presence of only minimal TGF-α/EGFR and c-ErbB2 signalling, and is likely to be directed towards endpoints other than proliferation, which may include cell survival. Similarly, autocrine induction of TGF-α by estrogen in such tumours is unlikely to be significant, since the effects of tamoxifen on this growth factor remain controversial.[85] Indeed, it is feasible that there is even inhibitory activity between these pathways, a phenomenon believed to result from estrogen/ERα suppression of the *EGFR*/c-*erbB2* genes.[86–88] We and others[89] have noted that this suppression is released by tamoxifen or toremifene treatment.

Breast cancer cells thus appear to possess potent mechanisms to limit any substantial EGFR/c-ErbB2-mediated signalling input under conditions of steroid-directed, tamoxifen-responsive growth.[90] This concept is certainly supported in vivo by the obvious inverse relationship noted between ERα and these receptor tyrosine kinase receptors.[11,80,81,91] In total, these data (together with in vitro evidence[92–94] indicate that TGF-α, EGFR, and c-ErbB2 signalling is unlikely to play an important role in driving the growth of tamoxifen-responsive cancer.

c-ErbB3/4 signalling elements

In marked contrast to EGFR and c-ErbB2, RT-PCR and immunocytochemical studies have demonstrated marked expression of the additional plasma membrane ErbB receptor tyrosine kinases c-ErbB3 and c-ErbB4 in the tumour epithelial cells comprising many tamoxifen-responsive breast cancers, with this expression being associated with the ERα-positive, lowly proliferative and well-differentiated phenotype (Figure 10.3a).[95–97] Moreover, our preliminary examination has indicated that expression of the mRNA for heregulin-β1 (the most potent ligand for the c-ErbB3 receptor when applied to tamoxifen-responsive breast cancer cells in vitro[98]) is also prominent in ERα-positive/c-ErbB3-positive clinical breast cancer material, possibly associated with both stromal and epithelial elements of tumours. While future examination of signalling mediated via c-ErbB3/4 in vivo will no doubt prove highly complex – with the possibility of multiple ligands, receptor hetero- and homodimerization of ErbB family members, and recruitment of several downstream signalling elements – there appears to be increasing evidence that this signalling network is important in tamoxifen-responsive breast cancer,[96] potentially enjoying close positive interactions with ERα/ERE signalling.[78]

Insulin-like growth factor signalling elements

The insulin-like growth factors IGF-I and IGF-II signal through a common ligand-activated

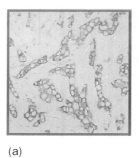

(a)

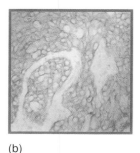

(b)

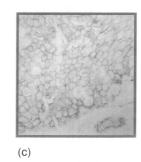

(c)

Figure 10.3 Immunocytochemical demonstration of ErbB receptors in clinical breast cancer. (a) SERM-responsive disease: increased c-ErbB3 expression. (b) SERM-resistant disease: increased EGFR expression. (c) SERM-resistant disease: increased c-ErbB2 expression.

transmembrane receptor tyrosine kinase, the insulin-like growth factor reactor IGF1-R (Figure 10.4).[39,99,100] This receptor comprises a disulfide-linked α_2–β_2 heterodimeric glycoproteinic complex, composed of two extracellular α chains providing the growth factor binding site and two transmembrane–intracellular β subunits possessing intrinsic tyrosine kinase activity.[39] The downstream signalling network recruited on receptor activation is IRS-1/PI3K/Akt (protein kinase B, PKB), with additional influences on the p21[Ras]/MAP kinase phosphorylation cascade – signalling ultimately impinging on a profile of nuclear transcription factors and thus cellular endpoints such as proliferation and survival. A family of IGF-binding

proteins (IGFBPs) and the mannose 6-phosphate/IGF-II receptor regulate IGF signalling by sequestration of IGFs in an inactive form and lysosomal degradation of IGF-II respectively. Perturbation of the IGF signalling network, which plays a role in both proliferation and cell survival, is common in breast cancer, and in particular may be important in the pathogenesis of steroid-hormone-dependent disease.[99,100] Thus, many ERα-positive, well-differentiated, and indolent breast carcinomas express considerable levels of the plasma-membrane-bound receptor for IGFs (IGF1-R) on their epithelial cells.[100] Indeed, 40-fold higher IGF1-R tyrosine kinase activity has been reported in the malignant breast versus its normal counterpart.[101] There is a strong correlation between IGF1-R and ERα expression, and the former receptor is also associated with better patient prognosis and an indolent clinical phenotype.[102,103] The dominant IGF1-R ligand, IGF-II, is generated predominantly from stromal cells in the vicinity of the malignant epithelial cells, although expression has been detected in several tumour epithelial cell lines in vitro.[103–105] Increased IGF-II expression again appears to correlate with low breast tumour grade.[106] The cancers also contain limited IGF-I expression, although in situ hybridization studies indicate that this is likely to be derived from stromal fibroblasts surrounding tumour–associated normal breast lobules, with additional systemic IGF-I input. Key downstream signalling elements of IGF signalling are also detectable in clinical disease (e.g. insulin receptor substrate 1 (IRS-1)[107] and PI3K[108]). Since IGF signalling has been demonstrated to be powerfully mitogenic in tamoxifen-responsive breast cancer cells in vitro,[35,109,110] it is certainly possible that this is a preferred pathway for the growth of tamoxifen-responsive breast cancer in vivo, although a definitive examination of this in relation to clinical response has yet to be carried out. There are likely to be substantial positive bidirectional interactions between IGF and ERα signalling driving the growth of such tumours,[100,111,112] a mechanism also obligatory for the growth of the normal breast, as demonstrated using IGF-I

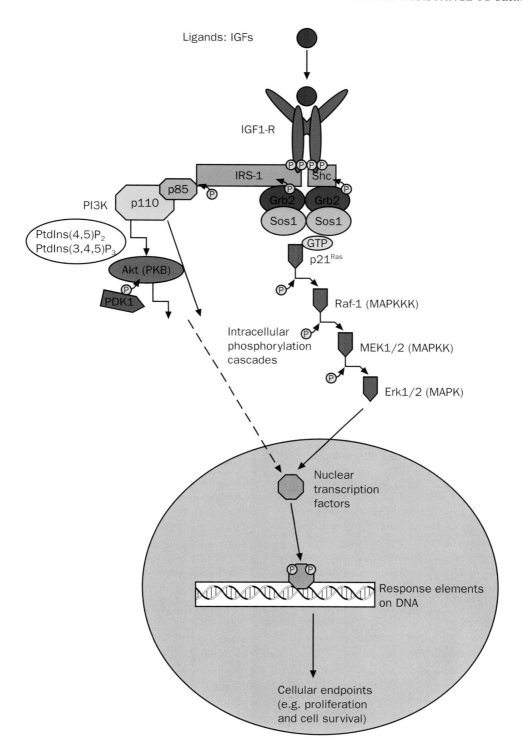

Figure 10.4 The insulin-like growth factor (IGF) signalling network.

and ERα (ERKO) gene knockout mice.[113,114] Growth synergy occurs between estradiol and IGF in vitro, together with IGF-mediated activation of the ERα protein (e.g. Akt-associated phosphorylation of Serine 167 in ER) and hence ERE transactivation.[100,111] The latter interaction is perhaps evidenced in clinical breast cancer by an association between stromal IGF-II and epithelial PgR expression,[115] and also by the association between IGF1-R mRNA and PgR that we have observed in the disease. Similarly, in vitro studies in endocrine-responsive breast cancer cells have demonstrated that tamoxifen (as well as droloxifene[59,116]) is capable of effecting a substantial reduction in IGF signalling. This is likely to occur via several mechanisms, including decreased IGF-II expression, inhibition of IGF-I-dependent growth, changes in IGFBPs, diminished activation/expression of IGFR and the downstream signal transduction elements IRS-1 and PI3K, and induction of relevant phosphatases that inhibit kinase activity.[100,117–121] Moreover, systemic levels of IGF-I fall during tamoxifen or droloxifene therapy – a feature that may also be contributory to the tumour-inhibitory effects of such agents.[59,116,122]

Intracellular signalling elements

Protein kinase C (PKC)

Growth factor activation of phospholipase C increases inositol lipid turnover, resulting in generation of the second messenger diacylglycerol and thereby activation of protein kinase C (PKC) isozymes, which are believed to interact with downstream signalling pathways such as the MAP kinase cascade.[123] The PKC family comprises at least 11 mammalian isozymes that play differential roles in cell growth regulation and differentiation.[124] While the subsequent downstream cascade initiated following activation of PKC is as yet highly controversial, the classical response element primed by such signalling is the 12-O-tetradecanoylphorbol-13-acetate (TPA) response element (TRE).[125,126] In addition, however, there is some evidence for positive effects of the δ isoform of PKC on ERE transactivation mediated via enhanced phosphorylation of serine 122 of ERα.[127]

Interestingly, our data indicate that PKCδ is the isoform of particular prominence in tamoxifen-responsive tumour cells in vitro and in comparable clinical breast cancer, where an association with increased duration of response and patient survival time is apparent.[128] Changes initiated during tamoxifen challenge have not as yet been addressed in vivo.

MAP kinase family members

Erk1 and 2 comprise one branch of an increasingly large, interwoven family of MAP kinases activated by a phosphorylation cascade initiated by ligand binding to ErbB receptor tyrosine kinases. Phosphorylated MAP kinases are believed to subsequently activate and increase the expression of several nuclear transcription factors, notably the AP-1 nuclear transcription factor complex, which again targets the TRE.[75,129] Interestingly, however, Erk1/2-mediated signalling is also capable of phosphorylation of the ERα,[79] with the serine 118 residue in the AF-1 region of the receptor being of some importance. Such ligand-independent phosphorylation results in significant transactivation of simple EREs experimentally. Our observation of low but nevertheless detectable activation of Erk1/2 in CR/PR tumour epithelial material on clinical presentation[130,131] implies that the Erk1/2 signal transduction cascade, while obviously highly regulated in responsive disease, is certainly available to crosstalk with ERα signalling. Indeed, our recent observation of decreased Erk1/2 activation as part of the clinical tamoxifen response profile indicates that such signalling is highly relevant to the growth of responsive disease. Further influences on both TRE and ERα signalling may occur with the parallel 'stress-activated' MAP kinase members JNK ('Jun N-terminal kinase') and p38.[132,133] For example, p38 may be activated during tamoxifen-induced apoptosis,[133] and indeed we have noted increased activation of p38 and JNK during the tumour regression that occurs on short-term clinical tamoxifen response. Evidence of increased activation of these latter MAP kinases at the time of disease presentation appears to predict for tamoxifen response, particularly in those ERα-positive patients whose tumours bear unusually elevated Erk1/2 activation.[131]

cAMP and protein kinase A (PKA)

ERα activation and estrogen-regulated gene expression can also be initiated experimentally by the signalling molecule cAMP. This event is mediated via ERα phosphorylation by protein kinase A (PKA).[134,135] Interestingly, PKA activity has been observed to be higher in clinical breast tumours than in normal breast.[136] Moreover, the mRNA for the PKA regulatory subunit Iα (RIα) has been associated with patient tamoxifen response, and levels have been observed to decline during therapy.[137]

AP-1

ERα is likely to take part in protein–protein interactions with the nuclear transcription factor complex AP-1 to augment transactivation from response elements other than the ERE, notably including the TRE.[138] In this light, there is certainly detectable nuclear expression of the key AP-1 components c-Fos and activated c-Jun in CR/PR tumours,[53,139,140] and so there remains the potential for such interactions in these tumours, albeit in a highly-regulated manner. AP-1 signalling is likely to be essential to such tumours, since changes in c-Fos expression closely mirror the profile of tumour response during tamoxifen therapy in the clinic.[53]

Negative growth factor signalling elements in CR/PR disease

Transforming growth factor β (TGF-β)

The TGF-β polypeptides belong to a family of pleiotropic growth and differentiation factors, and their production is inhibited by estrogens and inducible by tamoxifen. TGF-βs are produced by both normal and cancerous breast epithelial cells.[141] They are potent inhibitors of the normal breast epithelium, and can be growth-inhibitory to tumour cells in vitro, although such effects are more controversial within in vivo models. The profile of tumour TGF-β expression has not been fully examined

in relation to prediction of tamoxifen response in the clinic, while relationships with prognosis remain much debated.[142,143] However, several studies have demonstrated that patients exhibit increases in plasma and tumour levels of TGF-β1 and TGF-β2 following initial exposure to tamoxifen therapy, with increases in plasma TGF-β2 mirroring effective tamoxifen response.[144–147] Induction of TGF-β has similarly been observed with droloxifene and toremifene treatment.[18,59,148] However, the relevance of the association between SERM-mediated increases in TGF-βs and effective patient response remains controversial.[149] Indeed, some in vitro breast cancer model systems can paradoxically be tamoxifen-responsive yet apparently resistant to the inhibitory activity of TGF-βs.[150]

WHAT IS THE TUMOUR PHENOTYPIC PROFILE ASSOCIATED WITH DISEASE STABILIZATION ON TAMOXIFEN CHALLENGE?

About 20% of breast cancer patients exhibit stabilization of their disease as recorded after 6 months of tamoxifen therapy (i.e. static disease, SD).[151] Similar features have been reported for MCF-7 and ZR-75-1 human breast cancer xenograft model systems, where tamoxifen challenge or estrogen withdrawal are merely tumoristatic.[152] SD is commonly perceived to be clinically endocrine-responsive, since therapy prevents tumour progression and patients often enjoy a good survival.[151] However, in several ways, the breast cancer SD phenotype appears potentially less favourable than that of tumours from CR/PR patients. Thus, static disease is often of higher grade and elevated proliferative capacity compared with the tumours from CR/PR patients.[9,83,84] Moreover, we have noted a failure of tamoxifen in clinical SD to significantly decrease immunostaining of the proliferation marker Ki67, the cell survival factor Bcl-2, and the AP-1 component c-Fos.[31,53] Such events would perhaps serve to maintain tumour cell number, contributing towards the lack of substantial regression recorded at 6 months in such patients.

Estrogen receptor signalling elements in SD

Data regarding the expression of ERα/β and the associated signalling elements in SD is as yet sparse. However, there is certainly an importance for ERα-mediated cell growth and survival of breast cancer SD, since endocrine challenge effectively halts disease progression. Not surprisingly, therefore, SD frequently expresses significant levels of the ERα machinery necessary for tamoxifen response, together with estrogen-regulated expression of genes such as *PgR* and *pS2*. However, in parallel with the lack of significant remission, reductions in expression of ERα and estrogen-regulated genes during tamoxifen therapy are often very small.[31] These observations are in marked contrast with the significant downregulation often apparent in tumours from CR/PR patients, and are mirrored in MCF-7 cell xenograft studies, where tamoxifen effects on estrogen-regulated gene expression are reported to be relatively minor.[153]

Growth factor signalling elements in SD

In common with tumours obtained from CR/PR patients, there is some evidence for prominent c-ErbB3 and IGF signalling in clinical SD (and its relevant in vivo model systems), and again these pathways appear to interact with ERα signal transduction.[95,154] However, it is also likely that there is an increased role for TGF-α/EGFR/Erk1/2 signalling in SD. Thus, while EGFR/c-ErbB2 immunostaining is minimal in SD, enhanced expression of the EGFR ligand TGF-α[83] is commonly noted (about 70% of patients). This feature occurs in the presence of sustained activation of Erk1/2.[130,131] Such increased signalling input from this peptide growth factor may serve to protect against significant cell loss during therapy, and may interact with the ERα network, since SD growth is checked by tamoxifen challenge.

WHAT ARE THE TUMOUR PHENOTYPIC PROFILES ASSOCIATED WITH DE NOVO AND ACQUIRED RESISTANCE TO TAMOXIFEN CHALLENGE?

Unfortunately, clinical application of tamoxifen and other triphenylethylene derivatives has revealed that their beneficial actions are limited and can eventually be counteracted by the capacity of breast tumour cells to circumvent the need for steroid hormones, allowing them to continue to grow and progress despite such therapy. Thus, tamoxifen is ineffective in about 50% of patients on presentation (de novo tamoxifen resistance), while initially responsive tumours will inevitably progress despite such treatments (acquired tamoxifen resistance), resulting in patient relapse and ultimately death. Such tumours are for the most part cross-resistant to current triphenylethylene SERMs.[155–158] Loss of ERα or dislocation of growth from the receptor appears to be a feature of de novo tamoxifen-resistant disease. However, in acquired tamoxifen resistance, ERα paradoxically remains essential for tumour growth. What molecular changes, therefore, might underlie growth and enable the inhibitory qualities of tamoxifen to be circumvented in the various forms of SERM resistance? While there may be some role for aberrations within ERα signalling, there is an increasing body of phenotypic evidence to indicate that there are substantial genetic/epigenetic changes in growth factor signalling elements, cell cycle components, and tumour suppressor genes. In particular, autocrine TGF-α/EGFR signalling (including sustained downstream Erk1/2/PKCα/AP-1 activity) appears to become a dominant pathway in such tumours. In parallel, there is likely to be a somewhat diminished role for the principal pathways in hormone-responsive disease, c-ErbB3/4 and IGFR. Such signalling is reliant on a considerable stromal input of ligands, and the influence of stromal signals declines with progression to poorly-differentiated, endocrine unresponsive tumours.

Changes in ERα signalling elements in clinical de novo and acquired tamoxifen resistance

Loss of ERα in tamoxifen resistance

An ERα-negative protein status is a relatively common event comprising some 20–30% of breast tumours at presentation.[6,41,159–161] Absence of the ERα machinery necessary to respond to tamoxifen on presentation is generally (about 95% of cases) associated with de novo endocrine resistance in clinical breast cancer. ERα negativity in vitro (exemplified by the MDA-MB-231 and MDA-MB-436 breast cancer cell lines[163]) is similarly associated with de novo resistance to tamoxifen. In contrast, despite the likelihood that endocrine therapies specifically target the ERα-positive tumour cell population during the responsive phase of the disease, ERα negativity is only rarely manifested during antiestrogen therapy in breast cancer, and hence is generally not a feature of acquired tamoxifen resistance either in vitro or in vivo.[40] In comparison with tamoxifen-responsive disease, ERα-negative, de novo resistant breast cancers are higher in grade and more poorly differentiated, with an elevated proliferative capacity and increased nuclear pleomorphism.[9] They have a particular propensity to spread to unfavourable metastatic sites, with patients thus having very poor survival characteristics.[5,162,164–166]

The origins of the ERα-negative breast cancer phenotype at presentation are as yet unknown.[167] However, this phenotype is believed to present early in the life history of the disease, since an absence of ERα has been noted in poorly differentiated in situ disease. Mutations in the *ERα* gene resulting in an inability to transcribe ERα are likely to be extremely rare in breast cancer,[168] and indeed low levels of *ERα* mRNA are still detectable in ERα-negative tumours.[56] A number of potential mechanisms preventing efficient transcription or translation of the *ERα* gene, resulting in a lack of ERα expression, may exist. These mechanisms include (i) transcriptional inactivation by hypermethylation of the CpG island in the regulatory region of *ERα*,[169–171] (ii) altered expression of *trans*-acting factors aiding *ERα* transcription,[69] and (iii) abnormalities in *ERα* translation or synthesis of an unstable receptor protein.[167] Alternatively, increased ERα degradation has been reported in ERα-negative disease.[172] Finally, ERα-negative tumours may feasibly also arise from the selective outgrowth of a subpopulation of steroid-receptor-negative cells, which are likely to exist within the normal breast epithelium,[173,174] although such selective outgrowth is reported to be extremely infrequent in vivo.[175] Whatever the mechanism underlying the absence of ERα expression, regulation of these tumours is believed to be severed from the steroid hormone environment. Thus, in addition to such tumours being refractory to the inhibitory actions of tamoxifen, there is invariably an absence of estrogen-regulated gene expression (e.g. of *PgR* or *bcl-2*) on clinical presentation of ERα-negative disease.[11,28,54,56]

In the absence of any steroid hormone input, therefore, how might the growth of ERα-negative disease be sustained? As will be discussed below, such tumours appear to derive considerable growth input from aberrant peptide growth factor signalling,[80,81] with markedly exaggerated EGFR/c-ErbB2 signalling being heavily implicated in an autocrine signalling loop. In addition, evidence will be presented for genetic abnormalities within key cell survival and cell cycle regulatory elements that may contribute to their excessive proliferation and aggressive tumour growth.

Redundancy of ERα in tamoxifen resistance

Retention of ERα (albeit often at lower levels than observed in responding patients) is a common feature (about 30–40%) of de novo tamoxifen-unresponsive breast cancer.[40,162,165] ERα-positive, de novo endocrine-unresponsive breast cancers exhibit a high tumour grade and are poorly differentiated and highly proliferative, maintaining their growth despite tamoxifen therapy.[9] As with ERα-negative disease, they often spread to unfavourable metastatic sites, with patients thus having a poor prognosis.[5,162,164,165] There is clinical evidence that the growth of ERα-positive, de novo resistant disease is dislocated from ERα signalling, although this remains to be definitively tested by future clinical challenge with pure antiestrogens (agents reported to dramatically reduce ERα levels). Thus, responses to existing second-line endocrine agents are extremely rare in patients bearing such tumours.[3]

As will be discussed below, such dislocation of growth from a dependence on the normal ERα protein could be enabled by phenotypic/genotypic changes in ERα signalling or within crosstalking peptide growth factor pathways at points downstream of ERα, such as in cell cycle components/tumour suppressor genes. Extreme perturbation of upstream elements as well as aberrations within ERα-independent pathways might also enable the importance of ERα to be nullified. The tumours may arise from the proliferation of an aberrant, de novo unresponsive ERα-positive stem cell, or they may be derived by clonal selection of aberrations occurring within an endocrine-responsive phenotype during the early life history of the cancer. Whatever their aetiology, these aberrations must occur at such a cellular frequency as to enable the normal ERα to be redundant in tumour growth, hence explaining the lack of tamoxifen inhibition. The aberrations may be able to exert positive actions on estrogen-regulated genes such as *PgR*, since we have noted that expression is still detectable in about 60% of ERα-positive de novo tamoxifen-insensitive tumours, despite apparently non-functional ERα.

Continued use of ERα in tamoxifen resistance
Sadly, development of resistance is almost inevitable during tamoxifen treatment of ERα-positive patients who demonstrate an initial therapeutic sensitivity.[36,40,176,177] Disease relapse occurs after a median duration of remission of only about 18 months.[3] Increased tumour cellularity, proliferation, and grade, coupled with decreased apoptosis, are common features of clinical relapse.[53] Interestingly, most clinical breast tumours demonstrating acquired resistance maintain considerable ERα expression.[22,36,40,178] Various model systems of acquired resistance, including our MCF-7 sublines developed during long-term tamoxifen treatment or prolonged estrogen deprivation, further confirm the stability of ERα expression on the acquisition of many forms of endocrine resistance in breast cancer.[93,94,179,180]

There is a considerable amount of data indicating that ERα in acquired resistant breast cancer commonly remains functional[178] and moreover pivotal to the growth-regulation and gene-expression profile of breast tumours on their relapse, despite the presence of tamoxifen. Thus, frequent favourable responses (i.e. about 50%,[3] with a median duration of remission of 12 months) occur in the clinic on second-line endocrine therapeutic challenge of acquired resistant breast cancer with agents that serve to severely estrogen-deprive the tumour (notably recently including the use of pure antiestrogen treatment[181] and aromatase inhibitors[182,183]). We and others[179,184] have demonstrated that sensitivity to pure antiestrogen inhibition is a feature of acquired tamoxifen-resistant cell lines. Moreover, following their prominent inhibition by tamoxifen during the initial responsive phase of the disease, estrogen-regulated genes can be re-expressed on disease relapse in the clinic.

What might be the mechanisms that enable the inhibitory activity of tamoxifen to be circumvented on relapse despite an apparently retained importance for ERα evidenced by response to subsequent endocrine challenge? Phenotypic changes in ERα or growth factor signalling pathways may again be highly relevant. These changes may be induced/selected for during tamoxifen challenge of initially responsive breast cancer cells. In marked contrast to de novo resistant ERα-positive disease, the aberrant pathways in such acquired resistance must interact with, and remain dependent on, functional ERα in order to exhibit second-line responses. Such aberrations appear often to be able to exert positive actions on estrogen-regulated genes, since these are still detectable in a proportion (about 50%) of patients on relapse. The aberrations may even alter the cellular interpretation of tamoxifen so that an agonistic profile is prominent on relapse that is re-inhibited by challenge with an alternative endocrine agent. This agonism is perhaps evidenced by the increased growth rate, occasional tamoxifen withdrawal responses,[185] and the re-expression of estrogen-regulated genes on disease relapse in the clinic.[58] Indeed, the use of tamoxifen as a positive growth input in tumours has been elegantly demonstrated using breast cancer xenograft material.[186,187]

Finally, however, it should be remembered that 40–50% of initially responsive ERα-positive patients are completely resistant to second-line endocrine challenge. As with ERα-positive de novo resistance, it is feasible that there may be selection by tamoxifen therapy of an unresponsive ERα-positive subpopulation that is already present at a very low frequency in the responsive phase of the disease or alternatively may develop as part of a backdrop of mutational/adaptive events in the cancer cells during tamoxifen challenge. These cells may bear aberrations in the relevant crosstalking pathways downstream of ERα (e.g. in cell cycle components or tumour suppressor genes) or within ERα-independent pathways. It is also perhaps feasible that aberrations in signalling elements upstream of ERα might be so extreme as to enable entire growth dislocation from this receptor.

ERα variants, mutations, and ERβ in tamoxifen resistance

Tumour cells overexpressing certain ERα variants or mutations could feasibly escape inhibition by tamoxifen if their ligand-binding domain were compromised. If constitutively active, such aberrant forms might contribute to clinical tamoxifen resistance. Indeed, Zhang et al[188] have identified an ERα mutant with a substitution of tyrosine 537 with asparagine (Tyr537Asn) in clinical metastatic breast tumours. Experimental studies indicate that this mutant is constitutively active and is only minimally affected by antihormones. Levenson et al[189] have similarly identified a naturally occurring ERα mutant (codon 351 asparagine → tyrosine in the ligand-binding domain) that appears to confer increased estrogenic activity on raloxifene. Furthermore, the ERα δ5 variant has been localized at the mRNA level within clinical breast cancer. This variant is reported to exhibit constitutive activity in vitro, since it retains DNA-binding ability and AF-1 transcriptional activity,[190] and, since it lacks a major portion of the ligand-binding domain, has been predicted to escape SERM growth inhibition. In this light, Gallacchi et al[191] demonstrated that higher ratios of the ERα variant δ5 mRNA do appear to be associated with clinical acquired tamoxifen resistance. However, a significant role for such aberrations in de novo and acquired tamoxifen resistance appears in general unlikely from such mRNA studies.[66,192] Mutations are extremely rare in vivo[193] and the mRNA species are barely detectable yet apparently ubiquitous. Similarly, our own group has recently failed to demonstrate a relationship between expression of the ERα variant δ5 at a protein level and clinical de novo tamoxifen resistance. In summary, it is likely that such events at best contribute towards only a minority of tamoxifen-resistance cases.[194]

Unfortunately, there are virtually no clinical data available regarding the role of ERβ in tamoxifen resistance. Studies principally examining mRNA expression for this receptor have demonstrated that expression is generally very low, which may indicate a lack of significance in tumours for this receptor with regard to resistance. Nevertheless, our own group[63] and Speirs et al[195] have shown that *ERβ* mRNA expression does appear to be associated with increased tumour grade, while some increases in *ERβ* mRNA expression have been tentatively associated with the development of tamoxifen resistance.[62,196] In addition, the ERα : ERβ ratio may change through disease progression,[197,198] so that extremes are reached in ERα-negative disease, with its more obvious ERβ expression.[63] Such relationships remain highly controversial.[64] It is feasible that increased expression of the additional estrogen receptor ERβ may contribute to breast cancer tamoxifen resistance in a number of ways. ERβ is homologous to ERα in the ligand-binding domain (58%) and the DNA-binding domain (96%), while the A/B region, hinge, and F region are not well conserved.[199] Changes in the F domain would be predicted to significantly influence the control of the agonist/antagonist properties of tamoxifen under conditions of increased ERβ expression.[200] Such shifts in the balance of ERβ : ERα would potentially favour receptor heterodimerization. This would recruit a unique profile of response elements and modify the readout from response elements usually targeted by ERα homodimers, thereby potentially priming tumour growth in the presence of tamoxifen. In addition, different co-accessory proteins and crosstalking growth factor pathways would be predicted to interact with ERβ, enabling gene transactivation in the presence of tamoxifen.[197,201]

ERα co-accessory proteins in tamoxifen resistance

Alterations in the co-accessory protein ratio or activity in breast cancer cells are likely to significantly influence the agonistic/antagonistic properties of tamoxifen – a process that may contribute towards resistance to antihormonal agents such as tamoxifen.[202,203] In this light, changes in the co-accessory proteins N-CoR and SRC-1 have been observed following the acquisition of tamoxifen resistance both in a murine breast cancer model[204] and in the clinic.[71]

Modification of the ERE in tamoxifen resistance

Modification of the ERE by sequence variation, number, orientation, or spacing influences the binding affinity of the ligand/ERα complex as well as the transcriptional response to various ligands.[205–207] In vitro studies performed in the laboratory of McDonnell[206] have indicated that such changes may permit ERα agonism by antiestrogens such as tamoxifen. In addition, deletion and mutational analyses have revealed a specific *cis* element within the distal promoter of the progesterone receptor that modulates its

sensitivity to tamoxifen inhibition.[208] The relevance of these phenomena to tamoxifen resistance in vivo remains unknown.

Pharmacological changes in cellular levels and metabolic profile of tamoxifen

Impaired uptake and increased degradation of tamoxifen, the possibility of a drug-efflux pump, isomerization to estrogenic metabolites such as metabolite E and bisphenol, or accumulation of the less potent antiestrogenic *cis*-4-hydroxytamoxifen rather than the *trans* isomer are all mechanisms that have been suggested to result in diminished tamoxifen inhibition of ERα-mediated gene expression and hence tumour growth.[209] While these mechanisms have been implicated both in de novo and acquired resistance, their role in these processes has been convincingly questioned.[209-214] Similarly, the observation made by Pavlik et al[215] of excessive type II antiestrogen binding-site expression within some breast cancers, which could effectively partition tamoxifen away from the estrogen receptor, remains to be corroborated.

Changes in growth factor signalling elements in clinical de novo and acquired tamoxifen resistance

ErbB signalling elements

As detailed above, examination of the clinical and experimental phenotype of CR/PR tamoxifen-responsive disease points to a preference for c-ErbB3/4-mediated signalling in such tumours, with the pathway crosstalking with ERα in mitogenesis. In stark contrast, however, there appears to be a significant reduction in expression of the ErbB family members c-ErbB3/4 in ERα-negative and ERα-positive, de novo tamoxifen-unresponsive breast cancer versus responsive disease.[95] Moreover, there is increasing phenotypic evidence to indicate that substantial autocrine TGF-α/EGFR (and possibly c-ErbB2) signalling regulates growth of de novo and acquired tamoxifen resistant breast cancer.[11,80,81,83,84] Such aberrant growth factor signalling is likely to prime increased Erk1/2-mediated signalling. There is likely to be new crosstalk of such signalling with ERα in patients with acquired resistant disease, since many exhibit second-line responses. Indeed, Erk1/2 may phosphorylate AF-1 and hence activate ERα,[79] resulting in inappropriate gene transactivation and tamoxifen-resistant growth.

Ninety-five percent of ERα-negative, de novo tamoxifen-unresponsive breast cancers exhibit marked EGFR membrane immunostaining, while c-ErbB2 is overexpressed in about 40% (Figure 10.3b,c).[11,80,81,84] Such features are associated with aggressive disease and extremely poor patient survival characteristics in the clinic.[11,80,81,84] Importantly, a positive correlation can be demonstrated between the levels of proliferation and EGFR immunostaining in ERα-negative clinical material, with c-ErbB2 levels in ERα-negative/c-ErbB2-positive disease similarly being associated with Ki67 immunostaining.[80,81] As further confirmation of the importance of functional EGFR signalling, tumour epithelial expression of the EGFR ligand TGF-α is higher in EGFR-positive/ERα-negative tumours than in ERα-positive CR/PR disease.[80,81,83] Indeed, substantial positivity for TGF-α is a feature of about 70% of ERα-negative patients.

While substantial overexpression of c-ErbB2 and EGFR equivalent to that observed in ERα-negative patients does not generally underlie ERα-positive de novo tamoxifen resistance, nevertheless it is interesting that those patients (about 35%) who do show elevated expression of EGFR exhibit increased tumour mitotic activity and a poorer prognosis.[11,80,81,84] Our recent data indicate that where EGFR is elevated in ERα-positive clinical disease, it may be associated with ERβ co-expression, perhaps reflecting an inter-relationship of these elements in the circumvention of antihormonal sensitivity.[63] Rigorous exclusion of ERα-negative patients reveals that the relationship between c-ErbB2 overexpression and prognosis is more controversial in ERα-positive tumours, while associations with resistance may differ between antihormonal strategies.[11,80–82,216] However, elevated TGFα expression[83] is a feature commonly noted

(in about 90% of cases), where there is an association with proliferation.[83] These data again indicate that elevated expression of this peptide growth factor may be an autocrine driving force underlying the growth of ERα-positive, de novo tamoxifen-resistant tumours independently from their endocrine environment.[34–36,83]

As noted in de novo resistant disease, there is evidence of an increased importance for TGF-α/EGFR/c-ErbB2 in acquired resistance. We have observed that common tumour phenotypic features on tamoxifen relapse apparent with highly sensitive immunocytochemical assays include elevated tumour epithelial expression both of TGF-α and of EGFR,[35] although it is notable that the increases observed do not reach the levels seen in ERα-negative de novo resistance. Amplification of the c-erbB2 gene has also been observed.[217] These data complement in vitro gene-transfer studies[78,218–222] and the phenotypic profile observed in acquired tamoxifen-resistance models.[187,223–225] Enhanced EGFR/c-ErbB2 expression in acquired tamoxifen resistance may initially evolve during response to therapy as a consequence of the inverse relationship between such signalling and estrogen/ERα occupancy.[35,86–88,90] In this light, we have observed small increases in EGFR and c-ErbB2 expression during clinical response to tamoxifen in parallel with inhibition of ERα/ERE signalling.[35,58]

IGF signalling elements

There remains a controversial relationship between expression of IGF signalling elements and tamoxifen resistance. With regard to ERα-positive disease, the observation of IGF1-R upregulation observed occasionally in experimental tamoxifen resistance remain inconclusive.[225–227] Moreover, in vitro gene-transfer studies with IGF1-R or IRS-1 have demonstrated relationships with estrogen independence alone.[120] However, higher levels of IRS-1 have been reported to predict for a higher incidence of recurrence in ERα-positive patients,[107] while overexpression of Akt (PKB) is reported to protect against tamoxifen-induced apoptosis in vitro.[228]

For ERα-negative disease, IGF-II has been reported to be constitutively expressed in vitro.[229] In addition, IGFBP3 appears to be particularly prominent in ERα-negative, high S-phase, aneuploid tumours with an associated poor prognosis,[107,230] while increased IGF1-R expression has been associated with shortened disease-free survival in such patients.[102]

Fibroblast growth factor (FGF) signalling
The fibroblast growth factor (FGF) family is highly complex, with at least 10 genes encoding growth factor ligands for several FGF receptors. FGF-1 (acidic FGF) and FGF-2 (basic FGF) are perhaps the most ubiquitously expressed in clinical breast cancer.[231] There is a highly controversial relationship regarding FGF expression in normal breast versus cancer, growth factor source, and patient survival. Moreover, while FGF-2 signalling has been reported to interact with estrogen- and IGF-mediated growth in MCF-7 cells,[232] there is no literature monitoring FGF expression and response to tamoxifen. Overexpression of FGF-1 or FGF-4 has been related to acquisition of tamoxifen resistance in breast cancer model systems,[233–235] but this phenomena remains to be examined in the clinic. Since such overexpression is reported to allow development of tumours in ovariectomized animals treated with the pure antiestrogen fulvestrant,[234] it is likely that experimental FGF-mediated resistance occurs independently of ERα activation.

Intracellular signalling elements
PKC
In contrast to tamoxifen-responsive disease, the principle PKC isoform expressed in ERα-negative de novo unresponsive breast cancer cell lines appears to be PKCα,[236] with our recent observations furthermore indicating that PKCα is particularly prominent in ERα-negative, de novo resistant clinical disease. In contrast, we have observed only minimal expression of the PKCδ isozyme in such cells in vitro and in de novo tamoxifen-resistant breast cancer clinical material.[128] Morever, it has been demonstrated that transfection of PKCα into MCF-7 breast

cancer cells markedly enhances their proliferation, in parallel with diminished PKCδ and ERα content[237] and steroid hormone independence.[238] The PKC expression profile in acquired tamoxifen resistance in the clinic remains unknown.

MAP kinase family members
There is an increasing body of evidence to indicate that elevated activation of Erk1/2 is associated with de novo tamoxifen resistance, as exemplified by our own clinical studies, where we have also observed an association with poor survival and a shortened time to disease progression.[130,131] Indeed, hyperexpression/activity of MAP kinase has been noted in many breast cancers in vivo,[239] in parallel with additional intracellular molecules that comprise/regulate the MAP kinase signalling pathway. These include pp60[c-Src,240,241] Grb2,[242] RHAMM,[243] Ras,[244,245] Raf,[246] and PKC.[136,247] Since Erk1/2 is a key component of EGFR signalling,[248] it is perhaps not surprising that activation is particularly marked in 90% of ERα-negative, de novo tamoxifen-unresponsive tumours in the clinic.[130,131] There is similarly enhanced activity of Erk1/2 in about 80% of ERα-positive de novo progressive tumours that also demonstrate evidence of elevated TGF-α/EGFR signalling.[130,131]

With regard to acquired resistance, the reported ability of Erk1/2 to phosphorylate the AF-1 region of ERα and induce estrogen-regulated gene expression experimentally[79] might feasibly serve to sustain tamoxifen-resistant tumour growth if Erk1/2 activation were increased by aberrant growth factor signalling (Figure 10.5). Interestingly, therefore, elevated activation of Erk1/2 has been noted in acquired endocrine resistance in vitro,[222,249–251] including in our own panel of endocrine-resistant MCF-7 sublines. Moreover, we have recently observed increased Erk1/2 activation in clinical material at the time of acquisition of tamoxifen resistance and disease relapse in ERα-positive, initially responsive disease.

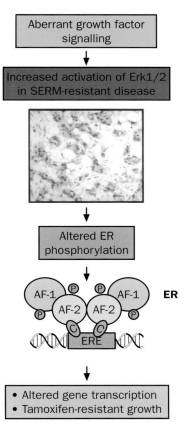

Figure 10.5 Aberrant growth factor signalling leading to increased activation of the MAP kinases Erk1/2 in altered ER phosphorylation, and tamoxifen-resistant tumour growth.

cAMP and PKA

Little is known regarding the role of the cAMP/PKA pathway in tamoxifen resistance. While experimental enhancement of the cAMP/PKA pathway may feasibly serve to increase the agonism of tamoxifen and promote tamoxifen resistance,[135] to date PKA expression has only been associated with an endocrine-responsive phenotype in the clinic.[137]

AP-1

Elevated expression/activity of key components of the AP-1 nuclear transcription factor complex appears to relate significantly to

tamoxifen resistance in clinical breast cancer. Thus, both c-Fos and activated c-Jun are expressed at high levels in ERα-negative and ERα-positive de novo tamoxifen resistance.[53,139,140] c-Jun overexpression has similarly been related to endocrine resistance in vitro.[252] Interestingly, increased expression/activation of AP-1 components appears to parallel TGF-α/EGFR overexpression in such tumours.[140] These data certainly indicate that enhanced AP-1 signalling may play a central role in the aberrant TGF-α/EGFR-mediated growth that appears obligatory to those tumours dislocated from ERα signalling. Indeed, at its extremes, such enhanced AP-1 signalling may inhibit ERα expression and estrogen-regulated gene transactivation.[253]

Similarly, it is likely that AP-1 is exaggerated in acquired tamoxifen resistance in the clinic.[53] We have observed increased c-Fos expression at the time of tamoxifen relapse of ERα-positive disease, data paralleling the increased AP-1 DNA-binding activity observed in acquired tamoxifen-resistant breast cancer cells in vitro[254] and in relapse material in vivo.[48] In addition, prolonged tamoxifen exposure has been reported to augment phorbol-ester-inducible TRE activity experimentally.[255,256] It is postulated that such enhanced AP-1 activity interacts positively with ERα signalling via protein–protein interactions to markedly increase transactivation of TRE-containing, growth-related genes, thereby allowing escape from tamoxifen inhibition and ultimately disease relapse (Figure 10.6). There may be additional modifying effects of ERβ expression on this profile, since both tamoxifen and raloxifene are reported to be potent transcriptional activators of TREs via interactions between AP-1 and this receptor.[257]

TGF-β signalling elements

TGF-β1 mRNA has paradoxically been reported in a small number of studies to be increased in highly proliferative, metastatic tumours[258] and in tamoxifen-unresponsive disease in the clinic.[149] Several in vitro studies appear to parallel these data for both TGF-β1 and TGF-β2.

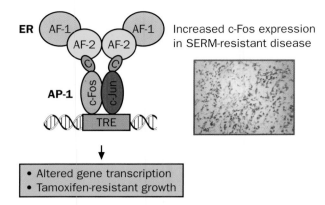

Figure 10.6 Increased c-Fos expression leading to tamoxifen-resistant tumour growth via AP-1/ER interaction.

Thus, Herman and Katzenellenbogen[259] noted that their tamoxifen-resistant MCF-7 subline produced more TGF-Bs and was resistant to exogenous TGF-βs. Increased expression is also seen in ERα-negative cell lines,[260] in LCC2 tamoxifen-resistant cells,[141,261] and in endocrine-unresponsive MCF-7 cells generated by v-Ha-*ras* transfection.[262] In addition, transfection of TGF-β1 into MCF-7 cells generated tumours in vivo that were estrogen-independent, with their growth being inhibited by an anti-pan-TGF-β neutralizing antibody, while tamoxifen resistance in LCC2 cells is reversible in vivo using such antibodies to target TGF-β2 overexpression.[141,261] In total, these data indicate that the ability of TGF-β to inhibit growth is likely to be lost, and that there may even be a switch to a positive influence of this growth factor, during disease progression.

Changes in cell cycle components and tumour suppressors in clinical de novo and acquired tamoxifen resistance

A highly proliferative profile is exhibited by most de novo resistant tumours in the clinic.[8,9] Thus, it is likely that key growth regulators are severely perturbed in such tumours, as evidenced by frequent genetic and epigenetic aberrations in cell cycle proteins and their regulators, as well as marked nuclear pleomorphism. The role of such changes in acquired resistance remains as yet unknown, although there is certainly increased proliferation on disease relapse.[53]

The *CCND1* gene encodes the cyclin D1 protein, which, when complexed to certain cyclin-dependent kinases (CDKs), controls cell cycle progression through G_1/S. Aberrant transcriptional/translational regulation of cyclin D1 is relatively common in breast tumours,[263] with cyclin D1 being overexpressed in about 50% of breast cancers and *CCND1* gene amplification occurring in 15–20%. *CCND1* amplification and overexpression of cyclin D1 have been directly related to ERα positivity (in agreement with its suggested role as an ERα cofactor)[264] and more controversially[265] with a poorer prognosis in breast cancer.[27,266] Thus, a high cyclin D1 level may be associated with a shortened endocrine response duration within the ERα-positive subgroup. Moreover, ectopic overexpression of cyclin D1 appears to allow unrestricted passage through the cell cycle and reverse the growth-inhibitory activity of tamoxifen in ERα-positive cells in vitro.[267] A similar association has been noted between cyclin E1 (a late G_1 cyclin again associated with progression through G_1/S) and an aggressive tumour phenotype and poor prognosis,[268] although the relationship is likely to be derived principally from ERα-negative disease.[269]

A variety of CDK inhibitors (CDIs) compete with cyclins for binding of CDKs to prevent progression through G_1/S, thus potentially acting as tumour suppressors. Loss of such mitogenic 'brakes' by genetic mutation or alternatively by post-transcriptional events such as increased degradation may prove to be a feature of some de novo tamoxifen-resistant tumours. Targets include members of the Cip/Kip protein family (notably p21[WAF1/Cip1] and p27[Kip1]), as well as the INK4 family (notably p16[INK4A]). While relationships with tamoxifen response remain to be substantiated, we have noted loss of p21 expression in poor-prognosis breast cancers in the clinic.[25] A similar relationship has been reported between low p27 expression, increased tumour grade, poorer outlook, and, additionally, hormone independence, although the relationship between p27 and prognosis using multivariate analysis remains controversial.[270–273] Inactivation of the *p16* gene by methylation has been observed in breast cancer, with an inverse relationship reported between p16[INK4A] and ERα gene expression.[274]

The p53 tumour suppressor protein functions in cell cycle control as a key mediator of differentiation, DNA repair, and apoptosis. p53 aberrations are relatively common in breast cancer (25–50% at a protein level and 15–35% at a DNA level), causing loss of normal p53 function or dominant-negative activity. As a consequence, there is disruption of the G_1/S checkpoint, loss of apoptosis in response to DNA damage, and ultimately increased genomic instability.[275] Prominent immunostaining identifies mutated p53, since the mutant protein has an extended half-life. Our co-examination of p53 and p21[WAF1] expression indicates the likelihood of such prominent p53 being non-functional as a tumour suppressor in poor-prognosis tumours.[25] Increased p53 staining associates with an aggressive, highly proliferative phenotype, ERα negativity, and poor patient survival. Aberrant p53 accumulation has, moreover, been reported to predict for poor clinical response to tamoxifen therapy,[23,24] with patients with gene mutations in codons that directly contact DNA or with mutations in the L3 domain showing the lowest response to tamoxifen.[276] Such prognostic data, however, remain controversial.[216] Finally, expression of the additional tumour suppressor gene *BRCA1* is often lower within ERα-negative cancers and occasionally genomically deleted.[26,277]

CONCLUDING REMARKS

It is apparent that considerable progress has already been made in identifying the signal transduction pathways that may be of central importance on SERM-responsive and -resistant breast cancer in the clinic, with substantial data available for tamoxifen, the SERM prototype in breast cancer. It is hoped that further expansion of our knowledge of these phenotypes using research technologies such as gene microarrays and proteomics, coupled with detailed pharmacological, cell biological, and molecular analysis of relevant model systems, will ultimately aid progress in many aspects of the clinical management of breast cancer. For example, more accurate stratification of patients for appropriate treatment should be feasible – a feature that will be essential if endocrine therapies are to be directed towards earlier stages of the disease, where treatment responses are not readily monitorable. In particular, however, since such knowledge contributes significantly towards the precise delineation of those signal transduction pathways involved in the development of de novo and acquired resistance, elucidation of novel targets for drug development should also be possible. Existing phenotypic data suggest that relevant strategies might be to inhibit steroid hormone receptor signalling more efficiently, or to nullify unwanted growth factor signalling and aberrant cell cycle regulation. In this light, several promising pharmacological agents are already in clinical trials.

Complete loss of estrogen-like activity of antiestrogens has recently been achieved through the development of steroidal 'pure' antiestrogens based on 7α substitutions of estradiol (fulvestrant[38,278] and ICI 164,384) currently in phase III breast cancer clinical trials. These compounds have been termed SERDs (selective estrogen receptor downregulators), since they increase ERα protein degradation and disrupt nucleocytoplasmic shuttling of the receptor and nuclear localization. The resultant dramatic loss of ERα protein (Figure 10.7) effectively blocks transactivation of ERα-regulated genes both in vitro and in clinical breast cancer,[279] and would be predicted to eliminate any ERα-mediated mitogenic 'cross-talk'. Not surprisingly, therefore, these agents are significantly more potent than tamoxifen at

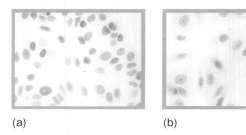

(a)   (b)

Figure 10.7 Inhibitory effect of fulvestrant (ICI 182,780, Faslodex) versus tamoxifen on ER protein in breast cancer in vitro: (a) tamoxifen; (b) fulvestrant.

promoting tumour remissions in several models of endocrine-sensitive and acquired resistant disease,[93,94,280,281] and, moreover, have efficacy in tamoxifen-refractory patients.[181] Such desirable ERα loss may also be a feature of 11β substitutions of estradiol,[282] as well as of the novel nonsteroidal benzopyran derivative EM-652 and its prodrug EM-800, which interestingly are reported to additionally be antagonistic to ERβ signalling.[283] There is similarly exciting progress with regard to targeting of aberrant growth factor receptor signalling – specifically that driven by the ErbB tyrosine kinase receptors c-ErbB2 and EGFR. Phase II clinical trials with a recombinant humanized antibody that produces anti-tumour effects by blocking the c-ErbB2 receptor (trastuzumab, Herceptin) performed on node-positive breast cancer patients showed an overall response rate of about 12%.[284] Preliminary data from Phase III studies indicate a 15% response rate in metastatic breast cancer treated using this antibody, with the agent demonstrating additive benefits with chemotherapy.[285,286] EGFR-selective tyrosine kinase inhibitors are in phase I/II clinical cancer trials, and have proved to be potent growth inhibitors in EGFR-overexpressing tumour cells in vitro and also capable of effectively instigating programmed cell death and inhibiting invasion.[287–289] Finally, the CDI flavopiridol (NSC 649890, HMR1275), reported to enable G_1 arrest and inhibit CDK2/4 in a range of breast cancer cells in

vitro,[290] is also in phase II clinical cancer trials. It is hoped that such agents might delay the appearance of, treat, or even reverse SERM resistance, thereby severely compromising the disease process.

REFERENCES

1. Mitlak BH, Cohen FJ. Selective estrogen receptor modulators: a look ahead. *Drugs* 1999; **57:** 653–63.

2. Baum M. Tamoxifen. *Endocr Rel Cancer* 1997; **4:** 237–43.

3. Cheung KL, Willsher PC, Pinder SE et al. Predictors of response to second-line endocrine therapy for breast cancer. *Breast Cancer Res Treat* 1997; **45:** 219–24.

4. Early Breast Cancer Trialists' Collaborative Group. Tamoxifen for early breast cancer: an overview of the randomised trials. *Lancet* 1998; **351:** 1451–67.

5. Nicholson RI, Wilson DW, Richards G et al. Biological and clinical aspects of oestrogen receptor measurements in rapidly progressing breast cancer. In: *Proceedings of IUPHAR 9th International Congress of Pharmacology*, Vol 3 (Paton W, Mitchell J, Turner P, eds). London: Macmillan, 1984: 75–9.

6. Williams MR, Todd JH, Nicholson RI et al. Survival patterns in hormone treated advanced breast cancer. *Br J Surg* 1986; **73:** 752–5.

7. Williams MR, Blamey RW, Todd JH et al. Histological grade in predicting response to endocrine treatment. *Breast Cancer Res Treat* 1986; **8:** 165–6.

8. Bouzubar N, Walker KJ, Griffiths K et al. Ki67 immunostaining in primary breast cancer: pathological and clinical associations. *Br J Cancer* 1989; **59:** 943–7.

9. Nicholson RI, Bouzubar N, Walker KJ et al. Hormone sensitivity in breast cancer: influence of heterogeneity of oestrogen receptor expression and cell proliferation. *Eur J Cancer* 1991; **27:** 908–13.

10. Locker AP, Birrell K, Bell JA et al. Ki67 immunoreactivity in breast carcinoma: relationships to prognostic variables and short term survival. *Eur J Surg Oncol* 1992; **18:** 224–9.

11. Nicholson RI, McClelland RA, Finlay P et al. Relationship between EGF-R, c-erbB-2 protein

expression and Ki67 immunostaining in breast cancer and hormone sensitivity. *Eur J Cancer* 1993; **29A:** 1018–23.

12. Skoog L, Rutqvist LE, Wilking N. Analysis of hormone receptors and proliferation fraction in fine-needle aspirates from primary breast carcinomas during chemotherapy or tamoxifen treatment. *Acta Oncol* 1992; **31:** 139–41.

13. Clarke RB, Laidlaw IJ, Jones LJ et al. Effect of tamoxifen on Ki67 labelling index in human breast tumours and its relationship to oestrogen and progesterone receptor status. *Br J Cancer* 1993; **67:** 606–11.

14. Maas RA, Bruning PF, Top B et al. Growth arrest associated changes of mRNA levels in breast cancer cells measured by semi-quantitative RT-PCR: potential early indicators of treatment response. *Cancer Lett* 1995; **97:** 107–16.

15. Keen JC, Dixon JM, Miller EP et al. The expression of Ki-S1 and BCL-2 and the response to primary tamoxifen therapy in elderly patients with breast cancer. *Breast Cancer Res Treat* 1997; **44:** 123–33.

16. Gee JMW, Robertson JFR, Ellis IO et al. Immunohistochemical analysis reveals a tumour suppressor-like role for the transcription factor AP-2 in invasive breast cancer. *J Pathol* 1999; **189:** 514–20.

17. Cameron DA, Keen JC, Dixon JM et al. Effective tamoxifen therapy of breast cancer involves both antiproliferative and pro-apoptotic changes. *Eur J Cancer* 2000; **36:** 845–51.

18. Warri AM, Huovinen RL, Laine AM et al. Apoptosis in toremifene-induced growth inhibition of human breast cancer cells in vivo and in vitro. *J Natl Cancer Inst* 1993; **85:** 1412–18.

19. Johnston SR, Boeddinghaus IM, Riddler S et al. Idoxifene antagonizes estradiol-dependent MCF-7 breast cancer xenograft growth through sustained induction of apoptosis. *Cancer Res* 1999; **59:** 3646–51.

20. Manning DL, Nicholson RI, Eaton CL. The role of oestrogens and growth factors in the aetiology of breast cancer. In: *Recent Advances in Endocrinology and Metabolism*, Vol 4 (Edwards CRW, Lincoln DW, eds). Edinburgh: Churchill Livingstone, 1992: 133–50.

21. Gee JMW, McClelland RA, Nicholson RI. Growth factors and endocrine sensitivity in breast cancer. In: *Molecular and Clinical Endocrinology* (Pasqualini JR, Katzenellenbogen

BS, eds). New York: Marcel Dekker, 1996: 169–97.

22. Nicholson RI, Gee JMW. Growth factors and modulation of endocrine response in breast cancer. In: *Hormones and Cancer* (Vedeckis WV, ed). Boston: Birkhäuser, 1996: 227–61.

23. Silvestrini R, Benini E, Veneroni S et al. p53 and bcl-2 expression correlates with clinical outcome in a series of node-positive breast cancer patients. *J Clin Oncol* 1996; **14:** 1604–10.

24. Berns EM, Klijn JG, van Putten WL et al. p53 protein accumulation predicts poor response to tamoxifen therapy of patients with recurrent breast cancer. *Clin Oncol* 1998; **16:** 121–7.

25. McClelland RA, Gee JM, O'Sullivan L et al. p21(WAF1) expression and endocrine response in breast cancer. *J Pathol* 1999; **188:** 126–32.

26. Seery LT, Knowlden JM, Gee JM et al. BRCA1 expression levels predict distant metastasis of sporadic breast cancers. *Int J Cancer* 1999; **84:** 258–62.

27. Kenny FS, Hui R, Musgrove EA et al. Overexpression of cyclin D1 messenger RNA predicts for poor prognosis in estrogen receptor-positive breast cancer. *Clin Cancer Res* 1999; **5:** 2069–76.

28. Gee JM, Robertson JF, Ellis IO et al. Immunocytochemical localization of BCL-2 protein in human breast cancers and its relationship to a series of prognostic markers and response to endocrine therapy. *Int J Cancer* 1994; **59:** 619–28.

29. Kobayashi S, Iwase H, Ito Y et al. Clinical significance of bcl-2 gene expression in human breast cancer tissues. *Breast Cancer Res Treat* 1997; **42:** 173–81.

30. Watts CK, Sweeney KJ, Warlters A et al. Antiestrogen regulation of cell cycle progression and cyclin D1 gene expression in MCF-7 human breast cancer cells. *Breast Cancer Res Treat* 1994; **31:** 95–105.

31. Kenny, FS, Willsher PC, Gee JMW et al. Change in expression of ER and bcl-2 predicts for quality and duration of response in endocrine sensitive breast cancer. *Eur J Cancer* 1998; **34:** S18.

32. Zhang GJ, Kimijima I, Onda M et al. Tamoxifen-induced apoptosis in breast cancer cells relates to down-regulation of bcl-2, but not bax and bcl-X(L), without alteration of p53 protein levels. *Clin Cancer Res* 1999; **5:** 2971–7.

33. Grasser WA, Pan LC, Thompson DD, Paralkar VM. Common mechanism for the estrogen

agonist and antagonist activities of droloxifene. *J Cell Biochem* 1997; **65:** 159–71.

34. Nicholson RI, McClelland RA, Robertson JF, Gee JM. Involvement of steroid hormone and growth factor cross-talk in endocrine response in breast cancer. *Endocr Rel Cancer* 1999; **6:** 373–87.

35. Nicholson RI, Hutcheson IR, Harper ME et al. Modulation of epidermal growth factor receptor in endocrine resistant, oestrogen receptor-positive breast cancer. *Endocr Relat Cancer* 2001; **8:** 175–82.

36. Nicholson RI, Gee JM. Oestrogen and growth factor cross-talk and endocrine insensitivity and acquired resistance in breast cancer. *Br J Cancer* 2000; **82:** 501–13.

37. Seery LT, Gee JMW, Dewhurst OL, Nicholson RI. Molecular mechanisms of antioestrogen action. In: *Pharmacological Handbook* (Oettel M, Schillinger E, eds). Berlin: Springer-Verlag, 1999: 201–20.

38. Wakeling AE, Bowler J. ICI 182,780, a new antioestrogen with clinical potential. *J Steroid Biochem Mol Biol* 1992; **43:** 173–7.

39. Favoni RE, De Cupis A. The role of polypeptide growth factors in human carcinomas: new targets for a novel pharmacological approach. *Pharmacol Rev* 2000; **52:** 179–206.

40. Robertson JF. Oestrogen receptor: a stable phenotype in breast cancer. *Br J Cancer* 1996; **73:** 5–12.

41. Robertson JF, Bates K, Pearson D et al. Comparison of two oestrogen receptor assays in the prediction of the clinical course of patients with advanced breast cancer. *Br J Cancer* 1992; **65:** 727–30.

42. Robertson JF, Cannon PM, Nicholson RI, Blamey RW. Oestrogen and progesterone receptors as prognostic variables in hormonally treated breast cancer. *Int J Biol Mark* 1996; **11:** 29–35.

43. Koenders PG, Beex LV, Langens R et al. Steroid hormone receptor activity of primary human breast cancer and pattern of first metastasis. The Breast Cancer Study Group. *Breast Cancer Res Treat* 1991; **18:** 27–32.

44. Leake R. Prediction of hormone sensitivity – the receptor years and onwards. *Endocr Rel Cancer* 1997; **4:** 289–96.

45. Berger U, Wilson P, McClelland RA et al. Correlation of immunocytochemically demonstrated estrogen receptor distribution and histopathologic features in primary breast cancer. *Hum Pathol* 1987; **18:** 1263–7.

46. Perry JJ, Berry DA, Weiss RB et al. High dose toremifene for estrogen and progesterone receptor negative metastatic breast cancer: a phase II trial of the Cancer and Leukemia Group B (CALGB). *Breast Cancer Res Treat* 1995; **36:** 35–40.

47. Vogel CL. Phase II and III clinical trials of toremifene for metastatic breast cancer. *Oncology (Huntingt)* 1998; **12**(3 Suppl 5): 9–13.

48. Johnston SR, Lu B, Scott GK et al. Increased activator protein-1 DNA binding and c-Jun NH2-terminal kinase activity in human breast tumors with acquired tamoxifen resistance. *Clin Cancer Res* 1999; **5:** 251–6.

49. Castagnetta L, Traina A, Di Carlo A et al. Heterogeneity of soluble and nuclear oestrogen receptor status of involved nodes in relation to primary breast cancer. *Eur J Cancer Clin Oncol* 1987; **23:** 31–5.

50. Rutqvist LE, Cedermark B, Glas U et al. The Stockholm trial on adjuvant tamoxifen in early breast cancer. Correlation between estrogen receptor level and treatment effect. *Breast Cancer Res Treat* 1987; **10:** 255–66.

51. Valavaara R, Tuominen J, Johansson R. Predictive value of tumor estrogen and progesterone receptor levels in postmenopausal women with advanced breast cancer treated with toremifene. *Cancer* 1990; **66:** 2264–9.

52. Jeng MH, Shupnik MA, Bender TP et al. Estrogen receptor expression and function in long-term estrogen-deprived human breast cancer cells. *Endocrinology* 1998; **139:** 4164–74.

53. Gee JM, Willsher PC, Kenny FS et al. Endocrine response and resistance in breast cancer: a role for the transcription factor Fos. *Int J Cancer* 1999; **84:** 54–61.

54. Manning DL, McClelland RA, Gee JM et al. The role of four oestrogen-responsive genes, pLIV1, pS2, pSYD3 and pSYD8, in predicting responsiveness to endocrine therapy in primary breast cancer. *Eur J Cancer* 1993; **29A:** 1462–8.

55. Wilson YG, Rhodes M, Ibrahim NB et al. Immunocytochemical staining of pS2 protein in fine-needle aspirate from breast cancer is an accurate guide to response to tamoxifen in patients aged over 70 years. *Br J Surg* 1994; **81:** 1155–8.

56. Knowlden JM, Gee JM, Bryant S et al. Use of reverse transcription–polymerase chain reaction methodology to detect estrogen-regulated gene

expression in small breast cancer specimens. *Clin Cancer Res* 1997; **3**: 2165–72.

57. McClelland RA, Manning DL, Gee JM et al. Oestrogen-regulated genes in breast cancer: association of pLIV1 with response to endocrine therapy. *Br J Cancer* 1998; **77**: 1653–6.

58. Willsher PC, Gee JMW, Blamey RW et al. Changes in ER, PgR and pS2 protein during tamoxifen therapy for primary breast cancer. *Breast Cancer Res Treat* 1996, **41**: 288.

59. Hasmann M, Rattel B, Loser R. Preclinical data for droloxifene. *Cancer Lett* 1994; **84**: 101–16.

60. Ravdin PM, Green S, Dorr TM et al. Prognostic significance of progesterone receptor levels in estrogen receptor-positive patients with metastatic breast cancer treated with tamoxifen: results of a prospective Southwest Oncology Group study. *J Clin Oncol* 1992; **10**: 1284–91.

61. Howell A, Harland RN, Barnes DM et al. Endocrine therapy for advanced carcinoma of the breast: relationship between the effect of tamoxifen upon concentrations of progesterone receptor and subsequent response to treatment. *Cancer Res* 1987; **47**: 300–4.

62. Speirs V, Malone C, Walton DS et al. Increased expression of estrogen receptor β mRNA in tamoxifen-resistant breast cancer patients. *Cancer Res* 1999; **59**: 5421–4.

63. Knowlden JM, Gee JM, Robertson JF et al. A possible divergent role for the oestrogen receptor α and β subtypes in clinical breast cancer. *Int J Cancer* 2000; **89**: 209–12.

64. Jarvinen TA, Pelto-Huikko M, Holli K, Isola J. Estrogen receptor beta is coexpressed with ERα and PR and associated with nodal status, grade, and proliferation rate in breast cancer. *Am J Pathol* 2000; **156**: 29–35.

65. Fuqua SA, Allred DC, Auchus RJ. Expression of estrogen receptor variants. *J Cell Biochem Suppl* 1993; **17G**: 194–7.

66. Dowsett M, Daffada A, Chan CM, Johnston SR. Oestrogen receptor mutants and variants in breast cancer. *Eur J Cancer* 1997; **33**: 1177–83.

67. Desai AJ, Luqmani YA, Walters JE et al. Presence of exon 5-deleted oestrogen receptor in human breast cancer: functional analysis and clinical significance. *Br J Cancer* 1997; **75**: 1173–84.

68. Balleine RL, Hunt SM, Clarke CL. Coexpression of alternatively spliced estrogen and progesterone receptor transcripts in human breast cancer. *J Clin Endocrinol Metab* 1999; **84**: 1370–7.

69. deConinck EC, McPherson LA, Weigel RJ. Transcriptional regulation of estrogen receptor in breast carcinomas. *Mol Cell Biol* 1995; **15**: 2191–6.

70. McPherson LA, Baichwal VR, Weigel RJ. Identification of ERF-1 as a member of the AP2 transcription factor family. *Proc Natl Acad Sci USA* 1997; **94**: 4342–7.

71. Berns EM, van Staveren IL, Klijn JG, Foekens JA. Predictive value of SRC-1 for tamoxifen response of recurrent breast cancer. *Breast Cancer Res Treat* 1998; **48**: 87–92.

72. Bautista S, Valles H, Walker RL et al. In breast cancer, amplification of the steroid receptor coactivator gene AIB1 is correlated with estrogen and progesterone receptor positivity. *Clin Cancer Res* 1998; **4**: 2925–9.

73. Lichtner RB, Harkins RN. Signal transduction by EGF receptor tyrosine kinase. In: *EGF Receptor in Tumor Growth and Progression (Ernst Schering Research Foundation Workshop 19)* (Lichtner RB, Harkins RN, eds). Berlin: Springer-Verlag, 1997: 3–17.

74. Martinez-Lacaci I, Bianco C, De Santis M, Salomon DS. Epidermal growth factor-related peptides and their cognate receptors in breast cancer. In: *Breast Cancer: Molecular Genetics, Pathogenesis and Therapeutics* (Bowcock AM, ed). Totowa, NJ: Humana Press, 1999: 31–57.

75. Davis RJ. Transcriptional regulation by MAP kinases. *Mol Reprod Dev* 1995; **42**: 459–67.

76. English J, Pearson G, Wilsbacher J et al. New insights into the control of MAP kinase pathways. *Exp Cell Res* 1999; **253**: 255–70.

77. Wells A. Molecules in focus EGF receptor. *Int J Biochem Cell Biol* 1999; **31**: 637–43.

78. Pietras RJ, Arboleda J, Reese DM et al. HER-2 tyrosine kinase pathway targets estrogen receptor and promotes hormone-independent growth in human breast cancer cells. *Oncogene* 1995; **10**: 2435–46.

79. Bunone G, Briand PA, Miksicek RJ, Picard D. Activation of the unliganded estrogen receptor by EGF involves the MAP kinase pathway and direct phosphorylation. *EMBO J* 1996; **15**: 2174–83.

80. Nicholson RI, Gee JMW, Harper ME et al. erbB signalling in clinical breast cancer: relationship to endocrine sensitivity. *Endocr Rel Cancer* 1997; **4**: 1–9.

81. Nicholson RI, Gee JMW, Jones H et al. erbB signalling and endocrine sensitivity of human

breast cancer. In: *EGF Receptor in Tumor Growth and Progression* (*Ernst Schering Research Foundation Workshop 19*) (Lichtner RB, Harkins RN eds). Berlin: Springer-Verlag, 1997: 105–28.

82. Houston SJ, Plunkett TA, Barnes DM et al. Overexpression of c-erbB2 is an independent marker of resistance to endocrine therapy in advanced breast cancer. *Br J Cancer* 1999; **79:** 1220–6.

83. Nicholson RI, McClelland RA, Gee JM et al. Transforming growth factor-α and endocrine sensitivity in breast cancer. *Cancer Res* 1994; **54:** 1684–9.

84. Nicholson RI, McClelland RA, Gee JM et al. Epidermal growth factor receptor expression in breast cancer: association with response to endocrine therapy. *Breast Cancer Res Treat* 1994; **29:** 117–25.

85. Noguchi S, Motomura K, Inaji H et al. Down-regulation of transforming growth factor-α by tamoxifen in human breast cancer. *Cancer* 1993; **72:** 131–6.

86. Dati C, Antoniotti S, Taverna D et al. Inhibition of c-erbB-2 oncogene expression by estrogens in human breast cancer cells. *Oncogene* 1990; **5:** 1001–6.

87. Chrysogelos SA, Yarden RI, Lauber AH, Murphy JM. Mechanisms of EGF receptor regulation in breast cancer cells. *Breast Cancer Res Treat* 1994; **31:** 227–36.

88. deFazio A, Chiew YE, McEvoy M et al. Antisense estrogen receptor RNA expression increases epidermal growth factor receptor gene expression in breast cancer cells. *Cell Growth Differ* 1997; **8:** 903–11.

89. Warri AM, Laine AM, Majasuo KE et al. Estrogen suppression of erbB2 expression is associated with increased growth rate of ZR-75-1 human breast cancer cells in vitro and in nude mice. *Int J Cancer* 1991; **49:** 616–23.

90. Yarden RI, Lauber AH, El-Ashry D, Chrysogelos SA. Bimodal regulation of epidermal growth factor receptor by estrogen in breast cancer cells. *Endocrinology* 1996; **137:** 2739–47.

91. Sharma AK, Horgan K, Douglas-Jones A et al. Dual immunocytochemical analysis of oestrogen and epidermal growth factor receptors in human breast cancer. *Br J Cancer* 1994; **69:** 1032–7.

92. Arteaga CL, Coronado E, Osborne CK. Blockade of the epidermal growth factor recep-tor inhibits transforming growth factor α-induced but not estrogen-induced growth of hormone-dependent human breast cancer. *Mol Endocrinol* 1988; **2:** 1064–9.

93. Nicholson RI, Gee JM, Manning DL et al. Responses to pure antiestrogens (ICI 164384, ICI 182780) in estrogen-sensitive and -resistant experimental and clinical breast cancer. *Ann NY Acad Sci* 1995; **12:** 148–63.

94. Nicholson RI, Gee JM, Francis AB et al. Observations arising from the use of pure antioestrogens on oestrogen-responsive (MCF-7) and oestrogen growth-independent (K3) human breast cancer cells. *Endocr Rel Cancer* 1995; **2:** 115–21.

95. Knowlden JM, Gee JM, Seery LT et al. c-erbB3 and c-erbB4 expression is a feature of the endocrine responsive phenotype in clinical breast cancer. *Oncogene* 1998; **17:** 1949–57.

96. Tang CK, Concepcion XZ, Milan M et al. Ribozyme-mediated down-regulation of ErbB-4 in estrogen receptor-positive breast cancer cells inhibits proliferation both in vitro and in vivo. *Cancer Res* 1999; **59:** 5315–22.

97. Kew TY, Bell JA, Pinder SE et al. c-erbB-4 protein expression in human breast cancer. *Br J Cancer* 2000; **82:** 1163–70.

98. Ram TG, Kokeny KE, Dilts CA, Ethier SP. Mitogenic activity of neu differentiation factor/heregulin mimics that of epidermal growth factor and insulin-like growth factor-I in human mammary epithelial cells. *J Cell Physiol* 1995; **163:** 589–96.

99. Ellis MJ. The insulin-like growth factor network and breast cancer. In: *Breast Cancer: Molecular Genetics, Pathogenesis and Therapeutics* (Bowcock AM, ed). Totowa, NJ: Humana Press, 1999: 121–42.

100. Surmacz E. Function of the IGF-1 receptor in breast cancer. *J Mammary Gland Biol Neoplasia* 2000; **5:** 95–105.

101. Resnik JL, Reichart DB, Huey K et al. Elevated insulin-like growth factor I receptor autophosphorylation and kinase activity in human breast cancer. *Cancer Res* 1998; **58:** 1159–64.

102. Railo MJ, von Smitten K, Pekonen F. The prognostic value of insulin-like growth factor-I in breast cancer patients. Results of a follow-up study on 126 patients. *Eur J Cancer* 1994; **30A:** 307–11.

103. Happerfield LC, Miles DW, Barnes DM et al. The localization of the insulin-like growth fac-

tor receptor 1 (IGFR-1) in benign and malignant breast tissue. *J Pathol* 1997; **183:** 412–17.

104. Peyrat JP, Bonneterre J. Type 1 IGF receptor in human breast diseases. *Breast Cancer Res Treat* 1992; **22:** 59–67.

105. Papa V, Gliozzo B, Clark GM et al. Insulin-like growth factor-I receptors are overexpressed and predict a low risk in human breast cancer. *Cancer Res* 1993; **53:** 3736–40.

106. Toropainen EM, Lipponen PK, Syrjanen KJ. Expression of insulin-like growth factor II in female breast cancer as related to established prognostic factors and long-term prognosis. *Anticancer Res* 1995; **15:** 2669–74.

107. Rocha RL, Hilsenbeck SG, Jackson JG et al. Insulin-like growth factor binding protein-3 and insulin receptor substrate-1 in breast cancer: correlation with clinical parameters and disease-free survival. *Clin Cancer Res* 1997; **3:** 103–9.

108. Gershtein ES, Shatskaya VA, Ermilova VD et al. Phosphatidylinositol 3-kinase expression in human breast cancer. *Clin Chim Acta* 1999; **287:** 59–67.

109. Osborne CK, Clemmons DR, Arteaga CL. Regulation of breast cancer growth by insulin-like growth factors. *J Steroid Biochem Mol Biol* 1990; **37:** 805–9.

110. De Leon DD, Wilson DM, Powers M, Rosenfeld RG. Effects of insulin-like growth factors (IGFs) and IGF receptor antibodies on the proliferation of human breast cancer cells. *Growth Factors* 1992; **6:** 327–36.

111. Lee AV, Weng CN, Jackson JG, Yee D. Activation of estrogen receptor-mediated gene transcription by IGF-I in human breast cancer cells. *J Endocrinol* 1997; **152:** 39–47.

112. Westley BR, Clayton SJ, Daws MR et al. Interactions between the oestrogen and insulin-like growth factor signalling pathways in the control of breast epithelial cell proliferation. *Biochem Soc Symp* 1998; **63:** 35–44.

113. Kleinberg DL, Feldman M, Ruan W. IGF-I: an essential factor in terminal end bud formation and ductal morphogenesis. *J Mammary Gland Biol Neoplasia* 2000; **5:** 7–17.

114. Couse JF, Korach KS. Estrogen receptor null mice: What have we learned and where will they lead us? *Endocr Rev* 1999; **20:** 358–417.

115. Giani C, Pinchera A, Rasmussen A et al. Stromal IGF-II messenger RNA in breast cancer: relationship with progesterone receptor expressed by malignant epithelial cells. *J Endocrinol Invest* 1998; **21:** 160–5.

116. Helle SI, Lonning PE. Insulin-like growth factors in breast cancer. *Acta Oncol* 1996; **35**(Suppl 5): 19–22.

117. Osborne CK, Coronado EB, Kitten LJ et al. Insulin-like growth factor-II (IGF-II): a potential autocrine/paracrine growth factor for human breast cancer acting via the IGF-I receptor. *Mol Endocrinol* 1989; **3:** 1701–9.

118. Freiss G, Rochefort H, Vignon F. Mechanisms of 4-hydroxytamoxifen anti-growth factor activity in breast cancer cells: alterations of growth factor receptor binding sites and tyrosine kinase activity. *Biochem Biophys Res Commun* 1990; **173:** 919–26.

119. Freiss G, Puech C, Vignon F. Extinction of insulin-like growth factor-I mitogenic signaling by antiestrogen-stimulated Fas-associated protein tyrosine phosphatase-1 in human breast cancer cells. *Mol Endocrinol* 1998; **12:** 568–79.

120. Guvakova MA, Surmacz E. Tamoxifen interferes with the insulin-like growth factor I receptor (IGF-1R) signaling pathway in breast cancer cells. *Cancer Res* 1997; **57:** 2606–10.

121. Molloy CA, May FE, Westley BR. Insulin receptor substrate-1 expression is regulated by estrogen in the MCF-7 human breast cancer cell line. *J Biol Chem* 2000; **275:** 12565–71.

122. Helle SI, Anker GB, Tally M et al. Influence of droloxifene on plasma levels of insulin-like growth factor (IGF)-I, pro-IGF-IIE, insulin-like growth factor binding protein (IGFBP)-1 and IGFBP-3 in breast cancer patients. *J Steroid Biochem Mol Biol* 1996; **57:** 167–71.

123. Newton AC. Regulation of protein kinase C. *Curr Opin Cell Biol* 1997; **9:** 161–7.

124. Kampfer S, Uberall F, Giselbrecht S et al. Characterization of PKC isozyme specific functions in cellular signaling. *Adv Enzyme Regul* 1998; **38:** 35–48.

125. Hata A, Akita Y, Konno Y et al. Direct evidence that the kinase activity of protein kinase C is involved in transcriptional activation through a TPA-responsive element. *FEBS Lett* 1989; **252:** 144–6.

126. Pfahl M. Nuclear receptor/AP-1 interaction. *Endocr Rev* 1993; **14:** 651–8.

127. Lahooti H, Thorsen T, Aakvaag A. Modulation of mouse estrogen receptor transcription activity by protein kinase C delta. *J Mol Endocrinol* 1998; **20:** 245–59.

128. Assender JW, Dutkowski CM, Francis AB et al. Insulin-like growth factor-1 activates protein kinase C-δ in endocrine responsive breast cancer. *Br J Cancer* (submitted).

129. Whitmarsh AJ, Davis RJ. Transcription factor AP-1 regulation by mitogen-activated protein kinase signal transduction pathways. *J Mol Med* 1996; **74:** 589–607.

130. Gee JM, Robertson JF, Ellis IO, Nicholson RI. Phosphorylation of ERK1/2 mitogen-activated protein kinase is associated with poor response to anti-hormonal therapy and decreased patient survival in clinical breast cancer. *Int J Cancer* 2001; **95:** 247–54.

131. Gee JM, Robertson JF, Ellis IO, Nicholson RI. Impact of activation of MAP kinase family members on endocrine response and survival in clinical breast cancer. *Eur J Cancer* 2000; **36**(Suppl 4): 105.

132. Paul A, Wilson S, Belham CM et al. Stress-activated protein kinases: activation, regulation and function. *Cell Signal* 1997; **9:** 403–10.

133. Zhang CC, Shapiro DJ. Activation of the p38 mitogen-activated protein kinase pathway by estrogen or by 4-hydroxytamoxifen is coupled to estrogen receptor-induced apoptosis. *J Biol Chem* 2000; **275:** 479–86.

134. Cho H, Aronica SM, Katzenellenbogen BS. Regulation of progesterone receptor gene expression in MCF-7 breast cancer cells: a comparison of the effects of cyclic adenosine 3',5'-monophosphate, estradiol, insulin-like growth factor-I, and serum factors. *Endocrinology* 1994; **134:** 658–64.

135. Fujimoto N, Katzenellenbogen BS. Alteration in the agonist/antagonist balance of antiestrogens by activation of protein kinase A signaling pathways in breast cancer cells: antiestrogen selectivity and promoter dependence. *Mol Endocrinol* 1994; **8:** 296–304.

136. Gordge PC, Hulme MJ, Clegg RA, Miller WR. Elevation of protein kinase A and protein kinase C activities in malignant as compared with normal human breast tissue. *Eur J Cancer* 1996; **32A:** 2120–6.

137. Miller WR, Hulme MJ, Bartlett JM et al. Changes in messenger RNA expression of protein kinase A regulatory subunit α in breast cancer patients treated with tamoxifen. *Clin Cancer Res* 1997; **3:** 2399–404.

138. Webb P, Lopez GN, Uht RM, Kushner PJ. Tamoxifen activation of the estrogen receptor/AP-1 pathway: potential origin for the cell-specific estrogen-like effects of antiestrogens. *Mol Endocrinol* 1995; **9:** 443–56.

139. Gee JM, Ellis IO, Robertson JF et al. Immunocytochemical localization of Fos protein in human breast cancers and its relationship to a series of prognostic markers and response to endocrine therapy. *Int J Cancer* 1995; **64:** 269–73.

140. Gee JM, Barroso AF, Ellis IO et al. Biological and clinical associations of c-jun activation in human breast cancer. *Int J Cancer* 2000; **89:** 177–86.

141. Koli KM, Arteaga CL. Transforming growth factor-β and breast cancer. In: *Breast Cancer: Molecular Genetics, Pathogenesis and Therapeutics* (Bowcock AM, ed). Totowa, NJ: Humana Press, 1999: 95–120.

142. Gorsch SM, Memoli VA, Stukel TA et al. Immunohistochemical staining for transforming growth factor β1 associates with disease progression in human breast cancer. *Cancer Res* 1992; **52:** 6949–52.

143. Auvinen P, Lipponen P, Johansson R, Syrjanen K. Prognostic significance of TGF-β1 and TGF-β2 expressions in female breast cancer. *Anticancer Res* 1995; **15:** 2627–31.

144. Butta A, MacLennan K, Flanders KC et al. Induction of transforming growth factor β1 in human breast cancer in vivo following tamoxifen treatment. *Cancer Res* 1992; **52:** 4261–4.

145. Kopp A, Jonat W, Schmahl M, Knabbe C. Transforming growth factor β2 (TGF-β2) levels in plasma of patients with metastatic breast cancer treated with tamoxifen. *Cancer Res* 1995; **55:** 4512–15.

146. Knabbe C, Kopp A, Hilgers W et al. Regulation and role of TGFβ production in breast cancer. *Ann NY Acad Sci* 1996; **784:** 263–76.

147. MacCallum J, Keen JC, Bartlett JM et al. Changes in expression of transforming growth factor β mRNA isoforms in patients undergoing tamoxifen therapy. *Br J Cancer* 1996; **74:** 474–8.

148. Knabbe C, Zugmaier G, Schmahl M et al. Induction of transforming growth factor β by the antiestrogens droloxifene, tamoxifen, and toremifene in MCF-7 cells. *Am J Clin Oncol* 1991; **14**(Suppl 2): S15–20.

149. Thompson AM, Kerr DJ, Steel CM. Transforming growth factor β1 is implicated in the failure of tamoxifen therapy in human breast cancer. *Br J Cancer* 1991; **63:** 609–14.

150. Koli KM, Ramsey TT, Ko Y et al. Blockade of

transforming growth factor-β signaling does not abrogate antiestrogen-induced growth inhibition of human breast carcinoma cells. *J Biol Chem* 1997; **272**: 8296–302.

151. Robertson JF, Willsher PC, Cheung KL, Blamey RW. The clinical relevance of static disease (no change) category for 6 months on endocrine therapy in patients with breast cancer. *Eur J Cancer* 1997; **33**: 1774–9.

152. Osborne CK, Coronado EB, Robinson JP. Human breast cancer in the athymic nude mouse: cytostatic effects of long-term antiestrogen therapy. *Eur J Cancer Clin Oncol* 1987; **23**: 1189–96.

153. Osborne CK, Coronado-Heinsohn EB, Hilsenbeck SG et al. Comparison of the effects of a pure steroidal antiestrogen with those of tamoxifen in a model of human breast cancer. *J Natl Cancer Inst* 1995; **87**: 746–50.

154. Lee AV, Jackson JG, Gooch JL et al. Enhancement of insulin-like growth factor signaling in human breast cancer: estrogen regulation of insulin receptor substrate-1 expression in vitro and in vivo. *Mol Endocrinol* 1999; **13**: 787–96.

155. Vogel CL, Shemano I, Schoenfelder J et al. Multicenter phase II efficacy trial of toremifene in tamoxifen-refractory patients with advanced breast cancer. *J Clin Oncol* 1993; **11**: 345–50.

156. Pyrhonen S, Valavaara R, Vuorinen J, Hajba A. High dose toremifene in advanced breast cancer resistant to or relapsed during tamoxifen treatment. *Breast Cancer Res Treat* 1994; **29**: 223–8.

157. Hamm JT. Phase I and II studies of toremifene. *Oncology (Huntingt)* 1997; **11**(5 Suppl 4): 19–22.

158. Buzdar AU, Hortobagyi GN. Tamoxifen and toremifene in breast cancer: comparison of safety and efficacy. *J Clin Oncol* 1998; **16**: 348–53.

159. Campbell FC, Blamey RW, Elston CW et al. Quantitative oestradiol receptor values in primary breast cancer and response of metastases to endocrine therapy. *Lancet* 1981; **ii**: 1317–19.

160. Nicholson RI, Colin P, Francis AB et al. Evaluation of an enzyme immunoassay for estrogen receptors in human breast cancers. *Cancer Res* 1986; **46**(8 Suppl): 4299s–302s.

161. Merkel DE, Osborne CK. Prognostic factors in breast cancer. *Hematol Oncol Clin North Am* 1989; **3**: 641–52.

162. Nicholson RI, McClelland RA, Gee JM. Steroid hormone receptors and their clinical significance in cancer. *J Clin Pathol* 1995; **48**: 890–5.

163. Thompson EW, Paik S, Brunner N et al. Association of increased basement membrane invasiveness with absence of estrogen receptor and expression of vimentin in human breast cancer cell lines. *J Cell Physiol* 1992; **150**: 534–44.

164. Blamey RW, Bishop HM, Blake JR et al. Relationship between primary breast tumor receptor status and patient survival. *Cancer* 1980; **46**(12 Suppl): 2765–9.

165. Williams MR, Todd JH, Ellis IO et al. Oestrogen receptors in primary and advanced breast cancer: an eight year review of 704 cases. *Br J Cancer* 1987; **55**: 67–73.

166. Robertson JF, Ellis IO, Pearson D et al. Biological factors of prognostic significance in locally advanced breast cancer. *Breast Cancer Res Treat* 1994; **29**: 259–64.

167. Ferguson AT, Davidson NE. Regulation of estrogen receptor α function in breast cancer. *Crit Rev Oncog* 1997; **8**: 29–46.

168. Ferguson AT, Lapidus RG, Davidson NE. The regulation of estrogen receptor expression and function in human breast cancer. In: *Biological and Hormonal Therapies of Cancer* (Foon KA, Muss HB, eds). Boston: Kluwer, 1998: 255–78.

169. Falette NS, Fuqua SA, Chamness GC et al. Estrogen receptor gene methylation in human breast tumors. *Cancer Res* 1990; **50**: 3974–8.

170. Ottaviano YL, Issa JP, Parl FF et al. Methylation of the estrogen receptor gene CpG island marks loss of estrogen receptor expression in human breast cancer cells. *Cancer Res* 1994; **54**: 2552–5.

171. Lapidus RG, Ferguson AT, Ottaviano YL et al. Methylation of estrogen and progesterone receptor gene 5′ CpG islands correlates with lack of estrogen and progesterone receptor gene expression in breast tumors. *Clin Cancer Res* 1996; **2**: 805–10.

172. Maeda K, Tsuzimura T, Nomura Y et al. Partial characterization of protease(s) in human breast cancer cytosols that can degrade estrogen and progesterone receptors selectively. *Cancer Res* 1984; **44**: 996–1001.

173. Walker KJ, Price-Thomas JM, Candlish W, Nicholson RI. Influence of the antioestrogen tamoxifen on normal breast tissue. *Br J Cancer* 1991; **64**: 764–8.

174. Walker KJ, McClelland RA, Candlish W et al. Heterogeneity of oestrogen receptor expression in normal and malignant breast tissue. *Eur J Cancer* 1992; **28**: 34–7.

175. Dowsett M. Endocrine resistance in advanced breast cancer. *Acta Oncol* 1996; **35**(Suppl 5): 91–5.

176. Patterson JS. Clinical aspects and development of antioestrogen therapy: a review of the endocrine effects of tamoxifen in animals and man. *J Endocrinol* 1981; **89:** 67–75.

177. Johnston SR. Acquired tamoxifen resistance in human breast cancer – potential mechanisms and clinical implications. *Anticancer Drugs* 1997; **8:** 911–30.

178. Johnston SR, Lu B, Dowsett M et al. Comparison of estrogen receptor DNA binding in untreated and acquired antiestrogen-resistant human breast tumors. *Cancer Res* 1997; **57:** 3723–7.

179. Herman ME, Katzenellenbogen BS. Response-specific antiestrogen resistance in a newly characterized MCF-7 human breast cancer cell line resulting from long-term exposure to *trans*-hydroxytamoxifen. *Steroid Biochem Mol Biol* 1996; **59:** 121–34.

180. Larsen SS, Madsen MW, Jensen BL, Lykkesfeldt AE. Resistance of human breast-cancer cells to the pure steroidal anti-estrogen ICI 182,780 is not associated with a general loss of estrogen-receptor expression or lack of estrogen responsiveness. *Int J Cancer* 1997; **72:** 1129–36.

181. Howell A, DeFriend D, Robertson J et al. Response to a specific antioestrogen (ICI 182780) in tamoxifen-resistant breast cancer. *Lancet* 1995; **345:** 29–30.

182. Blamey RW. The role of selective non-steroidal aromatase inhibitors in future treatment strategies. *Oncology* 1997; **54**(Suppl 2): 27–31.

183. Friedrichs K, Janicke F. Aromatase inhibitors – new possibilities in treatment of breast carcinoma. *Schweiz Rundsch Med Prax* 1998; **87:** 584–8.

184. Hu XF, Veroni M, De Luise M et al. Circumvention of tamoxifen resistance by the pure anti-estrogen ICI 182,780. *Int J Cancer* 1993; **55:** 873–6.

185. Howell A, Dodwell DJ, Anderson H, Redford J. Response after withdrawal of tamoxifen and progestogens in advanced breast cancer. *Ann Oncol* 1992; **3:** 611–17.

186. Gottardis MM, Jordan VC. Development of tamoxifen-stimulated growth of MCF-7 tumors in athymic mice after long-term antiestrogen administration. *Cancer Res* 1988; **48:** 5183–7.

187. Wolf DM, Jordan VC. Characterization of tamoxifen stimulated MCF-7 tumor variants grown in athymic mice. *Breast Cancer Res Treat* 1994; **31:** 117–27.

188. Zhang QX, Borg A, Wolf DM et al. An estrogen receptor mutant with strong hormone-independent activity from a metastatic breast cancer. *Cancer Res* 1997; **57:** 1244–9.

189. Levenson AS, Catherino WH, Jordan VC. Estrogenic activity is increased for an antiestrogen by a natural mutation of the estrogen receptor. *J Steroid Biochem Mol Biol* 1997; **60:** 261–8.

190. Fuqua SA, Wolf DM. Molecular aspects of estrogen receptor variants in breast cancer. *Breast Cancer Res Treat* 1995; **35:** 233–41.

191. Gallacchi P, Schoumacher F, Eppenberger-Castori S et al. Increased expression of estrogen-receptor exon-5-deletion variant in relapse tissues of human breast cancer. *Int J Cancer* 1998; **79:** 44–8.

192. Rea D, Parker MG. Effects of an exon 5 variant of the estrogen receptor in MCF-7 breast cancer cells. *Cancer Res* 1996; **56:** 1556–63.

193. Karnik PS, Kulkarni S, Liu XP et al. Estrogen receptor mutations in tamoxifen-resistant breast cancer. *Cancer Res* 1994; **54:** 349–53.

194. Daffada AA, Johnston SR, Smith IE et al. Exon 5 deletion variant estrogen receptor messenger RNA expression in relation to tamoxifen resistance and progesterone receptor/pS2 status in human breast cancer. *Cancer Res* 1995; **55:** 288–93.

195. Speirs V, Parkes AT, Kerin MJ et al. Coexpression of estrogen receptor α and β: poor prognostic factors in human breast cancer? *Cancer Res* 1999; **59:** 525–8.

196. Speirs V, Kerin MJ. Prognostic significance of oestrogen receptor β in breast cancer. *Br J Surg* 2000; **87:** 405–9.

197. Hansen RK, Fuqua SAW. The estrogen receptor and breast cancer. In: *Breast Cancer: Molecular Genetics, Pathogenesis and Therapeutics* (Bowcock AM, ed). Totowa, NJ: Humana Press, 1999: 1–30.

198. Leygue E, Dotzlaw H, Watson PH, Murphy LC. Expression of estrogen receptor β1, β2, and β5 messenger RNAs in human breast tissue. *Cancer Res* 1999; **59:** 1175–9.

199. Mosselman S, Polman J, Dijkema R. ER beta: identification and characterization of a novel human estrogen receptor. *FEBS Lett* 1996; **392:** 49–53.

200. Montano MM, Muller V, Trobaugh A,

Katzenellenbogen BS. The carboxy-terminal F domain of the human estrogen receptor: role in the transcriptional activity of the receptor and the effectiveness of antiestrogens as estrogen antagonists. *Mol Endocrinol* 1995; **9**: 814–25.

201. Kurebayashi J, Otsuki T, Kunisue H et al. Expression levels of estrogen receptor-α, estrogen receptor-β, coactivators, and corepressors in breast cancer. *Clin Cancer Res* 2000; **6**: 512–18.

202. Jackson TA, Richer JK, Bain DL et al. The partial agonist activity of antagonist-occupied steroid receptors is controlled by a novel hinge domain-binding coactivator L7/SPA and the corepressors N-CoR or SMRT. *Mol Endocrinol* 1997; **11**: 693–705.

203. Takimoto GS, Graham JD, Jackson TA et al. Tamoxifen resistant breast cancer: coregulators determine the direction of transcription by antagonist-occupied steroid receptors. *J Steroid Biochem Mol Biol* 1999; **69**: 45–50.

204. Lavinsky RM, Jepsen K, Heinzel T et al. Diverse signaling pathways modulate nuclear receptor recruitment of N-CoR and SMRT complexes. *Proc Natl Acad Sci USA* 1998; **95**: 2920–5.

205. Ponglikitmongkol M, White JH, Chambon P. Synergistic activation of transcription by the human estrogen receptor bound to tandem responsive elements. *EMBO J* 1990; **9**: 2221–31.

206. Dana SL, Hoener PA, Wheeler DA et al. Novel estrogen response elements identified by genetic selection in yeast are differentially responsive to estrogens and antiestrogens in mammalian cells. *Mol Endocrinol* 1994; **8**: 1193–207.

207. Tonetti DA, Jordan VC. Possible mechanisms in the emergence of tamoxifen-resistant breast cancer. *Anti Cancer Drugs* 1995; **6**: 498–507.

208. Montano MM, Kraus WL, Katzenellenbogen BS. Identification of a novel transferable cis element in the promoter of an estrogen-responsive gene that modulates sensitivity to hormone and antihormone. *Mol Endocrinol* 1997; **11**: 330–41.

209. Osborne CK. Tamoxifen metabolism as a mechanism for resistance. *Endocr Rel Cancer* 1995; **2**: 53–8.

210. Wiebe VJ, Osborne CK, Fuqua SA, DeGregorio MW. Tamoxifen resistance in breast cancer. *Crit Rev Oncol Hematol* 1993; **14**: 173–88.

211. Johnston SR, Haynes BP, Sacks NP et al. Effect of oestrogen receptor status and time on the intra-tumoural accumulation of tamoxifen and N-desmethyltamoxifen following short-term

212. Johnston SR, Haynes BP, Smith IE et al. Acquired tamoxifen resistance in human breast cancer and reduced intra-tumoral drug concentration. *Lancet* 1993; **342**: 1521–2.

213. Osborne CK, Jarman M, McCague R et al. The importance of tamoxifen metabolism in tamoxifen-stimulated breast tumor growth. *Cancer Chemother Pharmacol* 1994; **34**: 89–95.

214. MacCallum J, Cummings J, Dixon JM, Miller WR. Concentrations of tamoxifen and its major metabolites in hormone responsive and resistant breast tumours. *Br J Cancer* 2000; **82**: 1629–35.

215. Pavlik EJ, Nelson K, Srinivasan S et al. Resistance to tamoxifen with persisting sensitivity to estrogen: possible mediation by excessive antiestrogen binding site activity. *Cancer Res* 1992; **52**: 4106–12.

216. Elledge RM, Green S, Ciocca D et al. HER-2 expression and response to tamoxifen in estrogen receptor-positive breast cancer: a Southwest Oncology Group study. *Clin Cancer Res* 1998; **4**: 7–12.

217. Lonn U, Lonn S, Ingelman-Sundberg H et al. c-erb-b2/int-2 amplification appears faster in breast-cancer patients receiving second-line endocrine treatment. *Int J Cancer* 1996; **69**: 273–7.

218. Clarke R, Brunner N, Katz D et al. The effects of a constitutive expression of transforming growth factor-α on the growth of MCF-7 human breast cancer cells in vitro and in vivo. *Mol Endocrinol* 1989; **3**: 372–80.

219. Miller DL, el-Ashry D, Cheville AL et al. Emergence of MCF-7 cells overexpressing a transfected epidermal growth factor receptor (EGFR) under estrogen-depleted conditions: evidence for a role of EGFR in breast cancer growth and progression. *Cell Growth Differ* 1994; **5**: 1263–74.

220. van Agthoven T, van Agthoven TL, Portengen H et al. Ectopic expression of epidermal growth factor receptors induces hormone independence in ZR-75-1 human breast cancer cells. *Cancer Res* 1992; **52**: 5082–8.

221. Benz CC, Scott GK, Sarup JC et al. Estrogen-dependent, tamoxifen-resistant tumorigenic growth of MCF-7 cells transfected with HER2/neu. *Breast Cancer Res Treat* 1993; **24**: 85–95.

222. Kurokawa H, Lenferink AE, Simpson JF et al.

therapy in human primary breast cancer. *Breast Cancer Res Treat* 1993; **28**: 241–50.

Inhibition of HER2/neu (erbB-2) and mitogen-activated protein kinases enhances tamoxifen action against HER2-overexpressing, tamoxifen-resistant breast cancer cells. *Cancer Res* 2000; **60:** 5887–94.

223. Vickers PJ, Dickson RB, Shoemaker R, Cowan KH. A multidrug-resistant MCF-7 human breast cancer cell line which exhibits cross-resistance to antiestrogens and hormone-independent tumor growth in vivo. *Mol Endocrinol* 1988; **2:** 886–92.

224. van Agthoven T, van Agthoven TL, Dekker A et al. Induction of estrogen independence of ZR-75-1 human breast cancer cells by epigenetic alterations. *Mol Endocrinol* 1994; **8:** 1474–83.

225. van den Berg HW, Claffie D, Boylan M et al. Expression of receptors for epidermal growth factor and insulin-like growth factor I by ZR-75-1 human breast cancer cell variants is inversely related: the effect of steroid hormones on insulin-like growth factor I receptor expression. *Br J Cancer* 1996; **73:** 477–81.

226. Wiseman LR, Johnson MD, Wakeling AE et al. Type I IGF receptor and acquired tamoxifen resistance in oestrogen-responsive human breast cancer cells. *Eur J Cancer* 1993; **29A:** 2256–64.

227. Parisot JP, Hu XF, DeLuise M, Zalcberg JR. Altered expression of the IGF-1 receptor in a tamoxifen-resistant human breast cancer cell line. *Br J Cancer* 1999; **79:** 693–700.

228. Campbell RA, Bhat-Nakshatri P, Patel NM et al. Phosphatidylinositol 3-kinase/AKT-mediated activation of estrogen receptor α: a new model for anti-estrogen resistance. *J Biol Chem* 2001; **276:** 9817–24.

229. Brunner N, Moser C, Clarke R, Cullen K. IGF-I and IGF-II expression in human breast cancer xenografts: relationship to hormone independence. *Breast Cancer Res Treat* 1992; **22:** 39–45.

230. Rocha RL, Hilsenbeck SG, Jackson JG et al. Correlation of insulin-like growth factor-binding protein-3 messenger RNA with protein expression in primary breast cancer tissues: detection of higher levels in tumors with poor prognostic features. *J Natl Cancer Inst* 1996; **88:** 601–6.

231. Kern FG. The role of fibroblast growth factors in breast cancer pathogenesis and progression. In: *Breast Cancer: Molecular Genetics, Pathogenesis and Therapeutics* (Bowcock AM, ed). Totowa, NJ: Humana Press, 1999: 59–93.

232. Stewart AJ, Westley BR, May FE. Modulation of the proliferative response of breast cancer cells to growth factors by oestrogen. *Br J Cancer* 1992; **66:** 640–8.

233. Zhang L, Kharbanda S, Chen D et al. MCF-7 breast carcinoma cells overexpressing FGF-1 form vascularized, metastatic tumors in ovariectomized or tamoxifen-treated nude mice. *Oncogene* 1997; **15:** 2093–108.

234. McLeskey SW, Kurebayashi J, Honig SF et al. Fibroblast growth factor 4 transfection of MCF-7 cells produces cell lines that are tumorigenic and metastatic in ovariectomized or tamoxifen-treated athymic nude mice. *Cancer Res* 1993; **53:** 2168–77.

235. McLeskey SW, Zhang L, El-Ashry D et al. Tamoxifen-resistant fibroblast growth factor-transfected MCF-7 cells are cross-resistant in vivo to the antiestrogen ICI 182,780 and two aromatase inhibitors. *Clin Cancer Res* 1998; **4:** 697–711.

236. Morse-Gaudio M, Connolly JM, Rose DP. Protein kinase C and its isoforms in human breast cancer cells: relationship to the invasive phenotype. *Int J Oncol* 1998; **12:** 1349–54.

237. Ways DK, Kukoly CA, deVente J et al. MCF-7 breast cancer cells transfected with protein kinase C-α exhibit altered expression of other protein kinase C isoforms and display a more aggressive neoplastic phenotype. *J Clin Invest* 1995; **95:** 1906–15.

238. Tonetti DA, Chisamore MJ, Grdina W et al. Stable transfection of protein kinase C α cDNA in hormone-dependent breast cancer cell lines. *Br J Cancer* 2000; **83:** 782–91.

239. Sivaraman VS, Wang H, Nuovo GJ, Malbon CC. Hyperexpression of mitogen-activated protein kinase in human breast cancer. *J Clin Invest* 1997; **99:** 1478–83.

240. Lehrer S, O'Shaughnessy J, Song HK et al. Activity of pp60c-src protein kinase in human breast cancer. *Mt Sinai J Med* 1989; **56:** 83–5.

241. Lawrence DS, Niu J. Protein kinase inhibitors: the tyrosine-specific protein kinases. *Pharmacol Ther* 1998; **77:** 81–114.

242. Daly RJ, Binder MD, Sutherland RL. Overexpression of the Grb2 gene in human breast cancer cell lines. *Oncogene* 1994; **9:** 2723–7.

243. Wang C, Thor AD, Moore DH 2nd et al. The overexpression of RHAMM, a hyaluronan-binding protein that regulates ras signaling,

correlates with overexpression of mitogen-activated protein kinase and is a significant parameter in breast cancer progression. *Clin Cancer Res* 1998; **4**: 567–76.

244. Dati C, Muraca R, Tazartes O et al. c-erbB-2 and ras expression levels in breast cancer are correlated and show a co-operative association with unfavorable clinical outcome. *Int J Cancer* 1991; **47**: 833–8.

245. Bland KI, Konstadoulakis MM, Vezeridis MP, Wanebo HJ. Oncogene protein co-expression. Value of Ha-ras, c-myc, c-fos, and p53 as prognostic discriminants for breast carcinoma. *Ann Surg* 1995; **221**: 706–18; discussion 718–20.

246. Callans LS, Naama H, Khandelwal M et al. Raf-1 protein expression in human breast cancer cells. *Ann Surg Oncol* 1995; **2**: 38–42.

247. O'Brian C, Vogel VG, Singletary SE, Ward NE. Elevated protein kinase C expression in human breast tumor biopsies relative to normal breast tissue. *Cancer Res* 1989; **49**: 3215–17.

248. Boonstra J, Rijken P, Humbel B et al. The epidermal growth factor. *Cell Biol Int* 1995; **19**: 413–30.

249. Coutts AS, Murphy LC. Elevated mitogen-activated protein kinase activity in estrogen-nonresponsive human breast cancer cells. *Cancer Res* 1998; **58**: 4071–4.

250. Jeng MH, Yue W, Eischeid A et al. Role of MAP kinase in the enhanced cell proliferation of long-term estrogen deprived human breast cancer cells. *Breast Cancer Res Treat* 2000; **62**: 167–75.

251. Shim WS, Conaway M, Masamura S et al. Estradiol hypersensitivity and mitogen-activated protein kinase expression in long-term estrogen deprived human breast cancer cells in vivo. *Endocrinology* 2000; **141**: 396–405.

252. Smith LM, Wise SC, Hendricks DT et al. cJun overexpression in MCF-7 breast cancer cells produces a tumorigenic, invasive and hormone resistant phenotype. *Oncogene* 1999; **18**: 6063–70.

253. Doucas V, Yaniv M. Functional interaction between estrogen receptor and proto-oncogene products c-Jun and c-Fos. *C R Séances Soc Biol Fil* 1991; **185**: 464–74.

254. Dumont JA, Bitonti AJ, Wallace CD et al. Progression of MCF-7 breast cancer cells to antiestrogen-resistant phenotype is accompanied by elevated levels of AP-1 DNA-binding activity. *Cell Growth Differ* 1996; **7**: 351–9.

255. Astruc ME, Chabret C, Bali P et al. Prolonged treatment of breast cancer cells with antiestrogens increases the activating protein-1-mediated response: involvement of the estrogen receptor. *Endocrinology* 1995; **136**: 824–32.

256. Badia E, Duchesne MJ, Astruc M et al. Modulation of cellular response expression during prolonged treatment with antiestrogens. *C R Séances Soc Biol Fil* 1995; **189**: 755–64.

257. Paech K, Webb P, Kuiper GG et al. Differential ligand activation of estrogen receptors ERα and ERβ at AP1 sites. *Science* 1997; **277**: 1508–10.

258. Barrett-Lee P, Travers M, Luqmani Y, Coombes RC. Transcripts for transforming growth factors in human breast cancer: clinical correlates. *Br J Cancer* 1990; **61**: 612–17.

259. Herman ME, Katzenellenbogen BS. Alterations in transforming growth factor-α and -β production and cell responsiveness during the progression of MCF-7 human breast cancer cells to estrogen-autonomous growth. *Cancer Res* 1994; **54**: 5867–74.

260. Koli KM, Arteaga CL. Complex role of tumor cell transforming growth factor (TGF)-β on breast carcinoma progression. *J Mammary Gland Biol Neoplasia* 1996; **1**: 373–80.

261. Arteaga CL, Koli KM, Dugger TC, Clarke R. Reversal of tamoxifen resistance of human breast carcinomas in vivo by neutralizing antibodies to transforming growth factor-β. *J Natl Cancer Inst* 1999; **91**: 46–53.

262. Dickson RB, Kasid A, Huff KK et al. Activation of growth factor secretion in tumorigenic states of breast cancer induced by 17β-estradiol or v-Ha-ras oncogene. *Proc Natl Acad Sci USA* 1987; **84**: 837–41.

263. Hui R, Ball JR, Macmillan RD et al. EMS1 gene expression in primary breast cancer: relationship to cyclin D1 and oestrogen receptor expression and patient survival. *Oncogene* 1998; **17**: 1053–9.

264. Zwijsen RM, Wientjens E, Klompmaker R et al. CDK-independent activation of estrogen receptor by cyclin D1. *Cell* 1997; **88**: 405–15.

265. Barnes DM, Gillett CE. Cyclin D1 in breast cancer. *Breast Cancer Res Treat* 1998; **52**: 1–15.

266. Seshadri R, Lee CS, Hui R et al. Cyclin DI amplification is not associated with reduced overall survival in primary breast cancer but may predict early relapse in patients with features of good prognosis. *Clin Cancer Res* 1996; **2**: 1177–84.

267. Wilcken NRC, Prall OWJ, Musgrove EA, Sutherland RL. Inducible overexpression of cyclin D1 in breast cancer cells reverses the growth-inhibitory effects of antiestrogens. *Clin Cancer Res* 1997; **3**: 849–54.

268. Nielsen NH, Arnerlov C, Cajander S, Landberg G. Cyclin E expression and proliferation in breast cancer. *Anal Cell Pathol* 1998; **17**: 177–88.

269. Nielsen NH, Arnerlov C, Emdin SO, Landberg G. Cyclin E overexpression, a negative prognostic factor in breast cancer with strong correlation to oestrogen receptor status. *Br J Cancer* 1996; **74**: 874–80.

270. Fredersdorf S, Burns J, Milne AM et al. High level expression of p27(kip1) and cyclin D1 in some human breast cancer cells: inverse correlation between the expression of p27(kip1) and degree of malignancy in human breast and colorectal cancers. *Proc Natl Acad Sci USA* 1997; **94**: 6380–5.

271. Barbareschi M. p27 expression, a cyclin dependent kinase inhibitor in breast carcinoma. *Adv Clin Pathol* 1999; **3**: 119–27.

272. Leong AC, Hanby AM, Potts HW et al. Cell cycle proteins do not predict outcome in grade I infiltrating ductal carcinoma of the breast. *Int J Cancer* 2000; **89**: 26–31.

273. Lau R, Grimson R, Sansome C et al. Low levels of cell cycle inhibitor p27kip1 combined with high levels of Ki-67 predict shortened disease-free survival in T1 and T2 invasive breast carcinomas. *Int J Oncol* 2001; **18**: 17–23.

274. Hui R, Macmillan RD, Kenny FS et al. INK4a gene expression and methylation in primary breast cancer: overexpression of p16INK4a messenger RNA is a marker of poor prognosis. *Clin Cancer Res*. 2000; **6**: 2777–87.

275. Nicholson RI, Gee JMW, Seery LT et al. p53 protein expression in human breast cancer: relationship to tumour differentiation and endocrine response. In: *Scientific updates, Vol I: Prognostic and predictive value of p53* (Klijn JGM, ed). Elsevier Science, 1997.

276. Berns EM, Foekens JA, Vossen R et al. Complete sequencing of TP53 predicts poor response to systemic therapy of advanced breast cancer. *Cancer Res* 2000; **60**: 2155–62.

277. Schmutzler RK, Bierhoff E, Werkhausen T et al. Genomic deletions in the BRCA1, BRCA2 and TP53 regions associate with low expression of the estrogen receptor in sporadic breast carcinoma. *Int J Cancer* 1997; **74**: 322–5.

278. Howell A. Faslodex (ICI 182780): an oestrogen receptor downregulator. *Eur J Cancer* 2000; **36**: S87.

279. DeFriend DJ, Howell A, Nicholson RI et al. Investigation of a new pure antiestrogen (ICI 182780) in women with primary breast cancer. *Cancer Res* 1994; **54**: 408–14.

280. Gottardis MM, Jiang SY, Jeng MH, Jordan VC. Inhibition of tamoxifen-stimulated growth of an MCF-7 tumor variant in athymic mice by novel steroidal antiestrogens. *Cancer Res* 1989; **49**: 4090–3.

281. Brunner N, Frandsen TL, Holst-Hansen C et al. MCF7/LCC2: a 4-hydroxytamoxifen resistant human breast cancer variant that retains sensitivity to the steroidal antiestrogen ICI 182,780. *Cancer Res* 1993; **53**: 3229–32.

282. Van de Velde P, Nique F, Bouchoux F et al. RU 58,668, a new pure antiestrogen inducing a regression of human mammary carcinoma implanted in nude mice. *J Steroid Biochem Mol Biol* 1994; **48**: 187–96.

283. Tremblay A, Tremblay GB, Labrie C et al. EM-800, a novel antiestrogen, acts as a pure antagonist of the transcriptional functions of estrogen receptors α and β. *Endocrinology* 1998; **139**: 111–18.

284. Baselga J, Tripathy D, Mendelsohn J et al. Phase II study of weekly intravenous trastuzumab (Herceptin) in patients with HER2/neu-overexpressing metastatic breast cancer. *Semin Oncol* 1999; **26**(4 Suppl 12): 78–83.

285. Pegram MD, Lipton A, Hayes DF et al. Phase II study of receptor-enhanced chemosensitivity using recombinant humanized anti-p185HER2/neu monoclonal antibody plus cisplatin in patients with HER2/neu-overexpressing metastatic breast cancer refractory to chemotherapy treatment. *J Clin Oncol* 1998; **16**: 2659–71.

286. Baselga J. Clinical trials of single-agent trastuzumab. *Semin Oncol* 2000; **27**(5 Suppl 9): 20–6.

287. Wakeling AE, Barker AJ, Davies DH et al. Specific inhibition of epidermal growth factor receptor tyrosine kinase by 4-anilinoquinazolines. *Breast Cancer Res Treat* 1996; **38**: 67–73.

288. Jones HE, Dutkowski CM, Barrow D et al. New EGF-R selective tyrosine kinase inhibitor reveals variable growth responses in prostate carcinoma cell lines PC-3 and DU-145. *Int J Cancer* 1997; **71**: 1010–18.

289. Green S, Furr B. Prospects for the treatment of endocrine-responsive tumours. *Endocr Rel Cancer* 1999; **6**: 349–71.

290. Carlson BA, Dubay MM, Sausville EA et al. Flavopiridol induces G1 arrest with inhibition of cyclin-dependent kinase (CDK) 2 and CDK4 in human breast carcinoma cells. *Cancer Res* 1996; **56**: 2973–8.

11

Animal models of endocrine-responsive and -unresponsive breast cancers

Robert Clarke, Robert B Dickson

CONTENTS • **Introduction** • **Chemically induced models** • **Rodent mammary tumors with a viral etiology** • **Human breast tumor xenografts** • **Endocrine-responsive xenografts** • **Antiestrogen-resistant xenografts** • **Tamoxifen-stimulated xenografts** • **Endocrine-unresponsive xenografts** • **Gene transfer: xenograft and transgenic models** • **Hormonal response and resistance** • **Angiogenesis and metastasis** • **Conclusions and future prospects** • **Acknowledgments**

INTRODUCTION

Animal models are widely used in breast cancer research. For example, human breast cancer xenografts are often used to study the biology of breast cancer and to screen new endocrine and cytotoxic agents. Genetically manipulated animals, whether these have specific genes overexpressed (transgenic species) or eliminated (knockout or null species), can be used to study the effects of specific genes on carcinogenesis and the function of the normal mammary gland. The most common animal models for breast cancer occur in mice and rats. These fall into one of four categories: human breast cancer cell xenografts (mostly in immunodeficient mice), chemically induced mammary tumors (mostly in rats), virally induced mammary tumors in mice, and genetically manipulated animals (mostly mice).

Each of the rodent models has specific advantages and disadvantages. Most models for spontaneous breast cancer arise in mouse strains susceptible to mouse mammary tumor virus (MMTV)-induced mammary neoplasia, and some transgenic mouse models. For the chemically induced tumors, initiation events are induced by the carcinogen. In the human tumor xenografts, the malignant tissue is directly inoculated into host tissues. A major advantage of the xenografts is their human breast cancer origin, while a disadvantage of the rodent mammary models is their non-human origin.

The spontaneous and chemically induced models are particularly useful for chemoprevention studies. Full transformation of the mammary gland has either not occurred (young transgenic and MMTV-infected mice) or occurs within a reproducible time following carcinogenic insult (chemically induced tumors). Thus, the ability of experimental agents to either suppress or prevent full transformation can readily be explored. However, events that may occur during development or early life, and that lead to the initiation stage in carcinogenesis, may be difficult to address because genetic lesions may be present from conception (genetically manipulated models) or birth (MMTV). Xenografts provide a good model for the study of malignant progression in the human disease and the screening of drugs/therapies against established human tumors. However, the inherent problems associated with the use of genetically unstable cell lines or xenografts, and the largely homogenous biology of the cells, are clear limitations.

The use of these models remain a necessity, since in vitro models cannot adequately reproduce the complexity of the endocrinologic environment of the pituitary/adrenal/ovarian axis, tumor–host interactions, or the multistep nature of the metastatic cascade. However, even a well-justified requirement for the use of living animals imposes several ethical and scientific considerations. The use of animal models is heavily regulated, at both the institutional and governmental levels. Investigators are constantly required to refine, reduce, and re-evaluate their use of animals. Special training is required in the handling, care, and use of animals. Appropriate consideration must be given to the health and welfare of experimental animals (e.g. by providing adequate diet, space, health monitoring and hygiene).[1] For example, almost all mammary animal tumor models are sensitive to (i.e. inhibited by) caloric restriction.[2–4]

The use of animal models can prove among the most resource-demanding types of studies. Thus, a careful consideration of experimental design is essential. For example, sufficient numbers of animals must be used to provide adequate statistical power and to ensure the validity of the study,[5,6] but not such that there is unnecessary animal usage. Choice of the appropriate model, and a realistic assessment of its limitations, are critical for adequate and appropriate experimental design.[7]

CHEMICALLY INDUCED MODELS

Chemically induced tumors have been successfully used to demonstrate the antitumor and chemopreventive effects of endocrine agents[8–10] and vitamins.[11] Perhaps the most notable example of the use of chemically induced rodent models is their role in the preclinical development of the antiestrogen tamoxifen. The models remain in widespread use, particularly in the study of dietary and endocrine manipulations.

Chemically induced mammary tumor models have been available since the initial description by Huggins et al.[12] While the rat is the most widely used species, chemical carcinogens can also induce mammary tumors in mice.[13,14] Not all rodent strains are susceptible to the induction of mammary carcinogenesis by chemicals. For example, the Copenhagen rat[15] is essentially resistant, probably because of a dominant, autosomal allele on rat chromosome 2[16] that specifically inhibits the progression but not the initiation of mammary cells.[17] Among the most susceptible strains are Sprague–Dawley,[18] Buf/N,[19] Fischer 344,[20] Lewis,[21] and, to a lesser extent, Wistar–Furth.[20]

One of two carcinogens are most often used in the rat models – either 7,12-dimethylbenz[a]anthracene (DMBA), or N-methyl-N-nitrosourea (MNU). The former is an indirectly acting carcinogen, requiring metabolic activation that can occur within the liver or the mammary gland. The activation of DMBA has been reviewed.[22] MNU, which has been in use for almost 20 years,[23] is generally considered a direct carcinogen because there is no evidence of it requiring activation prior to inducing genetic damage. This difference can be important in the choice of carcinogen. Studies requiring the coadministration of carcinogen with another manipulation(s) are generally performed using MNU. This eliminates any potentially artifactual effect due to altered pharmacology or activation that could arise with DMBA.[22]

The dose of carcinogen and age of the rats are critical. The rats must be virgin, with the optimal age being 40–46 days. Rats that have completed a full-term pregnancy/lactation are less susceptible to carcinogenesis,[18] potentially modeling the effects of early pregnancy on lifetime breast cancer risk in humans.[24] This may reflect an endocrine-induced differentiation that reduces the number of target undifferentiated stem cells.[25]

The comparative biology of the rat models has been extensively reviewed,[18,26–28] and will be discussed only briefly here. Many of the mammary epithelial tumors that arise are well-differentiated adenocarcinomas. While these are histologically similar to a significant proportion of the lesions that arise in the human breast, other tumors can also arise. The endocrine dependence of these models has clear similarities and potential differences with the human disease. For example, the tumors are initially estrogen-dependent and respond to antiestrogens and ovariectomy. However, the concurrent prolactin dependence[29] may not fully reflect breast cancer in humans.[30] A high proportion of tumors induced by MNU exhibit *ras* activation. This mutational event is rare in breast cancer, although activation of signaling pathways downstream of *ras* is observed in the human disease.[31] Activation of *ras* may not be the primary effect of MNU, since MNU-induced tumors arise in cells that already possess an activated *ras*.[32,33] Thus, MNU may promote the survival and proliferation of these pre-existing mammary cells.

RODENT MAMMARY TUMORS WITH A VIRAL ETIOLOGY

Mouse strains that develop mammary tumors due to MMTV infections have been extensively used in breast cancer research. More recently, models using the polyoma WTA2 virus and the human adenovirus type 9 have been described.[34,35] There are similarities and differences among these virally driven models in terms of their biologies and endocrinologies. These have been described in detail elsewhere, and will be only briefly discussed here.

Neonatal female mice are infected with MMTV through their mother's milk. Infected female mice of susceptible strains develop preneoplastic hyperplastic alveolar nodules that arise from 4 weeks or more of age, with mammary tumors often appearing around 24–28 weeks of age.[4,36] Tumor incidence approaches 50% in virgin mice by about 35 weeks of age.[4] The tumors are estrogen- and prolactin-dependent and respond to antiestrogens[36,37] and retinoids.[37] Unlike the rat tumors, the histology of MMTV-driven mouse tumors does not strongly resemble that seen in many human breast tumors. Atypical lobular type A lesions appear similar to the hypoplastic alveolar nodules that arise in susceptible, MMTV-infected, mouse strains.[38] MMTV induces mammary tumors through insertional mutagenesis.[39] Proviral insertion is known to alter the expression of several fibroblast growth factors, including FGF-3, -4, and -8.[39,40] MMTV-induced oncogene activation has been reviewed in detail.[39,40]

Mouse polyoma virus infections can produce mammary hyperplasia, dysplasia, and mammary tumors by 6 weeks of age.[41] The initial epithelial hyperplasia is followed by dysplasia six weeks post inoculum, ductal adenocarcinomas arising with high incidence by 6–9 weeks post inoculum. These tumors are histologically comparable to mammary ductal adenocarcinomas in humans, but are ovarian-independent.[34,41]

Subcutaneous inoculation with human adenovirus type 9 produces benign mammary fibroadenomas, phyllodes-like tumors, and solid sarcomas by 3–5 months of age.[35,42] Tumors appear myoepithelial in origin, unlike other rodent and mouse mammary tumors, which are almost exclusively tumors of epithelial cells.[35] Tumorigenesis is inhibited by ovariectomy, indicating a likely estrogen dependence. These tumors may provide a useful model of mammary fibroadenomas, which are relatively common lesions in the human breast.[35]

HUMAN BREAST TUMOR XENOGRAFTS

The grafting of tissues into another host may be across species (xenograft) or to another animal of the same species (allograft). Immunocompromised rodents will maintain both allografts and xenografts. While tumor cells are more frequently transplanted, some normal tissue xenografts can also be successfully initiated. Generally, the biology of xenografts is comparable to that seen in vitro or in the original host, and this also appears to be true for breast cancer xenografts. Most xenografted cell lines exhibit comparable genetic stability in vivo as they do in vitro in the absence of any specific selective pressure. The stability of human tumor xenografts has been reviewed by Fodstad.[43] The removal of endocrine stimuli,[44] immunologic effectors or the imposition of other selective pressures (e.g. drug treatments). can produce phenotypic changes, and probably epigenetic changes, in some xenografts. This has proved an effective way to generate variant cell lines with desired phenotypes.

The ability to maintain human tumors in another immunodeficient species became widely available after the initial report of the ability of athymic nude mice to sustain human tumor xenografts.[45] Nude mice, which remain the most widely used recipients of human tumor xenografts, were identified in Glasgow, Scotland in 1962.[46] Lacking a thymus, B-cell maturation is defective but normal virgin B cells are present in nude mice. T-lymphocyte levels are very low or undetectable in most strains, as are responses to T-cell-dependent antigens. However, natural killer (NK)-cell activity is higher than that seen in wild-type mice This may contribute to the poor incidence of metastasis and the low take rate for breast tumors reported by some investigators.[47] Including the beige mutation (bg) with the nude mutation (nu) reduces NK-cell activity. Further adding the X-linked immunodeficiency mutation (xid) produces a triple-mutation-bearing strain (NIH-III) that is more immunocompromised than the single-mutant strains.[47] However, bg/nu and NIH-III mice have a clotting disorder, due to the beige mutation, which can be problematic when surgery is required (e.g. ovariectomy or mammary fat pad implantation).[47]

Perhaps the next most frequent xenograft recipient after the nude mouse is the scid mouse. These mice are homozygous for a severe combined immunodeficiency (scid) mutation that produces a defective V(D)J recombination. Scid mice cannot effectively join the cleaved variable region segments catalyzed by immunoglobulin V(D)J recombinase, and are essentially devoid of functional B and T cells.[48,49] Approximately 25% of primary breast tumors, when xenografted into scid mice, exhibit a sufficient growth rate to allow for repeated passage.[50]

Null mutations in the rag-1 and rag-2 genes produce a phenotype similar to that seen in scid mice, reflecting their loss of V(D)J recombination activity. Unlike several scid models, these mice do not become leaky with age. Mice bearing the non-obese diabetes mutation (NOD) also exhibit an unusual T-cell ontogeny. NOD/LtSz–rag-1null mice have recently been described.[51] These mice have an increased lifespan, reflecting the later onset of lymphomas, have no mature B or T cells, exhibit low levels of NK-cell activity, and can be infected with HIV. As other immunodeficient models are generated, their use as recipients for human breast cancer xenografts will likely be evaluated in detail. However, the most widely used xenografts are readily maintained in existing nude and scid mouse models.

Human breast cancer cell lines inoculated into nude mice represent the majority of human breast tumor xenograft models. However, there are relatively few xenografts that have been in regular and widespread use other than MCF-7 (endocrine-responsive), and MDA-MB-231 (endocrine-unresponsive) cells. In part, this reflects the low success rate for establishing human breast tumors either directly as xenografts or as stable established cell lines in vitro. Despite the ability to apply selective pressures resulting in variants with altered endocrine responsiveness,[44,52,53] most endocrine-responsive xenografts are phenotypically stable, at least with respect to biologically important characteristics (e.g. tumorigenicity, steroid hormone receptor expression, and hormone responsiveness) in the absence of selective pressures. Some minor phenotypic diversity is observed between laboratories, and is not surprising since some of these cell lines have been in continuous culture for more than 15 years.

ENDOCRINE-RESPONSIVE XENOGRAFTS

Relatively few human breast cancer xenografts exhibit an endocrine-responsive phenotype, and all are estrogen receptor (ER)-positive. We have previously defined two categories of endocrine-responsive cells: (a) estrogen-dependent and (b) estrogen-independent and estrogen-responsive.[54] Estrogen-dependent xenografts have an absolute requirement for the production of proliferating tumors in the mammary fat pads of ovariectomized immunodeficient mice. Estrogen-independent and estrogen-responsive tumors do not require estrogens, but exhibit a higher take rate and/or growth rate in the presence of estrogen supplementation. Generally, estrogen-responsive xenografts produce relatively well-differentiated adenocarcinomas,[55] are inhibited by antiestrogens,[56–60] and are poorly invasive and non-metastatic.[55] This early phenotype is exhibited despite the origin of these cell lines from malignant effusions in postmenopausal women.

Three endocrine-responsive human breast cancer cell lines account for most of the published studies. These are MCF-7, T47D, and ZR-75-1, and all are usually considered estrogen-dependent. Other models exist, but have been less well characterized.

Of the three main models, MCF-7 is by far the most widely used and best characterized.[61] MCF-7 cells were established by Soule et al,[62] and express receptors for several hormones and growth factors. The characteristics of MCF-7 cells have been reviewed in detail.[61,63] We and others have identified variants with altered estrogen dependence.[44,53,64] For example MCF7-MIII,[44] BSK-3,[44,53] and MCF7/LCC1[64] exhibit the estrogen-independent and estrogen-responsive phenotype. These variants form proliferating tumors in ovariectomized immunodeficient mice but grow more rapidly in the presence of

estrogen supplementation.[44,64] Analysis of the growth and endocrine responsiveness of the various endocrine-responsive xenografts has provided useful information[54,65–67] on the biology of malignant progression[54,65–67] and cross-resistance among antiestrogen therapies.[52,54]

T47D cells were established by Keydar et al,[68] and express ER, progesterone receptor (PgR) and androgen, glucocorticoid, and insulin receptors. Notable for their high levels of PgR and remarkable genetic and phenotypic instability,[69–72] it is not surprising that several T47D variants have been obtained. These represent the major in vitro human breast cancer models for the study of the antiproliferative effects of progestins and antiprogestins. While some variants are unstable and readily revert to the wild-type phenotype, the ER-negative, PgR-positive T47D$_{CO}$ variant has been stable for many years.[63]

ZR-75-1 cells were first described by Engel et al in 1978.[73] While the patient had been receiving tamoxifen, she did not respond.[73] Nonetheless, ZR-75-1 cells express both ER and PgR, are growth-stimulated by estrogens, and are growth-inhibited by antiestrogens in vitro.[63]

One xenograft model expresses an estrogen-inhibited phenotype: T61 tumors form proliferating xenografts in nude mice. However, estrogen supplementation inhibits tumorigenesis.[74] This may provide a model of high-dose estrogen therapy, which can produce responses in up to one-third of breast cancer patients. While this therapy has been largely replaced by the use of antiestrogens, T61 may provide critical insights into how estrogens affect proliferation in vivo.

Many studies of endocrine agents, or using endocrine-responsive xenografts, are performed in ovariectomized mice. These mice have low circulating estrogen concentrations that approximate the levels found in postmenopausal women.[75–77] Since the major endocrine-responsive human breast cancer cells lines were derived from tumors in postmenopausal women,[63] the endocrine environment of the ovariectomized mouse is appropriate. However, the need to remove the ovaries effectively eliminates the NIH-III (*bg/nu/xid*) model as a host because of the clotting problems that would arise in surgery. Estrogen-dependent models require estrogenic supplementation. We routinely use 60-day-release 0.72 mg 17β-estradiol pellets (Innovative Research of America, Sarasota, FL) placed subcutaneously in the interclavicular region.

ANTIESTROGEN-RESISTANT XENOGRAFTS

The study of acquired resistance has been greatly facilitated by the generation of several series of resistant variants. Most have been obtained by in vitro selection of the MCF-7 human breast cancer cell line. Almost all of these variants retain ER expression and show various patterns of resistance and cross-resistance. The R27 and LY2 variants were among the first stable antiestrogen-resistant variants reported. LY2 cells were generated following selection against the benzothiophene antiestrogen LY 117,018.[78] These cells exhibit some estrogen responsiveness, are cross-resistant to 4-hydroxytamoxifen[78,79] and ICI 164,384[79] and are nontumorigenic.[79] R27 cells were obtained following selection against tamoxifen in an anchorage-independent cloning assay.[80]

The MCF-7RR subline was obtained by selecting MCF-7 cells for their ability to grow in medium supplemented with 2% calf serum and 1 μM tamoxifen.[81] While their cross-resistance pattern among other antiestrogens is not reported, MCF-7RR cells exhibit retinoic acid cross-resistance.[82] Another MCF-7 variant, selected against 4-hydroxytamoxifen (MCF/TOT), has also been shown to exhibit cross-resistance to retinoic acid.[83]

Estrogen-independent and estrogen-responsive MCF-7/LCC1 cells were stepwise-selected against increasing concentrations of either 4-hydroxytamoxifen or fulvestrant (ICI 182,780, Faslodex). Cells that acquired resistance to 4-hydroxytamoxifen were designated MCF7/LCC2,[84] those resistant to fulvestrant being designated MCF7/LCC9.[84] MCF7/LCC2 cells retain estrogen-independent growth in vitro and in vivo,[52,85] and are not cross-resistant to the steroidal antiestrogens fulvestrant[52] and ICI 164,384.[85] These observations suggested that breast tumors that responded and then failed tamoxifen might respond to a second-line steroidal antiestrogen.[86] In a phase I trial of fulvestrant performed in tamoxifen responders who subsequently recurred, the overall response rate approached 70%. This is substantially higher than would be predicted if the patients had been treated with another triphenylethylene.[87] Using similar approaches, others have reported a MCF-7 variant (MCF-7/TAM^R-1) expressing a phenotype similar to that of MCF7/LCC2.[88]

MCF7/LCC9 cells (selected against fulvestrant) also retain ER and PgR expression, and exhibit an estrogen-independent and estrogen-responsive phenotype.[84] However, these cells also exhibit cross-resistance to tamoxifen, despite never having been exposed to the drug. Tamoxifen cross-resistance emerges at early passages during the selection, arising before stable fulvestrant resistance is apparent.[86] Others have selected MCF-7 cells against fulvestrant but have not seen tamoxifen cross-resistance.[89] The clinical relevance of these diverse phenotypes remain to be established.

A stepwise selection of the ZR-75-1 cells produced a resistant variant (ZR-75-9a1) that is not growth-inhibited or -stimulated by tamoxifen.[90] ZR-75-9a1 cells have lost expression of both ER and PgR. However, the phenotype is unstable unless maintained in the presence of the selective pressure.[90]

Overexpression of FGF-1, by transfection into MCF-7 cells, produces cells that generate highly vascularized, estrogen-independent, metastatic tumors.[91] Estrogen-independent growth is not affected by 4-hydroxytamoxifen, indicating the ability of FGF-1 overexpression to confer tamoxifen resistance. When FGF-4 is overexpressed, the cells become tamoxifen-stimulated in vivo.[91,92] Cells overexpressing either FGF-1 or FGF-4 remain responsive to the growth-inhibitory effects of fulvestrant in vitro but exhibit some reduction in responsiveness compared with controls.[93] The ability of overexpression of FGFs to produce these phenotypes may reflect the induction of both mitogenic and growth-inhibitory effects in breast cancer cells.[94,95]

FGF-4/kFGF-overexpressing tumors are inhibited by physiological doses of estrogen,[96,97] an inverse response relative to the parental MCF-7 cells.[59,60] Tumors inhibited by physiological estrogen concentrations may not arise frequently, since most breast tumors appear to contain physiological concentrations of estrogens, irrespective of menopausal status.[98] While pharmacological doses of estrogens produce remissions in hormone-responsive breast tumors,[99,100] estrogenic hormone replacement therapy is associated with a modest increase in the risk of breast cancer.[24]

TAMOXIFEN-STIMULATED XENOGRAFTS

While selection for antiestrogen resistance in vitro has proved useful, several investigators have also selected MCF-7 xenografts against tamoxifen and fulvestrant. In marked contrast to most of the in vitro models, these xenografts almost exclusively acquire a tamoxifen-stimulated phenotype.[56,60] Initially, the xenografts cease proliferating or regress. However, prolonged therapy produces tamoxifen-stimulated tumors that regress upon removal of tamoxifen.[56,60] The tamoxifen-stimulated tumors are not cross-resistant to the steroidal antiestrogens,[101] similar to the MCF7/LCC2 phenotype.[84] Resistance to fulvestrant arises, but takes longer than does the development of tamoxifen resistance,[101] perhaps reflecting the greater potency of fulvestrant relative to tamoxifen.[52] Tamoxifen-stimulated tumors also may arise in women, but with a relatively low frequency as assessed by tamoxifen-withdrawal responses. Objective responses to tamoxifen withdrawals rarely exceed 10%, with overall response rates of less than 20%.[102]

MCF-WES cells also exhibit a tamoxifen-stimulated phenotype. In contrast to the models requiring tamoxifen, these cells arose from an MCF-7 tumor growing in an ovariectomized nude mouse in the absence of tamoxifen selection.[103] Estrogen-independent and estrogen-responsive, MCF-WES cells are cross-resistant to fulvestrant.[103] A tamoxifen-stimulated MCF-7 cell population (MCF/TOT) has also been obtained by long-term exposure to 4-hydroxy-tamoxifen in vitro. However, the cells do not exhibit cross-resistance to ICI 164,384.[83]

ENDOCRINE-UNRESPONSIVE XENOGRAFTS

Most human breast tumor xenografts are ER- and PgR-negative. Consequently, these exhibit a typical de novo estrogen-unresponsive phenotype. Reflecting the biology of the human disease, several are more locally aggressive, and exhibit a significantly increased metastatic potential. Most give rise to poorly differentiated tumors, in contrast to most endocrine-responsive xenografts. MDA-MB-231 and MDA-MB-435 xenografts can produce distant metastases in an apparently reproducible manner, and with a sufficient incidence to be of use in the study of spontaneous metastasis.[104] The MDA-MB-435 model is sensitive to dietary manipulations.[105,106] We have isolated an ascites variant of these cells (MDA435/LCC6), which is sensitive to a variety of cytotoxic drugs with proven efficacy in the human disease.[107] Other estrogen-unresponsive xenografts have been described in detail elsewhere.[63,108]

GENE TRANSFER: XENOGRAFT AND TRANSGENIC MODELS

As progress is made in elucidating the molecular biochemical pathways involved in the hormonal sensitivity and resistance of breast cancer, it is essential to directly test mechanistic hypotheses in animal models. Four approaches have been taken to date. First, human breast cancer cell lines have been transfected with a specific gene(s) and then tested in the nude mouse for effects of the gene(s). Second, transgenic mice have been prepared with a particular gene expressed under a mammary-selective or -unselective promoter. Third, gene-knockout mice have been utilized. Finally, retroviral gene transfer has been used for in vivo applications; mammary epithelial cells are infected either in situ or in vitro, followed by their reimplantation and developmental regrowth in the mammary fat pad.[109,110] To date, transgenic and knockout mice have provided the most interesting models for the study of onset of hormone-dependent mammary tumors. Conversely, gene-transfected xenograft models of human breast cancer have been most informative for the process of progression of hormone-dependent tumors to hormone independence, tamoxifen resistance, and/or metastasis. Recent studies have also begin to combine these two different types of methodology. For example, gene-knockout nude mice may now be made that are deficient in a gene required for tumor progression, and different transgenic/knockout stains may be mated to study gene–gene interactions.

HORMONAL RESPONSE AND RESISTANCE

The role of estrogens in the onset of mammary tumorigenesis, as well as mechanisms of resistance to hormonal therapy, have begun to be studied in animal models by gene-knockout and gene-transfer methodologies. Landmark studies from the laboratories of Korach and O'Malley created knockout mice deficient for the estrogen and progesterone receptor genes, respectively. While early ductal morphogenesis of the mammary gland was abrogated by knockout of $ER\alpha$, lobulo-alveolar development of the gland was blocked by PgR knockout.[111] Results of $ER\beta$ knockout have clearly failed to demonstrate a role for this receptor in mouse mammary development.[112] However, this receptor is expressed at low/undetectable levels in the mouse mammary gland.[113] Studies where $ER\beta$ is knocked out in mice may be of limited use in predicting its function in other species, for example $ER\beta$ is readily detected in the rat mammary gland and human breast.[114,115]

The availability of these models has allowed the beginning of studies to evaluate the inter-

action of hormone signaling pathways with other carcinogenic insults in tumor onset. For example, the absence of $ER\alpha$ delays, but does not abrogate, mammary tumorigenesis induced by the wnt-1 transgene.[116] Even more striking, in the absence of PgR, mammary tumorigenesis induced by the carcinogen DMBA (in association with a pituitary isograft) reduced tumor incidence by 75%.[111]

Some of the more interesting results with a transgenic model of hormonal carcinogenesis of the mammary gland have relied upon the aromatase gene.[117–121] This could be considered broadly comparable to the double $ER\alpha/ER\beta$ knockout, with loss of all but any ligand-independent activation of ERs. Recent studies in MMTV-induced mouse mammary tumorigenesis have implicated aromatase as the gene activated at the $int5$ locus. Based on these findings, a transgenic mouse was generated whereby expression of aromatase was directed to the mammary glands under the enhancer/promoter influence of MMTV LTR sequences. In virgin females, this transgene led to hyperplasias, dysplasias, and mammary tumors. Administration of the aromatase inhibitor letrozole to these animals completely prevented these pathologies, supporting the use of an aromatase inhibitor as a breast cancer prevention strategy.[119]

Gene transfection and xenograft models have also addressed hormonal aspects of tumor onset and progression. First, transfection studies with $ER\alpha$ in ER-negative human breast cancer cells have yielded paradoxical responses; $ER\alpha$ inhibits proliferation and tumorigenesis. These data indicate that proliferative processes in ER-negative breast cancers may be quite different from those in ER-positive human breast cancer cells.[122] Other experiments have transfected the aromatase gene into ER-positive human breast cancer cells (MCF-7).[121] These cells produced sufficient estrogen to allow their growth in ovariectomized nude mice; again, aromatase inhibitors (letrozole and anastrozole) blocked the growth. Inhibition by aromatase inhibitors was more effective than that by tamoxifen in this model.

In other experiments with MCF-7 breast cancer cells, the mitogenic and angiogenic fibroblast growth factors were explored for their ability to allow breast tumors to overcome their regulation by the ER system.[96,97,123–125] These cells, when injected into nude mice, formed well-vascularized, metastatic tumors that were tamoxifen-stimulated. Tumor growth and metastasis, however, were insensitive to aromatase inhibitors and to the steroidal antiestrogen fulvestrant.

ANGIOGENESIS AND METASTASIS

The ultimate event that leads to mortality from breast cancer is metastasis. The relationships among this process and hormonal sensitivity/resistance in breast cancer are currently unclear. Both ER/PgR-positive and -negative tumors progress to metastasis, although the later are well known to be associated with poorer patient outcome. Three separate but apparently interactive cellular processes seem to occur to allow metastasis of the disease: tumor angiogenesis, loss of proper tissue compartmentalization (invasion), and survival in hostile environments. It is not yet fully established whether genetic or phenotypic changes underlie these alterations. However, several molecular determinants have been proposed to relate to each process. Loss of cell–cell attachment, altered cell substratum attachment, and altered cytoskeletal organization play a role in regulating cellular invasion. In addition, cell locomotion, proteolysis, and the ability to survive and proliferate at distant sites must also contribute. While acquisition of this group of characteristics is responsible for allowing a cancer to locally invade host tissue, the ability of a tumor to distribute itself to distant sites also requires the development of a tumor vasculature – the complex process of angiogenesis. Some studies have shown that metastatic alterations may have at least some genetic basis, and that distant metastases are more likely to exhibit dominance of a malignant clone than primary tumors.[125,126]

There has been a great deal of interest generated in recent years in the process of tumor angiogenesis. Since existing blood vessels must proliferate and then invade the tumor area as the tumor is proliferating and invading out, it is possible that antimetastatic drugs can be designed that attack both processes simultaneously. Seminal studies by Folkman's group have established that quantification of blood vessels in the area of in situ breast tumors has prognostic significance and is related to the metastatic capacity of the tumor.[126] The actual angiogenic regulatory molecules produced by breast tumors are not fully known. Growth factors of the FGF, vascular endothelial growth factor (VEGF), transforming growth factor β (TGFβ), pleiotropin, and hepatocyte growth factor (HGF) families are considered to be strong candidates for positive regulatory molecules, while angiostatin, endostatin, and thrombospondin are candidate negative regulatory molecules.[127,128]

Among the secreted growth factors, VEGF appears to be most clearly under estrogen regulation.[129] VEGF also appears to be a survival factor for the vascular endothelium;[130] a drug directed against one of its receptors (SU5416) is already in phase III clinical trials. Recent data demonstrate that the integrin $\alpha_v\beta_3$, which allows survival and proper extracellular adhesion of vascular endothelium, is required for angiogenesis; this integrin represents an attractive target for novel therapies.[131] Although a few studies have addressed the roles of these growth factors in animal models, considerable more work needs to be performed to clarify their roles in hormone sensitivity and resistance.

The principal cell–cell adhesion molecule thought to be involved in mammary epithelial differentiation, E-cadherin (also called uvomorulin or L-CAM), is now considered to be a tumor suppressor gene.[131–133] Cell–cell adhesion is thought to restrict motility and to promote differentiation. Loss of expression of E-cadherin is associated with a more motile, fibroblastic morphology in breast cancer, with increased production of matrix metalloproteinases, with increased local invasiveness, with ER and PgR negativity, and with poor prognosis of ductal carcinoma.[133] Thus, it is becoming increasingly clear that in breast cancer a subset of E-cadherin-negative or E-cadherin function-compromised cells can arise, some of which express the mesenchymal intermediate filament vimentin (along with epithelial keratins), and which express an even more strongly motile, invasive phenotype.[134]

Four types of mechanism seem to be responsible, in addition to its genetic inactivation, for functional compromise of E-cadherin in tumor progression: loss of expression, direct proteolysis, inactivational phosphorylation of E-cadherin, and inactivational phosphorylation of submembrane, E-cadherin-associated proteins plakoglobin and β-catenin. These phosphorylation events are triggered by the epidermal growth factor receptor (EGFR), the HGF receptor (HGFR), and ErbB2.[125] Such a dedifferentiated phenotype is associated with poor histologic grade in clinical breast cancer.[134,135] This type of malignant progression event has also been observed in studies of epidermal carcinogenesis in bladder cancer and in melanoma; it has also been termed an epithelial–mesenchymal transition (EMT) in these systems. The EMT is not restricted to cancer – it also occurs as a common process in embryogenesis.[136] More animal models need to be developed to more fully understand the EMT and its role in breast tumor progression and hormone resistance.

The metastatic process is initially characterized by local invasion, whereby the cancer migrates across the basement membrane and into the stromal area. This transition is likely to depend upon local proteolysis and tumor cell motility. Although several classes of proteolytic enzymes are thought to be critical, two collagen IV-selective degrading enzymes termed matrix metalloproteinases 2 and 9 (MMP-2 and -9; 72 kDa and 92 kDa gelatinases, respectively) are the subjects of much current study.[137,138] However, recent studies have demonstrated that MMP-3/stromelysin-1 can serve as a mammary tumor promoter in transgenic mice; its effects were reversed by co-expression of TIMP

(tissue inhibitor of metallproteinase)-1, a natural antagonist of MMP-3.[139] Other investigations have focused on production of plasmin (produced in the tumor area due to action on plasminogen of secreted plasminogen activator/urokinase, uPA), on cathepsin D, on cathepsin B, on cathepsin L, and on a newly discovered transmembrane epithelial serine proteinase termed matriptase. Recent animal model studies have demonstrated that uPA knockout slows tumor progression and metastasis. The possible roles of each of these proteinases are still under investigation; studies are particularly needed to define their hormonal interactions.[140–143]

uPA and MMPs (including a specialized MMP subfamily termed MT-MMP (for 'membrane type') that activates others in the same class) are the most widely studied enzymes for the development of antimetastatic therapies.[144] Peritumoral proteolysis may depend upon a balance between proteolytic enzymes and their inhibitors. The gelatinases may be indicators of poor prognosis; they are secreted by stromal and (to a lesser extent) by epithelial components in complexes with their endogenous inhibitors TIMP-1, TIMP-2, and TIMP-3.[137,145] In breast cancer, most MMPs (with the exception of MMP-7) are synthesized primarily in the stroma. MMPs are thought to promote tumor cell invasion after binding to tumor cell surface receptors. The TIMPs are suppressive of cellular invasion, but they are thought to have little potential as antimetastasis drugs, since their half-lives are rather short in vivo.[146,147] Other broad-spectrum antimetalloproteinase peptides and small molecules such as marimastat are also under drug development.[137] uPA and its inhibitor plasminogen activator inhibitor-1 (PAI-1) (and, to a lesser extent, PAI-2) are currently of pathologic significance as strong indicators of poor prognosis in breast cancer; they are primarily secreted by stromal cells adjacent to invasive breast cancer.[146,148] Both MMPs and uPA have been demonstrated to attach to cell surface receptors on tumor cells and to contribute to tumor cell invasion.[131,137] From this perspective, anti-uPA-receptor-directed peptides have antimetastic potential.[140] Another consequence of invasion is a complex basement membrane remodeling process that results in deposition of tenascin, an extracellular matrix molecule. However, induction of tenascin does not appear to contribute directly to metastasis.[147]

As noted earlier, another important event contributing to metastasis is the dedifferentiating cellular transition termed the EMT. Loss of expression of ER and PgR appears to be associated with poor differentiation and possibly with an EMT process in breast cancer.[135] Although the full molecular basis of the EMT remains unknown, it seems to be associated with an acquisition of primary defects in arrangement of desmosomal and cytoskeletal proteins, leading to increased motility.[149] Because expression of the enzyme PKC is reported to increase during malignant progression and resistance to chemotherapy, and since a primary substrate of PKC is an actin-filament-crosslinking protein thought to be involved in motility,[150,151] it is likely that PKC plays a role in the regulation of EMT. Gene-transfer experiments with *PKCα* have partially verified this hypothesis.[152] This enzyme also induces multiple matrix-degrading proteases via AP-1 transcription factor interactions, it regulates cell-substrate adhesion via NF-κB transcription factor interactions, and it regulates breast cancer cell adhesion and invasiveness.[151] Further animal model studies will clarify the relevance of these findings.

Cell–substratum attachment also seems critical both in differentiation[149] and in metastasis.[153,154] Expression of high levels of a sex-steroid-regulated, non-integrin, 67 kDa adhesion protein for laminin has been correlated with progression of breast and colon cancer.[155] Other studies have focused on the heterodimeric integrin class of attachment molecules as necessary for metastasis. Specifically, loss of expression or altered binding specificity of the integrins $\alpha_2\beta_1$, $\alpha_3\beta_1$, $\alpha_5\beta_1$, and $\alpha_6\beta_1$ seem to be important.[131] Overexpression of cadherin II,[156] a variant form of a non-integrin binding protein for hyaluronic acid (CD44) is of significant interest in this respect as well.[157] The process of cellular adhesion, in areas termed focal adhesions, signals the cell through a tyrosine kinase termed FAK (focal adhesion kinase) and through interactions with the actin cytoskeleton. The FAK kinase is upregulated in invasive breast cancer, and interacts with the Src kinase-mediated signal transduction pathways. Recent studies have suggested that FAK may be most important in the regulation of hormone-dependent breast cancer cells.[158,159] Further studies are required to clarify its interactions with hormone response.

Major questions still exist concerning mechanisms of organ site specificity for metastasis. The theory that the tumor 'seed' requires a properly nourishing 'soil' has been presented by Fidler, but the molecular basis of this phenomena is not yet clear, beyond the role of uPA, noted above. Another interesting and radiologically important phenomena is the calcification that breast tumors can induce in primary and metastatic sites. A hormone-like factor termed parathyroid hormone-related factor (PTHRP) has been characterized as the likely etiologic factor for calcification, but the relationship of PTHRP to hormonal stimulation is not yet clear. It should also be stated that our understanding of mechanisms involved in metastasis is still in its infancy, and many additional new candidate regulatory molecules such as the candidate tumor suppressors nm23, KAI-1 and KISS-1 are currently being explored.[154]

CONCLUSIONS AND FUTURE PROSPECTS

Animal models have played an important role in breast cancer research. This has included identifying many aspects of breast biology, and in the development of new therapies for the disease. Nonetheless, additional models are required. There are relatively few estrogen-dependent models of human origin, and few models that exhibit a strongly metastatic phenotype. Clearly, more models are needed.

In the future, transgenic and knockout models will continue to play an increasingly important role in breast cancer research. However, as with all experimental models, their advantages and disadvantages must be carefully considered. In the absence of a single model to accurately reflect all aspects of breast biology, investigators may have to select several. In this regard, there is a careful balance between adequately addressing a hypothesis and an appropriate use of animals for experimentation.[6]

ACKNOWLEDGMENTS

This work was supported in part by Grants NIH R01-CA/AG58022, NIH P30-CA51008, and NIH P50-CA58185 (Public Health Service), and USAMRMC (Department of Defense) BC980629, BC980586, and BC990358.

REFERENCES

1. Schiffer SP. Animal welfare and colony management in cancer research. *Breast Cancer Res Treat* 1997; **46:** 313–31.
2. Kritchevesky D, Weber MM, Klurfeld DM. Dietary fat versus caloric intake in initiation and promotion of 7,12-dimethylbenz(a)-anthracene-induced mammary tumorigenesis in rats. *Cancer Res* 1984; **44:** 3174–7.
3. Welsch CW. Enhancement of mammary tumorigenesis by dietary fat: review of potential mechanisms. *Am J Clin Nutr* 1987; **45:** 192–202.
4. Engelman RW, Day NK, Chen R-F et al. Calorie consumption level influences development of C3H/Ou breast adenocarcinoma with indifference to calorie source. *Proc Soc Exp Biol Med* 1990; **193:** 23–30.
5. Hanfelt J. Statistical approaches to experimental design and data analysis of in vivo studies. *Breast Cancer Res Treat* 1997; **46:** 279–302.
6. Clarke R. Issues in experimental design and endpoint analysis in the study of experimental cytotoxic agents in vivo in breast cancer and other models. *Breast Cancer Res Treat* 1997; **46:** 255–78.
7. Siemann DW. Rodent tumor models in experimental cancer therapy. In: *Rodent Tumor Models in Experimental Cancer Therapy* (Kallman, RF, ed). New York: Pergamon, 1987: 12–15.
8. Chan PC, Cohen LA. Effect of dietary fat, anti-estrogen and antiprolactin on the development of mammary tumors in rats. *J Natl Cancer Inst* 1974; **52:** 25–30.
9. Ip C, Ip MM. Serum estrogens and estrogen responsiveness in 7,12-dimethylbenz(a)anthracene-induced mammary tumors as influenced by dietary fat. *J Natl Cancer Inst* 1981; **66:** 291–5.
10. Zwiebel JA, Bano M, Nexo E et al. Partial purification of transforming growth factors from human milk. *Cancer Res* 1986; **46:** 933–9.
11. Lacroix A, Doskas C, Bhat PV. Inhibition of growth of established N-methyl-N-nitrosourea-induced mammary cancer in rats by retinoic acid and ovariectomy. *Cancer Res* 1990; **50:** 5731–4.
12. Huggins C, Grand LC, Brillantes FP. Mammary cancer induced by a single feeding of polynuclear hydrocarbons, and its suppression. *Nature* 1961; **189:** 204.
13. Medina D. Mammary tumorigenesis in chemical carcinogen-treated mice. II. Dependence on hormone stimulation for tumorigenesis. *J Natl Cancer Inst* 1974; **53:** 223–6.
14. Medina D. Mammary tumorigenesis in chemical carcinogen-treated mice. I. Incidence in BALB-c and C57BL mice. *J Natl Cancer Inst* 1974; **53:** 213–21.
15. Gould MN, Zhang R. Genetic regulation of mammary carcinogenesis in the rat by susceptibility and suppressor genes. *Environ Health Perspect* 1991; **93:** 161–7.
16. Hsu L-C, Kennan WS, Shepel LA et al. Genetic identification of *Mcs-1*, a rat mammary carcinoma suppressor gene. *Cancer Res* 1994; **54:** 2765–70.
17. Isaacs JT. A mammary cancer suppressor gene and its site of action in the rat. *Cancer Res* 1991; **51:** 1591–5.
18. Russo J, Gusterson BA, Rogers AE et al. Biology of disease: comparative study of human and rat mammary tumorigenesis. *Lab Invest* 1990; **62:** 244–78.
19. Sukumar S, Notario V, Martin-Zanca D, Barbacid M. Induction of mammary carcinomas in rats by nitroso-methylurea involves malignant activation of Ha-ras-1 locus by single point mutations. *Nature* 1983; **306:** 658–61.
20. Gould MN. Inheritance and site of expression of genes controlling susceptibility to mammary cancer in an inbred rat model. *Cancer Res* 1986; **46:** 1199–202.

21. Rivera EM, Vijayaraghavan S. Proliferation of ductal outgrowths by carcinogen-induced rat mammary tumors in gland-free mammary fat pads. *J Natl Cancer Inst* 1982; **69**: 517–25.

22. Clarke R. Animal models of breast cancer: experimental design and their use in nutrition and psychosocial research. *Breast Cancer Res Treat* 1997; **46**: 117–33.

23. Gullino PM, Pettigrew HM, Grantham FH. *N*-Nitrosomethylurea as a mammary gland carcinogen in rats. *J Natl Cancer Inst* 1975; **54**: 401.

24. Hulka BS, Stark AT. Breast cancer: cause and prevention. *Lancet* 1995; **346**: 883–7.

25. Raynaud A. Observations sur les modifications provoquées pas les hormones oestrogenes, du mode de développement des mamelons des foetus de souris. *C R Acad Sci Paris* 1955; **240**: 674–6.

26. Russo J, Russo IH. Experimentally induced mammary tumors in rats. *Breast Cancer Res Treat* 1996; **39**: 7–20.

27. Russo J, Russo IH. Biology of disease: biological and molecular bases of mammary carcinogenesis. *Lab Invest* 1987; **57**: 112–37.

28. Russo J, Russo I. Role of differentiation in the pathogenesis and prevention of breast cancer. *Endocr Rel Cancer* 1997; **4**: 7–21.

29. Manni A, Rainieri J, Arafah BM et al. Role of estrogen and prolactin in the growth and receptor levels of *N*-nitrosomethylurea-induced rat mammary tumors. *Cancer Res* 1982; **42**: 3492–5.

30. L'Hermite M, L'Hermite-Baleriaux M. Prolactin and breast cancer. *Eur J Cancer Clin Oncol* 1988; **24**: 955–8.

31. Clark GJ, Der CJ. Aberrant function of the Ras signal transduction pathway in human breast cancer. *Breast Cancer Res Treat* 1995; **35**: 133–44.

32. Cha RS, Thilly WG, Zarbl H. *N*-Nitroso-*N*-methylurea-induced rat mammary tumors arise from cells with preexisting oncogenic *Hras1* gene mutations. *Proc Natl Acad Sci USA* 1994; **91**: 3749–53.

33. Jin Z, Houle B, Mikheev AM et al. Alterations in *H-ras-1* promoter conformation during *N*-nitroso-*N*-methylurea-induced mammary carcinogenesis and pregnancy. *Cancer Res* 1996; **56**: 4927–35.

34. Fluck MM, Haslam SZ. Mammary tumors induced by polyomavirus. *Breast Cancer Res Treat* 1996; **39**: 45–56.

35. Javier R, Shenk T. Mammary tumors induced by adenovirus type-9: a role for the viral early region 4 gene. *Breast Cancer Res Treat* 1995; **39**: 57–67.

36. Welsch CW, Gribler C. Prophylaxis of spontaneously developing mammary carcinoma in C3H/HeJ female mice by prolactin. *Cancer Res* 1973; **33**: 2939–46.

37. Osborne MP, Telang NT, Kaur S, Bradlow HL. Influence of chemopreventive agents on estradiol metabolism and mammary preneoplasia in the C3H mouse. *Steroids* 1990; **55**: 114–19.

38. Wellings SR. A hypothesis of the origin of human breast cancer from the terminal ductal lobular unit. *Path Res Pract* 1980; **166**: 515–35.

39. Nusse R. Insertional mutagenesis in mouse mammary tumorigenesis. *Curr Top Microbiol Immunobiol* 1991; **171**: 43–65.

40. Callahan R. MMTV induced mutations in mouse mammary tumors: their potential relevance to human breast cancer. *Breast Cancer Res Treat* 1995; **39**: 33–44.

41. Haslam SZ, Wirth JJ, Counterman LJ, Fluck MM. Characterization of the mammary hyperplasia, dysplasia and neoplasia induced in athymic female adult mice by polyomavirus. *Oncogene* 1992; **7**: 1295–303.

42. Javier R, Raska K, MacDonald GJ, Shenk T. Human adenovirus type 9-induced rat mammary tumors. *J Virol* 1991; **65**: 3192–202.

43. Fodstad Ø. Limitations for studies in human tumor biology. In: *The Nude Mouse in Oncology Research* (Boven E, Winograd B, eds). Boca Raton, FL: CRC Press, 1991: 277–89.

44. Clarke R, Brünner N, Katzenellenbogen BS et al. Progression from hormone dependent to hormone independent growth in MCF-7 human breast cancer cells. *Proc Natl Acad Sci USA* 1989; **86**: 3649–53.

45. Rygaard J, Povlsen CO. Heterotransplantation of a human malignant tumour to 'nude' mice. *Acta Path Microbiol Scand* 1969; **77**: 758–60.

46. Pantelouris EM. Absence of thymus in a mutant mouse. *Nature* 1968; **217**: 370–1.

47. Clarke R. Human breast cancer cell line xenografts as models of breast cancer: the immunobiologies of recipient mice and the characteristics of several tumorigenic cell lines. *Breast Cancer Res Treat* 1996; **39**: 69–86.

48. Bosma MJ, Carroll AM. The SCID mouse mutant: definition, characterization, and potential uses. *Annu Rev Immunol* 1991; **9**: 323–50.

49. Ghetie MA, Gordon BE, Podar EM, Vitetta ES. Effect of sublethal irradiation of SCID mice on

growth of B-cell lymphoma xenografts and on efficacy of chemotherapy and/or immunotoxin therapy. *Lab Anim Sci* 1996; **46**: 305–9.

50. Sakakibara T, Xu Y, Bumpers HL et al. Growth and metastasis of surgical specimens of human breast carcinomas in SCID mice. *Cancer J Sci Am* 1996; **2**: 291–300.

51. Shultz LD, Lang PA, Christianson SW et al. NOD/LtSz-Rag1null mice: an immunodeficient and radioresistant model for engraftment of human hematolymphoid cells, HIV infection, and adoptive transfer of NOD mouse diabetogenic T cells. *J Immunol* 2000; **164**: 2496–507.

52. Brünner N, Frandsen TL, Holst-Hansen C et al. MCF7/LCC2: a 4-hydroxytamoxifen resistant human breast cancer variant which retains sensitivity to the steroidal antiestrogen ICI 182,780. *Cancer Res* 1993; **53**: 3229–32.

53. Katzenellenbogen BS, Kendra KL, Norman MJ, Berthois Y. Proliferation, hormonal responsiveness, and estrogen receptor content of MCF-7 human breast cancer cells grown in the short-term and long-term absence of estrogens. *Cancer Res* 1987; **47**: 4355–60.

54. Clarke R, Thompson EW, Leonessa F et al. *Breast Cancer Res Treat* 1993; **24**: 227–39.

55. Thompson EW, Brünner N, Torri J et al. The invasive and metastatic properties of hormone-independent and hormone-responsive variants of MCF-7 human breast cancer cells. *Clin Exp Metastasis* 1993; **11**: 15–26.

56. Osborne CK, Coronado EB, Robinson JP. Human breast cancer in athymic nude mice: cytostatic effects of long-term antiestrogen therapy. *Eur J Cancer Clin Oncol* 1987; **23**: 1189–96.

57. Gottardis MM, Jordan VC. Development of tamoxifen-stimulated growth of MCF-7 tumors in athymic mice after long-term antiestrogen administration. *Cancer Res* 1988; **48**: 5183–7.

58. Gottardis MM, Robinson SP, Satyaswaroop PG, Jordan VC. Contrasting actions of tamoxifen on endometrial and breast tumor growth in the athymic nude mouse. *Cancer Res* 1988; **48**: 812–15.

59. Brunner N, Bronzert D, Vindelov LL et al. Effect of growth and cell cycle kinetics of estradiol and tamoxifen on MCF-7 human breast cancer cells grown in vitro in nude mice. *Cancer Res* 1989; **49**: 1515–20.

60. Gottardis MM, Wagner RJ, Borden EC, Jordan VC. Differential ability of antiestrogens to stim-

ulate breast cancer cell (MCF-7) growth in vivo and in vitro. *Cancer Res* 1989; **49**: 4765–9.

61. Levinson AS, Jordan VC. MCF-7 the first hormone-responsive breast cancer cell line. *Cancer Res* 1997; **57**: 3071–8.

62. Soule HD, Vasquez J, Long A et al. A human cell line from a pleural effusion derived from a human breast carcinoma. *J Natl Cancer Inst* 1973; **51**: 1409–16.

63. Clarke R, Leonessa F, Brünner N, Thompson EW. In vitro models. In: *Diseases of the Breast*, 2nd edn (Harris JR, Lippman ME, Morrow M, Hellman S, eds). Philadelphia: Lippincott-Raven, 2000: 335–54.

64. Brünner N, Boulay V, Fojo A et al. Acquisition of hormone-independent growth in MCF-7 cells is accompanied by increased expression of estrogen-regulated genes but without detectable DNA amplifications. *Cancer Res* 1993; **53**: 283–90.

65. Clarke R, Dickson RB, Brünner N. The process of malignant progression in human breast cancer. *Ann Oncol* 1990; **1**: 401–7.

66. Clarke R, Skaar T, Baumann K et al. Hormonal carcinogenesis in breast cancer: cellular and molecular studies of malignant progression. *Breast Cancer Res Treat* 1994; **31**: 237–48.

67. Leonessa F, Boulay V, Wright A et al. The biology of breast tumor progression: acquisition of hormone-independence and resistance to cytotoxic drugs. *Acta Oncol* 1991; **31**: 115–23.

68. Keydar I, Chen L, Karby S et al. Establishment and characterization of a cell line of human carcinoma origin. *Eur J Cancer* 1979; **15**: 659–70.

69. Reddel RR, Alexander IE, Koga M et al. Genetic instability and the development of steroid hormone insensitivity in cultured T 47D human breast cancer cells. *Cancer Res* 1988; **48**: 4340–7.

70. Graham ML, Smith JA, Jewett PB, Horwitz KB. Heterogeneity of progesterone receptor content and remodeling by tamoxifen characterize subpopulations of cultured human breast cancer cells: analysis by quantitative dual parameter flow cytometry. *Cancer Res* 1992; **52**: 593–602.

71. Sartorius CA, Groshong SD, Miller LA et al. New T47D breast cancer cell lines for the independent study of progesterone B- and A-receptors: only antiprogestin-occupied B-receptors are switched to transcriptional agonists by cAMP. *Cancer Res* 1994; **54**: 3868–77.

72. Graham ML, Dalquist KE, Horwitz KB. Simultaneous measurement of progesterone

receptors and DNA indices by flow cytometry: analysis of breast cancer cell mixtures and genetic instability of the T47D line. *Cancer Res* 1989; **49:** 3943–9.

73. Engel LW, Young NA, Tralka TS et al. Establishment and characterization of three new continuous cell lines derived from human breast carcinomas. *Cancer Res* 1978; **38:** 3352–64.

74. Brünner N, Spang-Thomsen M, Cullen K. The T61 human breast cancer xenograft: an experimental model of estrogen therapy of breast cancer. *Breast Cancer Res Treat* 1996; **39:** 87–92.

75. Seibert K, Shafie SM, Triche TJ et al. Clonal variation of MCF-7 breast cancer cells in vitro and in athymic nude mice. *Cancer Res* 1983; **43:** 2223–39.

76. van Steenbrugge GJ, Groen M, van Kreuningen A et al. Transplantable human prostatic carcinoma (PC-82) in athymic nude mice (III). Effects of estrogens on the growth of the tumor. *Prostate* 1988; **12:** 157–61.

77. Brünner N, Svenstrup B, Spang-Thompsen M et al. Serum steroid levels in intact and endocrine ablated Balb\c nude mice and their intact litter mates. *J Steroid Biochem* 1986; **25:** 429–32.

78. Bronzert DA, Greene GL, Lippman ME. Selection and characterization of a breast cancer cell line resistant to the antiestrogen LY 117018. *Endocrinology* 1985; **117:** 1409–17.

79. Clarke R, Brünner N, Thompson EW et al. The inter-relationships between ovarian-independent growth, antiestrogen resistance and invasiveness in the malignant progression of human breast cancer. *J Endocrinol* 1989; **122:** 331–40.

80. Nawata H, Bronzert D, Lippman ME. Isolation and characterization of a tamoxifen resistant cell line derived from MCF-7 human breast cancer cells. *J Biol Chem* 1981; **256:** 5016–21.

81. Butler WB, Berlinski PJ, Hillman RM et al. Relation of in vitro properties to tumorigenicity for a series of sublines of the human breast cancer cell line MCF-7. *Cancer Res* 1986; **46:** 6339–48.

82. Butler WB, Fontana JA. Responses to retinoic acid of tamoxifen-sensitive and -resistant sublines of human breast cancer cell line MCF-7. *Cancer Res* 1992; **52:** 6164–7.

83. Herman ME, Katzenellenbogen BS. Response-specific antiestrogen resistance in a newly characterized MCF-7 human breast cancer cell line resulting from long-term exposure to trans-hydroxytamoxifen. *J Steroid Biochem Mol Biol* 1996; **59:** 121–34.

84. Brunner N, Boysen B, Jirus S et al. MCF7/LCC9: an antiestrogen-resistant MCF-7 variant in which acquired resistance to the steroidal antiestrogen ICI 182,780 confers an early cross-resistance to the nonsteroidal antiestrogen tamoxifen. *Cancer Res* 1997; **57:** 3486–93.

85. Coopman P, Garcia M, Brünner N et al. Antiproliferative and antiestrogenic effects of ICI 164,384 in 4-OH-tamoxifen-resistant human breast cancer cells. *Int J Cancer* 1994; **56:** 295–300.

86. Brünner N, Boysen B, Jirus S et al. MCF7/LCC9: an antiestrogen resistant MCF-7 variant in which acquired resistance to the steroidal antiestrogen ICI 182,780 confers an early crossresistance to the non-steroidal antiestrogen tamoxifen. *Cancer Res* 1997; **57:** 3486–93.

87. Howell A, DeFriend D, Robertson JFR et al. Response to a specific antioestrogen (ICI 182,780) in tamoxifen-resistant breast cancer. *Lancet* 1995; **345:** 29–30.

88. Lykkesfeldt AE, Madsen MW, Briand P. Altered expression of estrogen-regulated genes in a tamoxifen-resistant and ICI 164,384 and ICI 182,790 sensitive human breast cancer cell line, MCF-7/TAM^R-1. *Cancer Res* 1994; **54:** 1587–95.

89. Jensen BL, Skouv J, Lykkesfeldt AE. Differential regulation of specific genes in MCF-7 and the ICI 182,780-resistant cell line MCF-7182$^{R^-}$6. *Br J Cancer* 1999; **79:** 386–92.

90. van den Berg HW, Lynch M, Martin J et al. Characterization of a tamoxifen-resistant variant of the ZR-75-1 human breast cancer cell line (ZR-75-9a1) and stability of the resistant phenotype. *Br J Cancer* 1989; **59:** 522–6.

91. Zhang L, Kharbanda S, Chen D et al. MCF-7 breast carcinoma cells overexpressing FGF-1 form vascularized, metastatic tumors in ovariectomized or tamoxifen-treated nude mice. *Oncogene* 1997; **15:** 2093–108.

92. Kurebayashi J, McLeskey SW, Johnson MD et al. Quantitative demonstration of spontaneous metastasis by MCF-7 human breast cancer cells cotransfected with fibroblast growth factor 4 and LacZ. *Cancer Res* 1993; **53:** 2178–87.

93. McLeskey SW, Zhang L, El-Ashry D et al. Tamoxifen-resistant fibroblast growth factor-transfected MCF-7 cells are crossresistant in vivo to the antiestrogen ICI 182,780 and two aromatase inhibitors. *Clin Cancer Res* 1998; **4:** 697–711.

94. Wang H, Rubin M, Fenig E et al. Basic fibroblast growth factor causes growth arrest in MVF-7 human breast cancer cells while inducing both mitogenic and inhibitory G_1 events. *Cancer Res* 1997; **57:** 1750–7.

95. Fenig E, Wieder R, Paglin S et al. Basic fibroblast growth factor confers growth inhibition and mitogen-activated protein kinase activation in human breast cancer cells. *Clin Cancer Res* 1997; **3:** 135–42.

96. Mcleskey SW, Zhang L, Kharbanda S et al. Fibroblast growth factor-overexpressing models of angiogenesis and metastasis in breast cancer. *Breast Cancer Res Treat* 1996; **39:** 103–17.

97. McLeskey SW, Zhang L, Kharbanda S et al. Fibroblast growth factor overexpressing breast carcinoma cells as models for angiogenesis and metastasis. *Breast Cancer Res Treat* 1995; **39:** 103–17.

98. Pasqualini JR, Chetrite G, Nestour EL. Control and expression of oestrone sulphatase activities in human breast cancer. *J Endocrinol* 1996; **150:** S99–105.

99. Gockerman JP, Spremulli EN, Raney M, Logan T. Randomized comparison of tamoxifen versus diethylstilbestrol in estrogen receptor-positive or -unknown metastatic breast cancer: a southeastern cancer study group trial. *Cancer Treat Rep* 1986; **70:** 1199–203.

100. Kennedy BJ. Hormonal therapies in breast cancer. *Semin Oncol* 1974; **1:** 119–30.

101. Osborne CK, Coronado-Heinsohn EB, Hilsenbeck S et al. Comparison of the effects of a pure steroidal antiestrogen with those of tamoxifen in a model of human breast cancer. *J Natl Cancer Inst* 1995; **87:** 746–50.

102. Howell A, Dodwell DJ, Anderson H, Redford J. Response after withdrawal of tamoxifen and progestogens in advanced breast cancer. *Ann Oncol* 1992; **3:** 611–17.

103. Dumont JA, Bitoni AJ, Wallace CD et al. Progression of MCF-7 breast cancer cells to antiestrogen-resistant phenotype is accompanied by elevated levels of AP-1 DNA-binding activity. *Cell Growth Diff* 1996; **7:** 351–9.

104. Price JE, Polyzos A, Zhang RD, Daniels LM. Tumorigenicity and metastasis of human breast carcinoma cell lines in nude mice. *Cancer Res* 1990; **50:** 717–21.

105. Meschter CL, Connolly JM, Rose DP. Influence of regional location of the inoculation site and dietary fat on the pathology of MDA-MB-435 human breast cancer cell-derived tumors growing in nude mice. *Clin Exp Metastasis* 1992; **10:** 167–73.

106. Rose DP, Hatala MA, Connolly JM, Rayburn J. Effect of diets containing different levels of linoleic acid on human breast cancer growth and lung metastasis in nude mice. *Cancer Res* 1993; **53:** 4686–90.

107. Leonessa F, Green D, Licht T et al. MDA435/LCC6 and MDA435/LCC6^{MDR1}: ascites models of human breast cancer. *Br J Cancer* 1996; **73:** 154–61.

108. Clarke R. Animal models. In: *Diseases of the Breast*, 2nd edn (Harris JR, Lippman ME, Morrow M, Hellman S, eds). Philadelphia: Lippincott-Raven, 2000: 319–33.

109. Edwards PA. The use of transplanted mammary gland to study cancer signalling pathways. *Adv Exptl Med Biol* 2000; 480: 163–7.

110. Siegel PM, Hardy WR, Muller WL. Mammary gland neoplasia: insights from transgenic mouse models. *BioEssays* 2000; **22:** 554–63.

111. Lydon JP, Ge G, Kittrell FS et al. Murine mammary gland carcinogenesis is critically dependent on progesterone receptor function. *Cancer Res* 1999; **59:** 4276–84.

112. Course JF, Hewitt C, Korach KS. Receptor null mice reveal contrasting roles for estrogen receptor alpha and beta in reproductive tissues. *J Steroid Biochem Mol Biol* 2000; 74: 287–96.

113. Couse JF, Lindzey J, Grandien K et al. Tissue distribution and quantitative analysis of estrogen receptor-α (ERα) and estrogen receptor-β (ERβ) messenger ribonucleic acid in the wild-type and ERα-knockout mouse. *Endocrinology* 1997; **138:** 4613–21.

114. Enmark E, Pelto-Huikko M, Grandien K et al. Human estrogen receptor β-gene structure, chromosomal localization, and expression pattern. *J Clin Endocrinol Metab* 1997; **82:** 4258–65.

115. Saji S, Jensen EV, Nilsson S et al. Estrogen receptors α and β in the rodent mammary gland. *Proc Natl Acad Sci USA* 2000; **97:** 337–42.

116. Bocchinfusso WP, Hively WP, Couse JF et al. A mouse mammary tumor virus–Wnt-1 transgene induces mammary gland hyperplasia and tumorigenesis in mice lacking estrogen receptor-α. *Cancer Res* 1999; **59:** 1869–76.

117. Tekmal RR, Durgam VR. A novel in vitro and in vivo breast cancer model for testing inhibitors of estrogen biosynthesis and its action using mammary tumor cells with an acti-

vated int-5/aromatase gene. *Cancer Lett* 1997; **118**: 21–8.

118. Tekmal RR, Kirma N, Gill K, Fowler K. Aromatase overexpression and breast hyperplasia, an in vivo model – continued overexpression of aromatase is sufficient to maintain hyperplasia without circulating estrogens, and aromatase inhibitors abrogate these preneoplastic changes in mammary glands. *Endocr Rel Cancer* 1999; **6**: 307–14.

119. Brodie A, Lu Z, Liu Y et al. Preclinical studies using the intratumoral aromatase model for postmenopausal breast cancer. *Oncology* 1998; **12**: 36–40.

120. Sun XZ, Zhou D, Chen S. Autocrine and paracrine actions of breast tumor aromatase. A 3-dimensional cell culture system involving aromatase-transfected HCF-7 and T47D cells. *J Steroid Biochem Mol Biol* 1997; 63: 29–36.

121. Yue W, Wang J, Savinov A, Brodie A. Effect of aromatase inhibitors on growth of mammary tumors in a nude mouse model. *Cancer Res* 1995; **55**: 3073–7.

122. Dickson RB, Russo J. Biochemical control of breast development. In: *Diseases of the Breast*, 2nd edn (Harris JR, Lippman ME, Morrow M, Hellman S, eds). Philadelphia: Lippincott-Raven, 2000: 15–32.

123. Mcleskey SW, Zhang L, El-Ashry D et al. Tamoxifen-resistant fibroblast growth factor-transfected MCF-7 cells are cross-resistant in vivo to the antiestrogen ICI 182,780 and two aromatase inhibitors. *Clin Cancer Res* 1998; **4**: 697–711.

124. Zhang L, Kharbanda S, Chen D et al. MCF-7 breast carcinoma cells overexpressing FGF-1 form vascularized, metastatic tumors in ovariectomized or tamoxifen-treated nude mice. *Oncogene* 1997; **15**: 2093–108.

125. Zhang L, Kharbanda S, Mcleskey SW, Kern FG. Overexpression of fibroblast growth factor 1 in MCF-7 breast cancer cells facilitates tumor cell dissemination but does not support the development of macrometastases in the lungs or lymph nodes. *Cancer Res* 1999; **59**: 5023–9.

126. Weidner N, Semple JP, Welch WR, Folkman J. Tumor angiogenesis and metastasis – correlation in invasive breast carcinoma. *N Engl J Med* 1991; **324**: 1–8.

127. Meleakey S, Dickson RB. The role of angiogenesis in breast cancer progression. In: *Vascular Morphogenesis of the Reproductive System* (Augustin H, Rogers P, Smith S, Iruela-Arispe L, eds). NY: Springer Verlag, 2001: 41–62.

128. Valles AM, Tucker GC, Thiery JP, Boyer B. Alternative patterns of mitogenesis and cell scattering induced by acidic FGF as a function of cell density in a rat bladder carcinoma cell line. *Cell Regul* 1990; **1**: 975–88.

129. Hyder SM, Nawaz Z, Chiappetta C, Stancel GM. Identification of functional estrogen response elements in the gene coding for the potent angiogenic factor vascular endothelial growth factor. *Cancer Res* 2000; **60**: 3183–90.

130. Augustin HG, Kozian DH, Johnson RC. Differentiation of endothelial cells: analysis of the constitutive and activated endothelial cell phenotypes. *BioEssays* 1994; **16**: 901–6.

131. Rosfjord E, Dickson RB. Cell adhesion and metastasis In: *Contemporary Approaches to Breast Cancer* (Bowcock A, ed). Totowa, NJ: Humana Press, 1999: 285–304.

132. Navarro P, Gomez M, Pizarro A et al. A role for the E-cadherin cell–cell adhesion molecule during tumor progression of mouse epidermal carcinogenesis. *J Cell Biol* 1991; **115**: 517–33.

133. Gamallo C, Palacios J, Suarez A et al. Correlation of E-cadherin expression with differentiation grade and histological type in breast carcinoma. *Am J Pathol* 1993; **142**: 987–93.

134. Thomas PA, Kirschmann DA, Cerhan JR et al. Association between keratin and vimentin expression, malignant phenotype, and survival in postmenopausal breast cancer patients. *Clin Cancer Res* 1999; **5**: 2698–703.

135. Thompson EW, Paik S, Brunner N et al. Association of increased basement membrane invasiveness with absence of estrogen receptor and expression of vimentin in human breast cancer cell lines. *J Cell Physiol* 1992; **150**: 534–44.

136. Boyer B, Tucker GC, Valles AM et al. Rearrangements of desmosomal and cytoskeletal proteins during the transition from epithelial to fibroblastoid organization in cultured rat bladder carcinoma cells. *J Cell Biol* 1989; **109**: 1495–509.

137. Benaud C, Dickson RB, Thompson EW. Roles of matrix metalloproteases in mammary gland development and cancer. *Cancer Res Treat* 1998; **50**: 97–116.

138. Toi M, Ishigaki S, Tominaga T. Metalloproteinases and tissue inhibitors of metalloproteinases. *Breast Cancer Res Treat* 1998; **52**: 113–24.

139. Sternlicht MD, Lochter A, Sympson CJ et al.

The stromal proteinase MMP3/stromelysin-1 promotes mammary carcinogenesis. *Cell* 1999; **98:** 137–46.

140. Stephens RW, Brunner N, Janicke F, Schmitt M. The urokinase plasminogen activator system as a target for prognostic studies in breast cancer. *Breast Cancer Res Treat* 1998; **52:** 99–111.

141. Bianchi E, Cohen RL Thor AT et al. The uro-kinase receptor is expressed in invasive breast cancer but not in normal breast tissue. *Cancer Res* 1994; **54:** 861–6.

142. Sloan B. Cathepsin B and cystatins: evidence for a role in cancer progression. *Semin Cancer Biol* 1990; **1:** 137–52.

143. Lin CY, Sanders J, Johnson MD, Sang ZQ, Dickson RB. Molecular cloning of cDNA for matriptase, a matrix-degrading serine protease with trypsin-like activity. *J Biol Chem* 1999; **274:** 18231–6.

144. De Clerck YA, Perez N, Shimada H et al. Inhibition of invasion and metastasis in cells transfected with an inhibitor of metallopro-teinases. *Cancer Res* 1992; **52:** 701–8.

145. Coussens LM, Fingleton B, Matrisian LM. Matrix metalloproteinase inhibitors and cancer: trials and tribulations. *Science* 2002; 295: 2387–92.

146. Harbeck N, Thomssen C, Berger U et al. Invasion marker PAI-1 remains a strong prognostic factor after long-term follow-up both for primary breast cancer and following first relapse. *Breast Cancer Res Treat* 1999; **54:** 147–57.

147. Talts JF, Wirl G, Dictor M et al. Tenascin-C modulates tumor stroma and monocyte/macrophage recruitment but not tumor growth or metastasis in a mouse strain with sponta-neous mammary cancer. *J Cell Sci* 1999; **112:** 1855–64.

148. Bajau K, Noel A, Gerard RD et al. Absence of host plasminogen activator inhibitor-1 prevents cancer invasion and vascularization. *BMJ* 1998; **317:** 750.

149. Streuli CH, Bailey N, Bissell MJ. Control of mammary epithelial differentiation: basement membrane induces tissue-specific gene expres-sion in the absence of cell–cell interaction and morphological polarity. *J Cell Biol* 1991; **115:** 1383–95.

150. Johnson MD, Torri J, Lippman ME, Dickson RB. Regulation of motility and protease expression in PKC-mediated induction of MCF-7 breast cancer cell invasiveness. *Exp Cell Res* 1999; **247:** 105–13.

151. Hartwig JH, Thelen M, Rosen A et al. MARCKS is an actin filament crosslinking protein regu-lated by protein kinase C and calcium-calmod-ulin. *Nature* 1992; **356:** 618–22.

152. Ways DK, Kukoly CA, de Vente J et al. MCF-7 breast cancer cells transfected with protein kinase C-α exhibit altered expression of other protein kinase C isoforms and display a more aggressive neoplastic phenotype. *J Clin Invest* 1995; **95:** 1906–15.

153. Strange R, Li F, Friis RR et al. Mammary epithe-lial differentiation in vitro: minimum require-ments for a functional response to hormonal stimulation. *Cell Growth Differ* 1991; **2:** 549–59.

154. Welch DR, Rinker-Schaeffer CW. What defines a useful marker of metastasis in human cancer? *J Natl Cancer Inst* 1999; **91:** 1351–2.

155. Martignone S, Menard S, Bufalino R et al. Prognostic significance of the 67-kilodalton laminin receptor expression in human breast carcinomas. *J Natl Cancer Inst* 1993; **85:** 398–402.

156. Pishvaian MJ, Feltes CM, Thompson P et al. Cadherin-11 is expressed in invasive breast cancer cell lines. *Cancer Res* 1999; **59:** 947–52.

157. Bourguignon LY. CD44-mediated oncogenic signaling and cytoskeletal activation during mammary tumor progression. *J Mammary Gland Biol Neoplasia* 2001; **6:** 287–97.

158. Owens LV, Xu L, Craven RJ et al. Overexpression of the focal adhesion kinase (p125fak) in invasive human tumors. *Cancer Res* 1995; **55:** 2752–5.

159. Weiner T, Liu E, Craven R et al. Expression of focal adhesion kinase gene and invasive cancer. *Lancet* 1993; **342:** 1024–5.

12

Biological changes in primary breast cancer during antiestrogen therapies

Peter C Willsher, Frances Kenny, Julia MW Gee, Robert I Nicholson, John FR Robertson

CONTENTS • Introduction • Biological changes in breast cancers treated with tamoxifen • Biological changes in breast cancers treated with other SERMs • Biological changes in breast cancers treated with GLA and tamoxifen • Biological changes associated with the pure antiestrogen fulvestrant • Summary

INTRODUCTION

The effects of endocrine agents on breast cancer in a variety of animal models have been addressed in Chapter 11. The scientific literature contains extensive discussions regarding which biological factors in human primary breast cancer predict subsequent response to endocrine therapy, especially the antiestrogen tamoxifen. The Nottingham–Tenovus group have, for example, reported on a number of biological factors, including estrogen receptor (ER),[1,2] progesterone receptor (PgR),[2] Ki67,[3–5] epidermal growth factor receptor (EGFR),[4–6] p53,[4] Ras,[4,7] and cyclin D1.[8] In this chapter, we address not which biological factors predict therapeutic response but rather the biological changes that occur in human breast cancer during tamoxifen therapy, with a view to understanding (i) de novo progression, (ii) tamoxifen response, and (iii) acquired tamoxifen resistance.

The studies that address these biological effects have been relatively few, and have often reported only small numbers. Some of the reasons for this paucity of data are as follows:

- Primary medical therapy has been used more widely in some countries than others.
- Such studies are time-consuming – from explaining the reason for the study to patients and obtaining informed consent to the additional time needed to carry out repeat biopsies in busy outpatient clinics.
- Patients may withdraw informed consent at some point during the planned sequential tumour biopsy programme, making earlier biopsies of limited value.
- Sequential tumour biopsies may not be possible (e.g. for patients who attain a complete response or patients who died of comorbid diseases).
- The studies may take many years to collect sufficient biopsies. This is especially the case in acquired tamoxifen resistance, where the tumour initially responds to tamoxifen perhaps for many years before finally developing 'acquired' resistance.

This chapter will review the available literature in this area, but will focus on a prospective study (carried out jointly by the University of Nottingham and the Tenovus Institute, Cardiff), which represents one of the largest research programmes in this field.

In the Nottingham–Tenovus study, patients receiving initial tamoxifen therapy for primary breast cancer had sequential biopsies of the primary tumour. These biopsies were then examined for any changes in biological parameters occurring during treatment. The first 75 patients reported included elderly women (>70 years) with operable breast cancer or patients with locally advanced breast cancer. All received tamoxifen 20 mg/day, either within clinical trials[9,10] or by patient choice. No other anticancer therapy was administered during endocrine therapy. Clinical assessment of response was assessed after 6 months (UICC criteria[11]). All patients had the diagnosis confirmed by core cut biopsy and remained on tamoxifen until there was objective evidence of disease progression. When patients were reviewed after 6 weeks and at 6 months, a further biopsy of the primary tumour was requested. This study design uniquely allowed the 'natural history' of multiple biological features to be followed during response to hormone treatment, through to endocrine resistance. Further biopsy of the primary tumour was requested at the point of disease progression.

BIOLOGICAL CHANGES IN BREAST CANCERS TREATED WITH TAMOXIFEN

Changes in estrogen receptor and related proteins

Estrogen receptors
The most commonly assessed biological factor for any effect of hormone therapy has been ER. A number of retrospective studies claimed a greater tendency for ER-positive tumours to become ER-negative between sequential biopsies compared with when no treatment is received.[12–17] It was therefore proposed that tamoxifen resistance developed because the tumour became ER-negative. However, the

variety of patients and treatments included in these studies presented difficulties in drawing conclusions regarding the effect of specific therapies on ER.

Prospective studies are of more value in investigating this issue, especially if they are performed with the systematic aim of identifying the biological changes induced by hormone therapy. The reported studies that fulfil these criteria are summarized in Table 12.1. Several of these suggest that the ER status changes from positive to negative during tamoxifen treatment. This observation was reproduced when patients were given placebo or tamoxifen for 3, 7, and 14 days prior to mastectomy. Noguchi and colleagues[26] reported that with longer duration of therapy, ER levels became significantly lower than in the control group. Proposed explanations for the loss of ER levels include the selective death of ER-positive cells by hormone therapy with overgrowth of unaffected ER-negative cells, or downregulation of ER expression in all cells.[14,27] However, in all of these studies radioligand binding assays (RLBA) or dextran-coated charcoal (DCC) assays were used. Encarnacion and colleagues[22] subsequently showed that the presence of tamoxifen in tumour tissue results in a falsely low ER levels by such competitive binding assays. These authors took tumours from patients receiving tamoxifen and measured ER both by RLBA and ER immunocytochemical assays (ERICA), and found that the former resulted in a substantial false-negative rate. The ERICA method circumvents this problem of assay interference, making this method more accurate in examining the effects of tamoxifen on ER expression in breast cancer. Three studies that used ERICA are also shown in Table 12.1; all these studies show no significant change in ER with tamoxifen therapy. The weakness of these studies was the relatively short interval of tamoxifen therapy after which biopsies were taken. The tumours would still be responding to tamoxifen, and in these circumstances it was to be expected that they would continue to express ER.

In the Nottingham–Tenovus study, biopsies

Table 12.1 Prospective studies of change in ER status with tamoxifen therapy

Authors	Year	No. of cases	Sites of tumour[a]	ER assay[b]	Interval between biopsies	ER⁺ to ER⁻	ER⁻ to ER⁺
Namer et al[18]	1980	21	M-M	RLBA	1 week	6/13	0/8
Waseda et al[19]	1981	20	P-P	DCC	1–4 weeks	10/11	0/9
Taylor et al[20]	1982	8	?	DCC	>3 months	4/5	0/3
Montoya et al[21]	1992	17	P-P	DCC	1 week	10/15	0/2
Encarnacion et al[22]	1993	16	?	RLBA	>1 month	10/12	0/4
Robertson et al[23]	1991	23	P-P	ERICA	>4 months	3/17	0/6
Clarke et al[24]	1993	59	P-P	ERICA	3 weeks	No significant change	
Murray et al[25]	1994	10	M-M	ERICA	1 month	No significant change	

[a]M-M, tissue samples obtained sequentially from metastatic sites; P-P, tissue samples obtained sequentially from primary tumour.
[b]RLBA, radioligand binding assay; DCC, dextran-coated charcoal assay; ERICA, ER immunocytochemical assay.

were obtained up to 6 months on tamoxifen, and showed a significant decrease in the percentage of cells expressing ER at the 6-week and 6-month biopsies when compared with pretreatment ER expression using matched-pair analyses (Figure 12.1 and Table 12.2). Nevertheless, after 6 months of treatment, the majority of tumours that were initially found to be ER-positive retained ER expression. The initially ER-negative tumours remained negative throughout treatment. For the thirty-three patients who had biopsies at the time of disease progression, ER expression was not significantly different compared with pretreatment (Figure 12.1). Of interest, ER expression in this group was quite high, with a median of 40% of cells staining.

These data confirm that after 6 weeks of treatment with tamoxifen, there is a significant decrease in ER expression in primary breast cancer. The size of the decrease in ER seen in this study was greater than the results of short-term, presurgical studies where tamoxifen was given in the period between diagnosis and primary surgery and ER was measured by ERICA and not the DCC assay or RLBA.[23–25]

Furthermore this study of sequential tumour biopsies has shown that ER remains suppressed for up to 6 months on tamoxifen therapy. This observation raises the question as to whether this change represents either a selective growth of ER-negative clones or alternatively downregulation of ER expression within previously ER-positive cells. If the former were true, one would not expect to see the further decrease in ER between the 6-week and 6-month biopsies being associated with patients moving from static disease to objective response at these two time periods. Furthermore, if tamoxifen induced a selective growth of ER-negative clones, one might expect that at progression there would have been a further reduction or even total loss of ER expression. The fact that ER expression is maintained or even increased at the time of progression again suggests that the changes seen in ER expression are more likely due to alterations in its regulation.

More recently, a randomized neoadjuvant study comparing tamoxifen and the third-generation aromatase inhibitor vorozole has been reported.[28] This showed that ER expression was

Table 12.2 ER, PgR and pS2 percentage of cells for each biopsy for all patients

Biopsy	No. of cases	25th percentile	50th percentile	75th percentile	Comparison with pretreatment[a]
ER					
Pretreatment	75	20	60	80	—
6 weeks	53	2	50	70	$p = 0.002$, $Z = -3.74$
6 months	41	4	35	50	$p < 0.0001$, $Z = -4.42$
Progression	33	0	40	80	$p = 0.12$, $Z = -1.53$
PgR					
Pretreatment	69	1	10	50	—
6 weeks	49	0	5	30	$p = 0.17$, $Z = 1.42$
6 months	38	0	5	10	$p = 0.0007$, $Z = -3.39$
Progression	32	0	0	19	$p = 0.43$, $Z = 0.78$
pS2					
Pretreatment	65	0	2	30	—
6 weeks	47	1	15	40	$p = 0.057$, $Z = -1.90$
6 months	36	0	5	25	$p = 0.42$, $Z = -0.80$
Progression	24	0	3.5	33	$p = 0.98$, $Z = -0.03$

[a]Wilcoxon matched-pairs signed-ranks test.

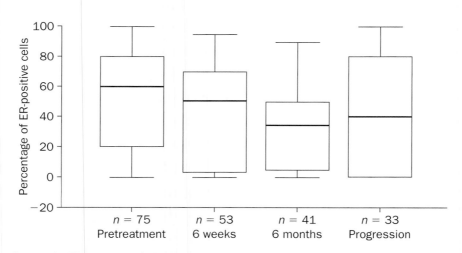

Figure 12.1 Change in ER expression during tamoxifen treatment for all cases. The median is shown as the bold horizontal line, the box length represents the interquartile range and the whiskers represent 'values within 1.5 box lengths from the 75th or 25th percentiles respectively'. Outliers are other values beyond this, shown as individual points.

decreased after 2 weeks and 12 weeks on tamoxifen.

Progesterone receptors

There are a small number of prospective studies that have investigated alterations in PgR status with tamoxifen treatment; these are summarized in Table 12.3. These studies are subject to the same assay and sample variability as the ER studies, but not the competition with tamoxifen for the assay.

The data presented in Table 12.3 suggest that there is an initial increase in PgR expression after commencement of tamoxifen therapy over the initial 2 weeks. This is followed by a fall in PgR level over subsequent weeks. These changes are only seen in ER-positive tumours. The rise in PgR expression after 2 weeks of tamoxifen was also recently reported in a large prospective randomized trial that compared 2–3 weeks of tamoxifen versus placebo 'tamoxifen' versus the pure antiestrogen fulvestrant (ICI 182,780, Faslodex).[30] These findings are also consistent with those of Noguchi and colleagues,[26] where PgR positivity showed a slight increase in the 3- and 7-day tamoxifen groups, but returned to the level of the control group after 21 days of tamoxifen. Since PgR is known

to be an expression of functional estrogenic stimulus, this bimodal change in PgR expression with tamoxifen treatment is consistent with the in vitro finding of a dose–response activity of tamoxifen. At low levels, tamoxifen is an estrogen agonist, and as tissue levels rise it functions as an antiestrogen.[26] In the Nottingham–Tenovus study, the matched-pair analyses showed a non-significant reduction in PgR expression after 6 weeks, but a highly significant reduction in expression after 6 months of tamoxifen therapy (Figure 12.2 and Table 12.2). At the time of progression, PgR levels were low, with a median of 0% for the 32 cases. A matched-pair comparison with pretreatment biopsies did not show any significant difference. Figure 12.2 shows that at the time of tamoxifen resistance, some tumours express PgR in a high proportion of cells – up to 90%.

Previously published work has shown that PgR tends to be upregulated during the initial phase of tamoxifen therapy (Table 12.3). The studies described in Table 12.3 examined changes in PgR during tamoxifen therapy that lasted for only between 1 and 3 weeks. Noguchi et al[26] showed that upregulation of PgR occurred in the first week of therapy, but that

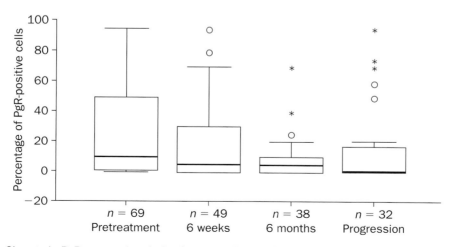

Figure 12.2 Change in PgR expression during hormone therapy for all cases.

Table 12.3 Prospective studies of change in PgR status with tamoxifen therapy

Authors	Year	No. of cases	Tumour sites[a]	Assay method[b]	Interval between biopsies	PgR$^+$ to PgR$^-$	PgR$^-$ to PgR$^+$
Namer et al[18]	1980	23	M-M	RLBA	1 week	2/11	3/12[c]
Waseda et al[19]	1981	8	P-P	DCC	1–2 weeks	PgR increase in 5/6[c]	
		3	P-P	DCC	3 weeks	PgR decrease in 3/3[c]	
Howell et al[29]	1987	52	P-P	ISO	2 weeks	PgR increase in 21	
Montoya et al[21]	1992	17	P-P	DCC	1 week	1/13	2/4
Clarke et al[24]	1993	59	P-P	PRICA	3 weeks	No significant change	

[a]M-M, tissue samples obtained sequentially from metastatic site; P-P, tissue samples obtained sequentially from primary tumour.
[b]RLBA, radioligand binding assay; DCC, dextran-coated charcoal assay; ISO, isoelectric focusing; PgR, progesterone receptor; PRICA, progesterone receptor immunocytochemical assay.
[c]Change in PgR status occurred only in ER-positive tumours.

PgR levels had returned to pretreatment levels by 3 weeks. In the Nottingham–Tenovus study, biopsies were taken well after this (6 weeks), and it would be expected that any initial rise would be reversed by this time. The subsequent reduction in PgR expression at 6 months is consistent with the reduced levels of ER expressed after that duration of tamoxifen therapy.

Harper-Wynne and colleagues[28] compared tamoxifen versus vorozole as neoadjuvant therapy, and showed a non-significant rise in PgR on tamoxifen after 2 weeks of treatment compared with a significant reduction on vorozole. The change in PgR expression was significantly different between the tamoxifen- and the vorozole-treated tumours. By 12 weeks, PgR expression in the tamoxifen-treated tumours had fallen, but this did not reach statistical significance.

pS2

pS2 is an estrogen-regulated protein, and so, like PgR, one might expect a bimodal pattern of change during tamoxifen therapy. In the first reported study of this effect, Chesser et al[31] took fine-needle aspiration (FNA) samples from 27 primary tumours prior to and after 2–6 months of tamoxifen treatment. Of the 27 tumours, 15 showed an increase in pS2 expression. In the Nottingham–Tenovus study, after 6 weeks of tamoxifen therapy, pS2 expression was seen to increase from a median of 2% at pretreatment to 15%. In the overall analysis, this change was of borderline significance ($p = 0.057$) (Table 12.2). However, in the patients who had initial response/static disease, this increase in expression was highly significant ($p = 0.017$). After 6 months of therapy, pS2 expression fell to levels similar to pretreatment.

With respect to pS2, the Nottingham–Tenovus study confirms that a significant proportion of tumours show an increase in pS2 expression after 6 weeks of tamoxifen therapy. This finding contrasts with the absence of increase at 6 weeks for PgR. Since both PgR and pS2 are estrogen-induced proteins, the previous suggestion that PgR induction relates to the initial partial agonist effect of tamoxifen would apply equally to the increase seen in pS2. The persistence of pS2 upregulation at 6 weeks (compared with PgR) may be related to the longer half-life of the pS2 protein. In vitro studies show that this may well be the case (RI Nicholson, unpublished work). After 6 months, pS2 fell to similar levels as pretreatment, in parallel with ER and PgR.

Changes in growth factor receptors and ligands

The potential crosstalk between markers of the type 1 growth factor family and the ER pathway is discussed in detail in Chapter 9. Several studies have examined these interactions in humans treated with tamoxifen.

Epidermal growth factor receptor

In a study of 70 patients who received tamoxifen, EGFR expression was monitored by immunohistochemistry, comparing pretreatment and relapse biopsies. No significant change was identified, irrespective of response.[32] Likewise, the Nottingham–Tenovus study showed similar findings, with EGFR expression remaining remarkably consistent during the first 6 months of hormone therapy, irrespective of clinical response and ER status.

The median of 5% cells and interquartile ranges were virtually unchanged for the pretreatment, 6-week, and 6-month biopsies.

c-ErbB2

The presence of c-ErbB2 (HER2/Neu) in ER-positive primary breast cancers has been reported to correlate with hormone-receptor negativity in human breast cancer.[33] Reports of a relationship between c-ErbB2 expression and lack of hormone sensitivity, both in advanced disease and in the adjuvant setting, have been less consistent.[33,34] The effect of tamoxifen on c-ErbB2 expression is therefore of some interest. Short-term tamoxifen prior to mastectomy has been shown to increase *cytoplasmic* expression of c-ErbB2.[35] This suggests that cytoplasmic expression was induced by the treatment and that c-ErbB2 may be under estrogen regulation. However, the same authors have also reported a larger immunohistochemical study comparing pretreatment biopsies with specimens obtained at the time of development of secondary resistance in 70 patients receiving tamoxifen, and they did not demonstrate any significant change in c-ErbB2 expression.[32]

In the Nottingham–Tenovus study, a trend (Figure 12.3) was observed for an increase in the proportion of tumours classified as c-ErbB2 cytoplasmic-positive during the first 6 months

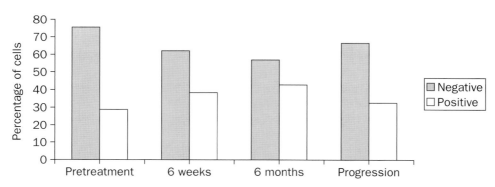

Figure 12.3 Proportion of tumours with positive or negative cytoplasmic c-ErbB2 staining for each biopsy during hormone therapy for all cases.

of hormone therapy, rising from 24% at pre-treatment to 43% at 6 months. Matched-pair analysis comparing pretreatment and 6-week biopsies for 49 cases shows that 12 of the 39 negative tumours became positive ($p = 0.076$). This change was statistically significant in those with initial response/static disease ($p = 0.035$). The tendency for cytoplasmic c-ErbB2 expression to be increased at 6 weeks, and the finding that this change was largely confined to the ER-positive and initial response/static subgroups, is further evidence to support the suggestion that c-ErbB2 is estrogen-regulated. Therefore both an in vitro study[36] and the clinical biopsy studies have shown that c-ErbB2 is estrogen-regulated to some extent. Estrogens are seen to inhibit c-ErbB2 expression, while tamoxifen shows a tendency to upregulate expression in the cytoplasm.[37,38] In contrast to the changes seen in *cytoplasmic* expression, the *membrane* expression of c-ErbB2 showed no pattern of change during tamoxifen therapy or on relapse. This latter finding questions whether the change in cytoplasmic staining is of functional importance in the growth and control of breast cancers.

Of biological importance, a profound reduction in the two growth factor receptors discussed (EGFR and c-ErbB2) has not been identified during hormone response. If such a reduction in expression were an important mechanism of hormone response, then this might be expected to be identified in these studies, particularly in responding tumours. Equally important was the finding that, on using antibodies to c-ErbB2 and EGFR, no significant induction of these growth factor receptors was noted at the time of acquired tamoxifen resistance. However, antibodies are now available for the activated phosphorylated forms of these receptors – their downstream signalling molecules.[39,40] Further studies in this direction are clearly warranted before concluding that these pathways are not involved either in tamoxifen response or in acquired tamoxifen resistance.

Transforming growth factor α

Noguchi and colleagues[41] examined the effect of tamoxifen on the mitogenic growth factor transforming growth factor α (TGF-α). An enzyme immunoassay method was used to compare TGF-α levels in FNA samples obtained from primary breast cancer both prior to and after a median of 10 days of tamoxifen therapy. TGF-α levels were significantly downregulated in 10 patients with ER-positive tumours after tamoxifen treatment. In contrast, there was no significant change in TGF-α levels in tumours from either a group of 10 patients who had not received tamoxifen or a further group of 10 patients who were treated with tamoxifen but had ER-negative tumours. The authors suggest that TGF-α is estrogen-regulated in the presence of a functional ER. In ER-negative tumours, TGF-α may be more important as a growth factor because it is produced independently of estrogens. They conclude that TGF-α downregulation may be involved, at least in part, in the growth-inhibitory mechanism of tamoxifen. A report by Gregory and colleagues[42] in which TGF-α was assayed by radioimmunoassay also showed lower TGF-α levels in tumours from patients who had received tamoxifen compared with controls.

The Nottingham–Tenovus study did not show significant changes in the immunohistochemical expression of TGF-α during tamoxifen treatment. No clear pattern of change was evident in either response/static disease patients or initial progression patients. Biopsies performed on the development of hormone resistance following an initial response/static disease were not significantly different in TGF-α expression to those at pretreatment. Only a small number of biopsies (6 cases) were available for comparison of biopsies performed during response (i.e. at 6 weeks or 6 months) and acquired resistance. In all of these cases, TGF-α expression was considered to be increased at the time of progression.

The Nottingham–Tenovus study was the first immunohistochemical study to investigate changes in TGF-α expression during prolonged tamoxifen therapy. A report of 21 patients given 7 days of preoperative fulvestrant showed no significant change in immunohistochemical staining for TGF-α.[43] This study of prolonged tamoxifen therapy has also not shown any significant reduction in TGF-α expression after 6 weeks of tamoxifen. While a reduction in the median percentage of cells was evident after 6 months, this also was not statistically significant. The findings of these two immunohistochemical studies are inconsistent with the two reports using different methods mentioned above. This suggests that, at least for TGF-α, methodological differences between studies have to be taken into account in interpreting the literature on the effect of tamoxifen on TGF-α.

Changes in the proliferation markers Ki67 and MIB1

It may be anticipated that any anticancer therapy will result in downregulation of markers associated with cellular proliferation. To examine this, a study was performed in patients with operable breast cancer randomized after diagnostic biopsy to receive tamoxifen or placebo.[24] A second sample was obtained from the mastectomy, performed after a median 21 days. In the 59 patients in the tamoxifen-treated group there was a significant decrease in Ki67 antigen expression between diagnostic and mastectomy specimens. No significant change was seen in a comparison group who received placebo. A further study of pre- and post-tamoxifen Tru-cut biopsies showed a significant reduction in Ki67 staining in 8 of 9 ER-positive tumours and no significant change in 9 ER-negative tumours.[36] This finding would be consistent with a greater reduction in proliferation and higher response rate in ER-positive tumours. However, no response data were provided, so this hypothesis could not be confirmed as the basis of these studies. More recently, it has been reported that tamoxifen produced a significant decrease in Ki67 expression after 2 and 12 weeks of treatment.[28] There were significant decreases in Ki67 at 2 weeks and in the tumour volume (i.e. tumour response) at 12 weeks.

The Nottingham–Tenovus study used the MIB1 antibody to assess expression of the Ki67 antigen. Overall, the expression of MIB1 decreased during hormone therapy (Figure 12.4). Expression fell from a median of 5% cells pretreatment to a median of 0% in both the 6-week ($p = 0.23$) and 6-month biopsies

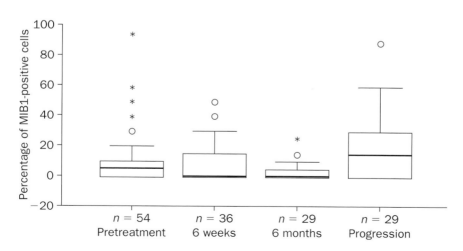

Figure 12.4 Change in MIB1 expression during hormone treatment for all cases.

($p = 0.068$). A statistically significant reduction in MIB1 staining was identified after 6 months of treatment for the patients in the initial response/static disease group ($p = 0.026$) and the ER-positive group ($p = 0.047$).

Figure 12.4 also shows a tendency for MIB1 expression to increase at the time of progression. In the overall group, the median of 0% pretreatment increased to 15% at relapse. However, it should be noted that the number of biopsies at progression is only half the number of pretreatment biopsies. This undoubtedly reflects a bias towards tumours that exhibited a shorter duration of response; the precise ER-positive tumours that would be expected to have a higher expression of Ki67 (i.e. the increased expression of Ki67 at progression) may in part be explained by this 'selection' bias.

Since MIB1 is a marker of proliferating cells, the changes seen in MIB1 expression are consistent with the biological behaviour of the tumours at the time of biopsy. Specifically, reduced expression was seen during response to tamoxifen therapy, and increased expression at the development of endocrine resistance. While these are interesting findings, and are consistent with a reduction in proliferating cells associated with tamoxifen therapy, they do not provide insight into the mechanisms of endocrine resistance.

Changes in the nuclear transcription factor c-Fos

The Nottingham–Tenovus study was the first to examine for changes in c-Fos protein expression during tamoxifen therapy.[44] It showed that expression is reduced from a median of 26% cells positive pretreatment to 20% after 6 weeks of tamoxifen therapy and to a median of 12% after 6 months, but these trends were not significant. Subsequent studies have reported that c-Fos expression appears to be increased at the development of endocrine resistance, with a median of 40% cells compared with 25% pretreatment.[45]

From what is known of c-*fos* in malignant proliferation, it could be anticipated not only that c-Fos protein levels would fall during tamoxifen therapy but also that these levels would be up-regulated at the time of tumour progression. The data from the Nottingham–Tenovus study show that c-Fos appears to be changing appropriately to the clinical situation, and its significance in predicting response from pretreatment expression[44] suggests that c-Fos may be an important factor in mediating ER control of cellular growth in breast cancer. The lack of statistical significance for any change suggests that either the inclusion of more patients or a more sensitive assay, such as for c-*fos* message (mRNA) may be of benefit in defining the importance of *changes* in c-Fos in endocrine response.

Changes in the apoptosis-related protein Bcl-2

Bcl-2 protein is considered as a 'cell survival factor' in that it is thought to be protective for apoptosis. Despite this, it has been reported that Bcl-2 expression is increased in ER-positive cancers.[7] Furthermore, it might have been expected that loss of Bcl-2 expression would render cells susceptible to the apoptoptic response to hormone therapy, and hence would be more likely to occur in responding tumours. In the Nottingham–Tenovus study, however, the opposite of this was in fact identified. Analysis of the initial response/static disease patients showed that, compared with pretreatment biopsies (median 60% cells), there was a tendency to increased expression in the 6-week biopsies (median 70%). Of note *all* the tumours showing an increase in Bcl-2 expression in the 6-week biopsy went on to have an initial response/static disease at the 6-month assessment. This initial upregulation of Bcl-2 occurring in ER-positive tumours is supported by similar results reported by Johnston and colleagues.[36] The seemingly contradictory change in Bcl-2 expression, together with the previous report of a correlation between high levels of Bcl-2 expression and endocrine response,[7] suggests that Bcl-2 may not play an important role in endocrine response. Rather, *bcl-2* should be considered as an estrogen-regulated gene and therefore a marker of ER functionality. Further work in this area in breast cancer should consider other apoptosis-related genes, or use alternative methods of detection for function of *bcl-2* during hormone therapy.

Changes in other biological markers

Few studies have examined the effect of systemic therapy on the expression of a variety of antigens in primary breast cancer. Robertson and colleagues[23] found no significant change in a number of biological features (115D8, DF3, NCRC 11, CEA, and ploidy) in 33 patients in whom Tru-cut biopsies had been performed prior to and after 1–4 months of tamoxifen therapy. A further study of 38 patients treated with combined chemotherapy and hormone therapy showed no significant change between pre- and post-treatment biopsies for the antigens mucin 1, cytokeratin, B72.3, Leu-M1, and β-glycoprotein.[46] In this study, the percentage of tumours showing lactalbumin expression was increased from 40% to 60% after therapy. The authors suggest that this may be a reflection of increase in tumour differentiation, but drew no firm conclusions.

Immunohistochemical features of secondary hormone resistance

One of the main objectives of the Nottingham–Tenovus study was to identify the phenotypic features of tumours at the time when a change occurred from a state of control with tamoxifen to one of clinical progression, i.e. at the development of acquired hormone resistance. In particular, efforts were made to identify any differences between pretreatment and progression biopsies in patients showing an initial response or static disease.

In a previous study, high levels of ER expression at the time of development of acquired resistance were reported by Johnston and colleagues.[47] A more recent report[48] compared biopsies from pretreatment and acquired resistance in 18 tamoxifen-treated patients, using an immunohistochemical assay. No difference in expression of ER, PgR, or pS2 was identified. Specifically, the majority of tumours were seen to express these antigens at the time of secondary resistance. The results from the Nottingham–Tenovus study support this finding by showing that loss of ER expression is not a major feature of acquired endocrine resistance. In the biopsies performed at secondary resistance (i.e. after a period of response), half of the tumours expressed ER in over 50% of cells and one-quarter expressed over 80% of cells positive for ER (Figure 12.5). These findings exclude loss of ER as a significant mechanism of *acquired* endocrine resistance, and confirm that ER expression is a stable phenotype.[49]

The levels of PgR and pS2 expression at the development of acquired resistance (Figure 12.5 and Table 12.2) are consistent with the presence of a functional ER at the time of relapse. The return of this function of the ER at the time of loss of the apparent growth-inhibitory effects of tamoxifen is interesting and requires interpretation. One possible reason for this observation is the development of autonomy, where cellular proliferation is independent of the normal inhibitory effects of the tamoxifen–ER complex. Alternatively, the activity of the tamoxifen–ER complex may have altered to become growth-stimulatory – as is its function in the endometrium. The mechanisms of tamoxifen resistance are discussed in Chapters 9 and 10.

Bcl-2 expression in the acquired-resistance biopsies is remarkably similar to pretreatment levels (Figure 12.5). This is suggestive of a relative lack of importance of Bcl-2 in breast cancer in relation to the mechanisms of resistance acquisition. Of more interest is the finding of an absence of increase in EGFR expression at the development of acquired resistance (median 3%, Figure 12.6). A single, abstracted report[50] has previously shown no difference between pretreatment and progression biopsies in 70

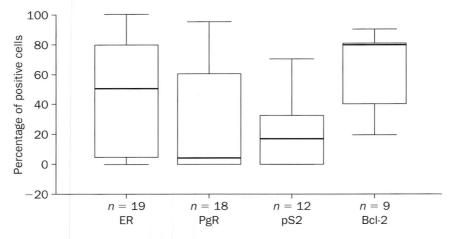

Figure 12.5   Expression of ER, PgR, pS2 and Bcl-2 in acquired-resistance biopsies.

patients. The Nottingham–Tenovus study confirms this finding and shows that the selective outgrowth of EGFR-positive cells either during tamoxifen treatment or at acquired resistance does not occur. Also c-ErbB2 staining in secondary progression biopsies did not show any significant increase in the proportion of c-ErbB2-positive tumours (Figure 12.3). These findings suggest that upregulation of the EGFR (c-ErbB1) and c-ErbB2 growth factors may not be a mechanism of acquired tamoxifen resistance. However, these results should be interpretated with caution, since there are in vitro data suggesting that in MCF-7 breast cancer cells with acquired tamoxifen-resistance, there is increased expression of EGFR and c-ErbB2 compared with the parental MGF-7 cell line.[43] Furthermore, activated forms of EGFR and c-ErbB2 also showed increased expression in these tamoxifen-resistant MCF7 cells. Future studies on these human breast cancer biopsies should investigate whether there is an increased expression of activated EGFR and c-ErbB2 on acquired tamoxifen resistance.

The lack of any significant difference in TGF-α expression between pretreatment and relapse biopsies suggests that increased levels of TGF-α at relapse are a return to the basal levels of expression for a given tumour. This finding is in contrast to de novo hormone resistance in ER-positive tumours, where TGF-α expression is associated with hormone insensitivity.[6] However, it should be noted that TGF-α is not the only ligand for EGFR. It does not appear that an upregulation of TGF-α is a mechanism of secondary resistance.

The tendency for MIB1 expression to increase at the time of acquired resistance (Figure 12.6) is of interest, since it is consistent with the clinical observation that tumour growth and hence proliferation has returned after a period of suppression. However, as noted above, these early results may be due to a selection bias of the type of tumours that have a shorter duration of response and therefore progress earlier. Data from the Nottingham–Tenovus study suggest that c-Fos may be upregulated at the time of acquired endocrine resistance. The median of 43% at secondary progression compared with 25% pretreatment is consistent with the increased proliferation shown by the MIB1 data. Since c-Fos is inducible in vitro by both growth factors and estrogens, upregulation of c-Fos at the time of secondary resistance would not help to determine the relative importance for either growth factor or estrogenic pathways in the development of acquired endocrine resistance.

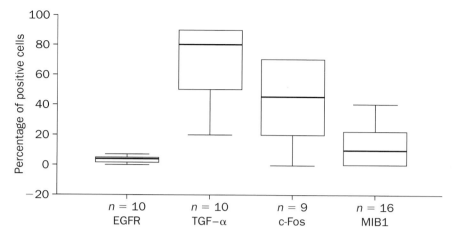

Figure 12.6 Expression of EGFR, TGF-α, c-Fos, and MIB1 in acquired-resistance biopsies.

BIOLOGICAL CHANGES IN BREAST CANCERS TREATED WITH OTHER SERMs

Studies of other tamoxifen-like antiestrogens, i.e. selective estrogen receptor modulators (SERMs), have been reported. These have been mainly presurgical studies where patients awaiting surgery have been treated with a SERM (or placebo) rather than studies of primary medical therapy. Biopsies have been obtained before starting therapy (e.g. as part of the diagnostic process), and the effect of the SERM has been assessed by comparing this with the tumour resected at surgery. Studies have been reported on idoxifene and more recently raloxifene.

The idoxifene study was a placebo-controlled trial in 77 postmenopausal patients, of whom 57 were evaluable.[51] Patients were evaluable if they had ER-positive tumours as assessed in the pretreatment core biopsy along with tumour present in the post-treatment biopsy. The tumours treated with idoxifene (for 14–21 days) showed a significant reduction in ER and Ki67 compared with tumours that were exposed to placebo. These results are similar to those from studies of tamoxifen, noted above. There was a non-significant increase in PgR in idoxifene-treated tumours. Robertson and colleagues[30] also reported an increase in PgR in tamoxifen-treated tumours, although in this study the increase in PgR was highly significant. More recently, Harper-Wynne and colleagues[28] reported a non-significant increase in PgR expression after 2 weeks of tamoxifen. Although in each of these studies the SERM was compared with the effect of placebo, any comparison between the SERMs involves cross-study comparisons. It is therefore difficult, for example, to draw any inference about whether the apparent difference in degree of increase in PgR by idoxifene and tamoxifen may be a useful surrogate marker for differences in the agonistic properties of these two drugs. Interestingly, idoxifene had no effect on apoptosis. This is similar to the findings with both tamoxifen[28,30] and the pure antiestrogen fulvestrant[30] given over similar time periods, and contrasts with previous non-randomized studies that suggested that tamoxifen and fulvestrant did induce apoptosis.[52]

A similar presurgical study comparing raloxifene (at two doses) with placebo has been reported.[53] One hundred and sixty seven patients with primary operable breast cancer (stage I or II) were randomized to receive placebo or raloxifene at 60 or 600 mg/day. Both doses of raloxifene were associated with significant decreases in tumour ER and Ki67 expression compared with placebo. Neither dose of raloxifene had any significant effect on either PgR or apoptosis. The reported effects of raloxifene are consistent with those reported for other SERMs. Furthermore, the lack of effect on apoptosis after 2 weeks of raloxifene treatment is consistent with data noted above on tamoxifen, idoxifene, and fulvestrant.

BIOLOGICAL CHANGES IN BREAST CANCERS TREATED WITH GLA AND TAMOXIFEN

Introduction

Over recent years much interest has been directed at the potential role of the polyunsaturated essential fatty acids (EFAs) in the inhibition of carcinogenesis, in particular eicosapentaenoic acid (EPA) of the *n*-3 series and γ-linolenic acid (GLA) of the *n*-6 series. Numerous in vitro and animal studies have shown that EFAs possess a variety of anticancer properties yet have the advantage of not inducing damage to normal cells (reviewed by Jiang et al[54]). More recently, pilot clinical trials have reported treatment with EFAs to result in improvement in symptoms, useful tumour regression and in some cases a significant prolongation of survival in several advanced human malignancies.[55-59]

Action of EFAs on hormone receptors

A number of mechanisms have been identified by which EFAs exert their antitumour action. These include direct cytotoxicity via liberation of lipid peroxides and free radicals, inhibition of angiogenesis, induction of apoptosis, and upregulation of antimetastatic cell adhesion molecules.[54] EFAs have also been implicated as playing a central role as modulators of steroid hormone receptor signalling.[60]

A number of animal studies conducted during the 1980s have shown EFAs to be capable of

modulating the structure and function of steroid hormone receptors, including ER.[61-65] Given the experimental capacity of EFAs to modulate the structure and function of steroid hormone receptors, of particular interest in the tamoxifen plus GLA study has been to examine whether GLA exerts an influence additional to that of tamoxifen on the inhibition of clinical breast cancer growth via the ER pathway. In a follow-on study from the main sequential biopsy study described earlier, the Nottingham–Tenovus group assessed the clinical and biological effects of GLA in addition to primary tamoxifen in patients with breast cancer.[66] The group hypothesized that tamoxifen plus GLA might produce a greater ER downregulation than tamoxifen alone and that this might be associated with a better clinical outcome. This hypothesis was based on a study showing that in tumours treated with tamoxifen, the degree of decrease in ER expression correlated with clinical outcome.[67]

Phase II clinical study of tamoxifen plus GLA

Thirty-eight patients with elderly primary, locally advanced, or metastatic breast cancer (in all of whom primary endocrine therapy was indicated as appropriate initial treatment) consented to take 8 capsules of high-dose oral GLA per day (total 2.8 g) in addition to primary tamoxifen 20 mg once daily; 47 patients who had received tamoxifen alone 20 mg once daily as first-line therapy were used as historical controls. The two treatment groups were closely matched for stage of disease and initial ER expression (Table 12.4). Repeat tumour core biopsies were obtained with patient consent at 6 weeks and 6 months of therapy and at the time of progressive disease.

Clinical response
The tamoxifen plus GLA cases were found to achieve a significantly faster clinical response compared with the tamoxifen-alone controls (objective response versus static disease), evident by 6 weeks of treatment ($p = 0.016$) and

Table 12.4 Patient features at study entry for the phase II study of tamoxifen plus γ-linolenic acid (GLA)

	Numbers of patients	
	Tamoxifen alone	Tamoxifen + GLA
Elderly primary	26 (55%)	20 (53%)
Locally advanced	17 (36%)	14 (39%)
Metastatic	4 (9%)	4 (10%)
ER-positive (*H*-score > 0)	42 (89%)	34 (89%)
ER-negative (*H*-score = 0)	5 (11%)	4 (11%)
Premenopausal	2 (4%)	2 (5%)

H-score is a recognized reflection of oestrogen receptor, reflecting both the intensity and proportion of positive staining cells in the tumour.[68]

Table 12.5 Quality of response at 6 weeks, 3 months and 6 months by treatment group

	Complete response	Partial response	Static disease	Progression	
6 weeks					
Tamoxifen alone	0	4 (9%)	40 (85%)	3 (6%)	$p = 0.010$
Tamoxifen + GLA	0	12 (31%)	26 (68%)	0	($\chi^2 = 9.1$; 2 df)
3 months					
Tamoxifen alone	0	6 (13%)	38 (81%)	3 (6%)	$p = 0.016$
Tamoxifen + GLA	2 (5%)	14 (37%)	21 (55%)	1 (3%)	($\chi^2 = 10.3$; 3 df)
6 months					
Tamoxifen alone	2 (4%)	14 (30%)	23 (49%)	8 (17%)	$p = 0.27$
Tamoxifen + GLA	6 (16%)	10 (26%)	14 (37%)	8 (21%)	($\chi^2 = 3.95$; 3 df)

maintained at 3 months ($p = 0.010$) (Table 12.5). By 6 months of therapy, 16% of the tamoxifen plus GLA cases had achieved a complete response compared with 4% of the tamoxifen-alone controls, and there remained proportionately more tamoxifen plus GLA than tamoxifen-alone objective responders (42% versus 34%). Statistical significance was lost, however, because a greater number of the tamoxifen-alone group had now achieved a partial response after earlier static disease.[66]

Changes in expression of ER

There were paired ER data for 30 tamoxifen plus GLA cases and 32 tamoxifen-alone cases from initial to 6-week biopsy, and for 21 and 27 cases, respectively, from initial to 6-month biopsy. In the ER-positive cases, there were significant 6-week and 6-month reductions in ER expression in both of the treatment arms (Figure 12.7). In the ER-positive responders with acquired-resistance biopsies (4 tamoxifen plus GLA and 16 tamoxifen alone), ER expression was found to be maintained at a level similar to that at 6 months. None of the originally ER-positive tumours became negative at the time of progression. There was a significantly greater fall in ER expression in the tamoxifen plus GLA objective responders than in the tamoxifen-alone counterparts from both the initial to 6-week biopsy ($p = 0.026$, Mann–Whitney U) and the initial to 6-month biopsy

($p = 0.019$, Mann–Whitney U). In contrast, there was no statistical difference found in the extent of ER change between the static disease cases of the two treatment groups or the few de novo ER-positive progressors.

Change in expression of Bcl-2

All of the 38 tamoxifen plus GLA cases and 35 of the tamoxifen-alone cases had a pretreatment Bcl-2 H-score (Bcl-2 H-score[68] range 5–205). Pretreatment Bcl-2 expression was positively correlated with pretreatment ER expression ($r_S = 0.473$, $p < 0.001$). There were paired Bcl-2 data for 36 tamoxifen plus GLA cases and 26 tamoxifen-alone cases from initial to 6-week biopsy, and for 23 and 24 cases, respectively,

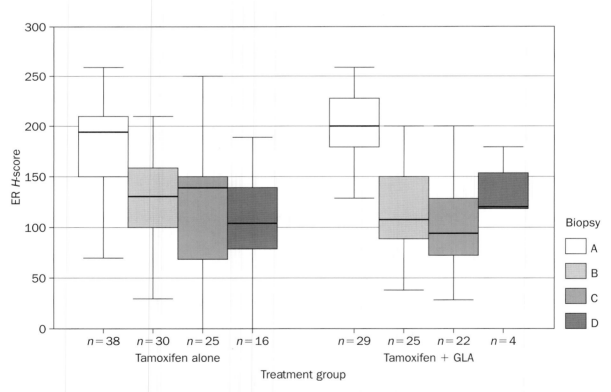

Figure 12.7 Change in ER expression from sequential biopsies during treatment in ER-positive responders (objective response plus static disease cases). ER H-score: A = initial; B = 6-week; C = 6-month; D = progression. Tamoxifen alone: A versus B, $p = 0.0002$; A versus C, $p = 0.0002$; A versus D, $p = 0.018$. Tamoxifen plus GLA: A versus B, $p < 0.0001$; A versus C, $p < 0.0001$; A versus D, $p = 0.068$. (Wilcoxon matched-pairs.)

from initial to 6-month biopsy. The tamoxifen plus GLA responders (objective response plus static disease cases) displayed a significant reduction in 6-week Bcl-2 expression that did not occur in the tamoxifen-alone responders (Figure 12.8) nor in the 7 of 8 tamoxifen plus GLA de novo progressors with paired Bcl-2 data available (data not shown). In contrast to the 6-week fall in Bcl-2 found in the tamoxifen plus GLA responders, there was a tendency for an increase in Bcl-2 at 6 weeks in the tamoxifen responders prior to a subsequent fall in expression by 6 months on therapy.

Interpretation of results

Combined treatment with GLA and tamoxifen resulted in a faster clinical response along with greater reduction of expression of ER and the ER-regulated protein Bcl-2 compared with treatment with tamoxifen alone. These findings suggest that the antiproliferative actions of GLA in breast cancer may involve downregulation of the ER apparatus. Borras and LeClercq[69] have previously demonstrated a dose-dependent downregulatory effect of n-6 EFA metabolites on growth and ER expression in the ER-positive breast cancer cell line MCF-7. Previous kinetic studies have shown that EFAs bind to an entity on the hormone receptor separate from the hormone-binding site, thus inhibiting subsequent ligand binding via induction of a conformational change in the receptor molecule.[65,70,71] Vallette et al[64] investigated the influence of unsaturated fatty acids on the

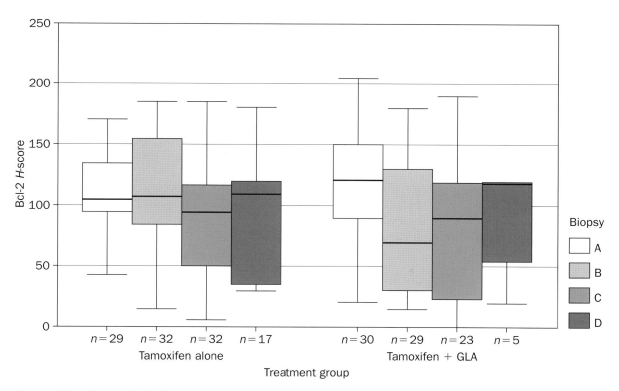

Figure 12.8 Change in Bcl-2 expression from sequential biopsies during treatment in responders (objective response plus static disease cases). Bcl-2 H-score: A = initial; B = 6-week; C = 6-month; D = progression. Tamoxifen alone: A versus B, $p = 0.32$; A versus C, $p = 0.048$; A versus D, $p = 0.92$. Tamoxifen plus GLA: A versus B, $p = 0.001$; A versus C, $p = 0.0079$; A versus D, $p = 0.043$. (Wilcoxon matched pairs.)

binding of estradiol to ERs in the uterine tissue of juvenile rats. They found estradiol binding to be either reduced or potentiated, depending on the relative concentrations of estradiol and EFA present. From these dynamic binding patterns, the authors have proposed that for high estradiol concentrations, EFAs may induce a conformational change in the receptor that results in irreversible covalent binding of estradiol to components of the receptor protein. In the Nottingham–Tenovus study, it is possible that in the presence of GLA, a similar covalent link is formed between tamoxifen and ER, with resultant attenuation of receptor activity. Further studies are necessary to confirm these hypotheses.

The findings of a significant 6-week reduction in Bcl-2 expression in the tamoxifen plus GLA cases is of particular interest. The *bcl-2* proto-oncogene is associated with prolonged cell survival and prevention of apoptosis.[72] Expression of Bcl-2 in breast cancer has been shown to be under estrogen regulation and to be correlated with ER positivity.[7] As discussed earlier, a number of investigations have identified a transient increase in the expression of estrogen-inducible gene products, including Bcl-2, in tamoxifen-treated breast cancers, followed by subsequent downregulation with continued therapy. This transient upregulatory effect is thought to be attributable to early agonist activity of tamoxifen before higher steady-state tissue levels are reached. In the present study, the addition of GLA appears to have attenuated this transient tamoxifen-induced upregulation of Bcl-2. These findings raise the possibility that earlier induction of apoptotic cell death may be an underlying mechanism of the faster clinical response seen in the tamoxifen plus GLA cases. This hypothesis is in keeping with in vitro studies, which have identified apoptosis to be an underlying mode of EFA-induced cell death in a variety of cancer cell lines,[73–76] including ER-positive breast cancer.[77] The modulatory effects of GLA on ER and ER-regulated gene function and the possibility of an additive or synergistic inhibitory effect of GLA with tamoxifen via enhanced downregula-

tion of the ER pathway require further investigation.

BIOLOGICAL CHANGES ASSOCIATED WITH THE PURE ANTIESTROGEN FULVESTRANT

The results of both experimental studies and the early clinical studies have suggested that the pure antiestrogen fulvestrant (ICI 182,780, Faslodex) may be therapeutically more effective than currently available antiestrogen therapies. The clinical and experimental data are discussed in Chapters 5 and 9 respectively. There are two studies of the biological effects of fulvestrant on human breast cancer. Both are presurgical studies but their design and detail were quite different. The first was a study using the short-acting formulation of fulvestrant, which was given at one of two doses (6 or 18 mg) for 1 week prior to primary surgery.[78] There was a third 'no-treatment' control group as distinct from a placebo control group. This was an open randomized study in postmenopausal women with newly diagnosed, primary, operable breast cancer. There were no significant differences between the treatment groups with respect to pre-study ER and PgR levels. Among tumours known to be ER-positive, pre-study treatment with fulvestrant produced a significant decrease in ER expression compared with the control group. Furthermore, the decrease in ER was significantly greater with the 18 mg dose compared with the 6 mg dose. This study reported that ER was downregulated by short-acting fulvestrant in a dose-dependent manner. PgR was also downregulated. The proliferation antigen Ki67 was also downregulated on fulvestrant. Further investigations of these same tumour biopsies showed that 7–14 days of short-acting fulvestrant had no effect on either EGFR or TGF-α expression in the tumour.

The biological effects of short acting fulvestrant given prior to surgery in the above study have been compared with the biological effects of tamoxifen.[79] This was a comparison between studies and not a randomized comparison.

Nevertheless, the data was reported to show that short-acting fulvestrant decreased the expression of ER significantly more than tamoxifen did. There was a different response in PgR expression between tumours treated with fulvestrant and those treated with tamoxifen. Fulvestrant caused a significant decrease in PgR, while tamoxifen promoted an increase in PgR expression.

The formulation of fulvestrant that was developed and has been used in the clinical trials programme is a long-acting formulation known as Faslodex. There has been a presurgical study in 201 post-menopausal women, again with newly diagnosed primary breast cancer.[30] This was a partially blind, randomized, multicentre study where patients were randomized to one of five groups: tamoxifen tablets or placebo ('tamoxifen') tablets for 14–21 days or to Faslodex at one of three doses (50, 125, or 250 mg). The primary objective of the study was to compare the effects on ER, PgR, Ki67, and apoptotic index in each of the five groups.

Faslodex resulted in a dose-related reduction of ER index. All doses of Faslodex caused a significant reduction of ER index when compared with placebo.[30] The reduction in ER index was of greater significance for Faslodex 250 mg (which is the dose being used in current clinical trials) when compared with tamoxifen ($p = 0.02$). These data suggest that the pure antiestrogen Faslodex may be more potent in its effect on the ER pathway than tamoxifen. This is further supported by the fact that the median changes in PgR index showed decreases for all doses of Faslodex, while tamoxifen showed an increase (in keeping with its known agonistic properties) and placebo showed little change. Indeed, PgR was significantly reduced by all doses of Faslodex compared with tamoxifen, and by Faslodex 125 mg when compared with placebo. These data suggest that Faslodex may have a novel effect on ER, distinct from that of tamoxifen and other SERMs. The downregulation of PgR by Faslodex supports the conclusion that, unlike tamoxifen, Faslodex is devoid of estrogen agonist activity in humans.

Changes in Ki67 were not significantly different between tamoxifen and Faslodex, although it should be noted that the reduction in Ki67 was numerically greater with Faslodex 250 mg compared with tamoxifen. Ki67 was, however, significantly reduced both by Faslodex 125 mg and Faslodex 250 mg when compared with placebo. There have been suggestions that antiestrogens exert their antitumour effect not solely through reducing proliferation (e.g. as measured by Ki67) but also by increasing cell death (i.e. apoptosis). One publication has even suggested that the effect of fulvestrant on apoptosis was greater than that of tamoxifen.[52] However, these data on the effects of fulvestrant and tamoxifen on apoptosis came from two different studies – one investigating long-acting fulvestrant (i.e. Faslodex)[30] and the other comparing short-acting fulvestrant.[78] In the randomized study where Faslodex at one of three doses was compared with tamoxifen or placebo there was no significant increase in the apoptotic index in tumours treated with Faslodex (at any of the three doses) or tamoxifen compared with placebo.[30] As noted above, it is interesting that presurgical studies of idoxifene[51] and of raloxifene[53] also failed to show any effect of these antiestrogens on apoptosis in human primary breast cancer.

However, more recently, a retrospective analysis of the data from the presurgical study comparing Faslodex (three doses), tamoxifen, and placebo has identified a composite measurement of both proliferation and apoptosis called 'cell turnover index' (CTI). Faslodex significantly reduced CTI compared with both placebo ($p = 0.0003$) and tamoxifen ($p = 0.026$). In comparison, tamoxifen did not reduce CTI compared with placebo.[80] Further prospective studies that support CTI as a useful endpoint are now required.

SUMMARY

It would appear that antiestrogens do reduce ER and Ki67 expression in human breast cancer. It would appear from the studies of

GLA plus tamoxifen and the studies of the pure antiestrogen fulvestrant that the degree of reduction can be increased from that seen with tamoxifen and other SERMs. The PgR data from the presurgical study of Faslodex has suggested that it may have a novel effect on ER, distinct from that of tamoxifen and other SERMs, and that it may be devoid of agonistic activity. Furthermore, these studies have also made us re-assess whether antiestrogens do induce apoptosis in human breast cancer.

Data on biological changes at the time of acquired hormone resistance are much scarcer. Nevertheless, it would appear that tumours do not undergo major phenotypic changes at acquired tamoxifen resistance (e.g. changing from ER-positive to ER-negative). It would appear that more subtle changes in the growth-stimulatory pathways (which crosstalk with the ER pathway) are responsible for tumours developing acquired tamoxifen resistance. The clinical data showing that few tumours that are resistant to tamoxifen respond to other SERMs suggest that the molecular basis for resistance to tamoxifen and other SERMs is similar in human breast cancer.

However, a significant number of tumours that develop acquired tamoxifen resistance will respond to subsequent endocrine manoeuvres such as an aromatase inhibitor (e.g. anastrozole or letrozole) or the pure antiestrogen fulvestrant. Furthermore, in experimental systems, inhibitors of some of these biological pathways (e.g. tyrosine kinase inhibitors such as Iressa) have been reported to be effective in treating tumours that have developed acquired tamoxifen resistance.[81] These findings support the importance of crosstalk between ER and growth factor pathways and the fact that when tumours have developed acquired tamoxifen resistance, inhibition of the ER pathway and/or selected growth factor pathways can result in further inhibition of tumour growth. Future studies of acquired endocrine resistance must be directed to elucidate these biological changes.

REFERENCES

1. Williams MR, Todd JH, Ellis IO et al. Oestrogen receptors in primary and advanced breast cancer. *Br J Cancer* 1987; **55**: 67–73.
2. Robertson JFR, Cannon P, Nicholson RI, Blamey RW. Oestrogen and progesterone receptors as prognostic variables in hormonally treated breast cancer. *Int J Biol Markers* 1996; **11**: 29–33.
3. Nicholson RI, Bouzubar N, Walker KJ et al. Hormone sensitivity in breast cancer: influence of heterogeneity of oestrogen receptor expression and cell proliferation. *Eur J Cancer* 1991; **27**: 908–13.
4. Archer SG, Eliopoulos A, Spandidos D et al. Expression of ras-p21, p53 and c-erbB-2 in advanced breast cancer and response to first line hormonal therapy. *Br J Cancer* 1995; **72**: 1259–66.
5. Nicholson RI, McCelland RM, Finlay P et al. Relationship between EGF-R, c-erb-B2 protein expression and Ki67 immunostaining in breast cancer and hormone sensitivity. *Eur J Cancer* 1993; **29A**: 1018–23.
6. Nicholson RI, McClelland RA, Gee JMW et al. Transforming growth factor α and endocrine sensitivity in breast cancer. *Cancer Res* 1994; **54**: 1684–9.
7. Gee JMW, Robertson JFR, Ellis IO et al. Immunocytochemical localization of BCL-2 protein in human breast cancers and its relationship to a series of prognostic markers and response to endocrine therapy. *Int J Cancer* 1994; **59**: 619–28.
8. Kenny FS, Hui R, Musgrove EA et al. Overexpression of cyclin D1 messenger RNA predicts for poor prognosis in estrogen receptor positive breast cancer. *Clin Cancer Res* 1999; **5**: 2069–76.
9. Willsher PC, Robertson JFR, Chan SY et al. Locally advanced breast cancer: randomised trial of multimodal therapy versus initial hormone therapy. *Eur J Cancer* 1997; **33**: 45–9.
10. Willsher PC, Robertson JFR, Jackson L et al. Investigation of primary tamoxifen therapy for elderly patients with operable breast cancer. *Breast* 1997; **6**: 150–4.
11. Hayward JL, Carbone PP, Henson JC et al. Assessment of response to treatment in advanced breast cancer. *Cancer* 1977; **39**: 1289–93.
12. Peetz ME, Nunley DL, Moseley S et al. Multiple simultaneous and sequential estrogen receptor values in patients with breast cancer. *Am J Surg* 1982; **143**: 591–4.

13. Harland RNL, Barnes DM, Howell A et al. Variation of receptor status in cancer of the breast. *Br J Cancer* 1983; **47**: 511–15.

14. Raemaekers JM, Beex LV, Koenders AJ et al. Concordance and discordance of estrogen and progesterone receptor content in sequential biopsies of patients with advanced breast cancer: relation to survival. *Eur J Cancer Clin Oncol* 1984; **20**: 1011–18.

15. Crawford DJ, Cowan S, Fitch R et al. Stability of oestrogen receptor status in sequential biopsies from patients with breast cancer. *Br J Cancer* 1987; **56**: 137–40.

16. Allegra JC, Barlock A, Huff KK, Lippman ME. Changes in multiple or sequential estrogen receptor determinations in breast cancer. *Cancer* 1980; **45**: 792–4.

17. King RJB, Stewart JF, Millis RR et al. Quantitative comparison of estradiol and progesterone receptor contents of primary and metastatic human breast tumors in relation to response to endocrine treatment. *Breast Cancer Res Treat* 1982; **2**: 339–46.

18. Namer M, Laianne C, Baulieu EE. Increase of progesterone receptor by tamoxifen as a hormonal challenge test in breast cancer. *Cancer Res* 1980; **40**: 1750–2.

19. Waseda N, Kato Y, Imura H, Kurata M. Effects of tamoxifen estrogen and progesterone receptors in human breast cancer. *Cancer Res* 1981; **41**: 1984–8.

20. Taylor RE, Powles TJ, Humphries J et al. Effects of endocrine therapy on steroid-receptor content of breast cancer. *Br J Cancer* 1982; **45**: 80–5.

21. Montoya F, Barbazan MJ, Schneider J et al. Variations in estrogen and progesterone receptor levels after short-term tamoxifen treatment in breasts carcinoma. *Oncology* 1992; **49**: 422–5.

22. Encarnacion CA, Ciocca DR, McGuire WL et al. Measurement of steroid hormone receptors in breast cancer patients on tamoxifen. *Breast Cancer Res Treat* 1993; **26**: 237–46.

23. Robertson JFR, Ellis IO, Nicholson RI et al. Cellular effects of tamoxifen in primary breast cancer. *Breast Cancer Res Treat* 1991; **20**: 117–23.

24. Clarke RB, Laidlaw IJ, Jones LJ et al. Effect of tamoxifen on Ki67 labelling index in human breast tumours and its relationship to oestrogen and progesterone receptor status. *Br J Cancer* 1993; **67**: 606–11.

25. Murray PA, Gomm J, Ricketts D et al. The effect of endocrine therapy on the levels of oestrogen and progesterone receptor and transforming growth factor-β1 in metastatic human breast cancer: an immunocytochemical study. *Eur J Cancer* 1994; **30A**: 1218–22.

26. Noguchi S, Miyauchi K, Nishizawa Y, Koyama H. Induction of progesterone receptor with tamoxifen in human breast cancer with special reference to its behaviour over time. *Cancer* 1988; **61**: 1345–9.

27. Toma S, Leonassa F, Paidaens R. The effects of therapy on estrogen receptors in breast cancer. *J Steroid Biochem* 1985; **23**: 1105–9.

28. Harper-Wynne CL, Sacks NPM, Shenton K et al. Comparison of the systemic and intratumoral effects of tamoxifen and the aromatase inhibitor Vorazole, on postmenopausal patients with primary breast cancer. *J Clin Oncol* 2002; **20**: 1026–35.

29. Howell A, Harland RNI, Barnes DM et al. Endocrine therapy for advanced carcinoma of the breast: relationship between the effect of tamoxifen upon concentrations of progesterone receptor and subsequent response to treatment. *Cancer Res* 1987; **47**: 300–4.

30. Robertson JF, Nicholson RI, Bundred NJ et al. Comparison of the short-term biological effects of 7α-[9-(4,4,5,5,5-pentafluoropentylsulfinyl)-nonyl]estra-1,3,5(10)-triene-3,17β-diol (Faslodex) versus tamoxifen in postmenopausal women with primary breast cancer. *Cancer Res* 2001; **61**: 6739–46.

31. Chesser TJS, Rhodes MA, Ibrahim NB, Cawthorn S. Induction of pS2 protein in breast cancers treated by tamoxifen correlates with clinical response. In: *Proceedings of British Association of Surgical Oncology 48th Scientific Meeting*, July 1994: Abst 34.

32. Newby JC, Johnston SRD, Smith IE, Dowsett M. Change in expression of epidermal growth factor receptor and c-erbB2 during the development of tamoxifen resistance. *Breast* 1995; **4**: 256 (Abst).

33. Tagliabue E, Menard S, Robertson JFR, Harris L. c-erbB2 expression in primary breast cancer. *Int J Biol Markers* 1999; **14**: 16–26.

34. Yamauchi H, Stearns V, Hayes DF. When is a tumor marker ready for prime time? A case study of c-erbB-2 as a predictive factor in breast cancer. *J Clin Oncol* 2001; **19**: 2334–56.

35. Johnston SRD, McLennan KA, Sacks NM et al. Tamoxifen induces the expression of cytoplasmic c-erbB2 immunoreactivity in oestrogen-receptor

positive breast carcinoma in-vivo. *Breast* 1993; **2:** 93–9.

36. Johnston SRD, MacLennan KA, Sacks NPM et al. Modulation of Bcl-2 and Ki-67 expression in oestrogen receptor-positive human breast cancer by tamoxifen. *Eur J Cancer* 1994; **30A:** 1663–9.

37. Dati C, Andoniotti S, Taverna D et al. Inhibition of c-erbB2 oncogene expression by estrogens in human breast cancer cells. *Oncogene* 1990; **5:** 1001–6.

38. Antoniotti S, Maggiora P, Dati C, DeBortoli M. Tamoxifen up-regulates c-erbB expression in oestrogen-responsive breast cancer cells in-vitro. *Eur J Cancer* 1992; **28:** 318–21.

39. Thor AD, Liu S, Edgerton S et al. Activation (tyrosine phosphorylation) of ErbB-2 (HER-2/neu): study of incidence and correlation with outcome in breast carcinoma. *J Clin Oncol* 2000; **18:** 3230–9.

40. Gee JM, Robertson JF, Ellis IO, Nicholson RI. Phosphorylation of ERK 1/2 mitogen-activated protein kinase is associated with poor response to anti-hormonal therapy and decreased patient survival in clinical breast cancer. *Int J Cancer* 2001; **95:** 247–54.

41. Noguchi S, Motomura K, Inaji H et al. Down-regulation of transforming growth factor-α by tamoxifen in human breast cancer. *Cancer* 1993; **72:** 131–6.

42. Gregory H, Thomas CE, Willshire IR et al. Epidermal and transforming growth factor α in patients with breast tumours. *Br J Cancer* 1989; **59:** 605–9.

43. McClelland RA, Gee JMW, Francis AB et al. Short-term effects of pure anti-oestrogen ICI 182780 treatment on oestrogen receptor, epidermal growth factor receptor and transforming growth factor-alpha protein expression in human breast cancer. *Eur J Cancer* 1996; **32A:** 413–16.

44. Gee JMW, Ellis IO, Robertson JFR et al. Immunocytochemical localization of fos protein in human breast cancers and its relationship to a series of prognostic markers and response to endocrine therapy. *Int J Cancer* 1995; **64:** 269–73.

45. Gee MMW, Willsher PC, Kenny FS et al. Endocrine response and resistance in breast cancer: a role for the transcription factor FOS. *Int J Cancer* 1999; **84:** 54–61.

46. Kennedy S, Merino MJ, Swain SM, Lippman ME. The effects of hormonal and chemotherapy on tumoral and nonneoplastic breast tissue. *Hum Pathol* 1990; **21:** 192–8.

47. Johnston SRD, Hayes BP, Smith IE et al. Acquired tamoxifen resistance in human breast cancer and reduced intra-tumoral drug concentration. *Lancet* 1994; **ii:** 1521–2.

48. Johnston SRD, Saccani-Jotti G, Smith IE et al. Changes in estrogen receptor, progesterone receptor, and pS2 expression in tamoxifen-resistant human breast cancer. *Cancer Res* 1995; **55:** 3331–8.

49. Robertson JFR. Oestrogen receptor in breast cancer – a stable phenotype. *Br J Cancer* 1996; **73:** 5–12.

50. Newby JC, Johnston SRD, Smith IE, Dowsett M. Change in expression of epidermal growth factor receptor and cerbB2 during the development of Tamoxifen resistance. *The Breast* 1995; **4:** 256.

51. Dowsett M, Dixon JM, Horgan K et al. Antiproliferative effects of idoxifene in a placebo-controlled trial in primary breast cancer. *Clin Cancer Res* 2000; **6:** 2260–7.

52. Ellis PA, Saccani-Jotti G, Clarke R et al. Induction of apoptosis by tamoxifen and ICI 182780 in primary breast cancer. *Int J Cancer* 1997; **72:** 608–13.

53. Dowsett M, Lu Y, Hills M et al. Effect of raloxifene on Ki67 and apoptosis. *Breast Cancer Res Treat* 1999; **57:** 31 (Abst 26).

54. Jiang WG, Bryce RP, Horrobin DF. Essential fatty acids: molecular and cellular basis of their anti-cancer action and clinical implications. *Crit Rev Oncol Hematol* 1998; **27:** 179–209.

55. Van der Merwe CF, Booyens J, Katzeff IE. Oral γ-linolenic acid in 21 patients with untreatable malignancy – an ongoing pilot open clinical-trial. *Br J Clin Pract* 1987; **41:** 907–15.

56. Van der Merwe CF, Booyens J, Joubert HF et al. The effect of γ-linolenic acid, an in vitro cytostatic substance contained in evening primrose oil, on primary liver cancer – a double-blind placebo controlled trial. *Prostaglandins* 1990; **40:** 199–202.

57. Lockwood K, Moesgaard S, Hanioka T, Folkers K. Apparent partial remission of breast cancer in high-risk patients supplemented with nutritional antioxidants, essential fatty acids and coenzyme q(10). *Mol Asp Med* 1994; **15:** 231–40.

58. Das UN, Prasad VVSK, Reddy DR. Local application of γ-linolenic acid in the treatment of human gliomas. *Cancer Lett* 1995; **94:** 147–55.

59. Fearon KCH, Falconer JS, Ross JA et al. An open-label phase I/II dose-escalation study of the treatment of pancreatic cancer using lithium-γ-linolenate. *Anticancer Res* 1996; **16:** 867–74.

60. Nunez EA. Fatty acids as modulators of the steroid hormone message. *Prostaglandins Leukot Essent Fatty Acids* 1993; **48:** 63–70.

61. Clerc-Hoffman F, Vallette G, Secco-Millet C et al. Inhibition of the uterine binding of estrogens by unsaturated fatty acids in the immature rat. *C R Acad Sci Paris* 1983; **296:** 53–8.

62. Mitsuhashi N, Takano A, Kato J. Inhibition of the binding of R-5020 and rat uterine progesterone receptors by long-chain fatty acids. *Endocrinol Jpn* 1986; **33:** 251–6.

63. Mitsuhashi N, Mizuno M, Miyagawa A, Kato J. Inhibitory effect of fatty acids on the binding of androgen receptor and R1881. *Endocrinol Jpn* 1988; **35:** 93–6.

64. Vallette G, Christeff N, Bogard C et al. Dynamic pattern of estradiol binding to uterine receptors of the rat. *J Biol Chem* 1988; **263:** 3639–45.

65. Vallette G, Vanet A, Sumida C, Nunez E. Modulatory effects of unsaturated fatty acids on the binding of glucocorticoid receptors. *Endocrinology* 1991; **129:** 1363–9.

66. Kenny FS, Pinder SE, Ellis IO et al. Gamma linolenic acid with tamoxifen as primary therapy for breast cancer. *Int J Cancer* 2000; **85:** 643–8.

67. Kenny FS, Willsher PC, Gee JMW et al. Change in expression of ER, bcl-2 and MIB-1 on primary tamoxifen and relation to response in ER positive breast cancer. *Breast Cancer Res Treat* 2000; **65:** 135–44.

68. Nicholson RI, Colin P, Francis AB et al. Evaluation of an enzyme immunoassay for estrogen receptors in human breast cancers. *Cancer Res* 1986; **46:** 4299s–302s.

69. Borras M, Leclercq G. Modulatory effect of non-esterified fatty acids on structure and binding characteristics of estrogen receptor from MCF-7 human breast cancer cells. *J Receptor Res* 1992; **12:** 463–84.

70. Hwang P. Interaction of unsaturated fatty acids with anti-oestrogen-binding sites. *J Biochem* 1987; **243:** 359–64.

71. Kato J. Arachidonic acid as a possible modulator of estrogen, progestin, androgen and glucocorticoid receptors in the central and peripheral tissues. *J Steroid Biochem* 1989; **34:** 219–27.

72. Reed JC. Bcl-2 and the regulation of programmed cell death. *J Cell Biol* 1994; **124:** 1–6.

73. De Kock M, Lottering ML, Grobler CJS et al. The induction of apoptosis in human cervical carcinoma (HeLa) cells by γ-linolenic acid. *Prostaglandins Leukot Essent Fatty Acids* 1996; **55:** 403–11.

74. Lai PBS, Ross JA, Fearon KCH et al. Cell cycle arrest and induction of apoptosis in pancreatic cancer cells exposed to eicosapentaenoic acid in vitro. *Br J Cancer* 1996; **74:** 1375–83.

75. Seegers JC, De Kock M, Lottering M-L et al. Effects of γ-linolenic acid and arachidonic acid on cell cycle progression and apoptosis induction in normal and transformed cells. *Prostaglandins Leukot Essent Fatty Acids* 1997; **56:** 271–80.

76. Hawkins RA, Sangster K, Arends MJ. Apoptotic death of pancreatic cancer cells induced by polyunsaturated fatty acids varies with double bond number and involves an oxidative mechanism. *J Pathol* 1998; **185:** 61–70.

77. Hawkins RA, Sangster K, Arends MJ. The apoptosis-inducing effects of polyunsaturated fatty acids (PUFAs) on benign and malignant breast cells in vitro. *Breast* 1999; **8:** 16–20.

78. DeFriend DJ, Howell A, Nicholson RI et al. Investigation of a new pure antiestrogen (ICI 182780) in women with primary breast cancer. *Cancer Res* 1994; **54:** 408–14.

79. Nicholson RI, Gee JMW, Eaton CL et al. Pure antioestrogens in breast cancer: experimental and clinical observations. In: *Sex hormones and antihormones in endocrine dependent pathology: basic and clinical aspects* (Motta M, Serio M, eds) Elsevier Science, Exerpta Medicine, International Congress Series 1064, Amsterdam, 1994: 347–60.

80. Bundred N, Anderson E, Nicholson RI et al. ICI 182,780 (Faslodex) an Estrogen Receptor Downregulator reduces cell turnover index more effectively than tamoxifen. *Proc Am Soc Clin Oncol* 2001; **20:** 416a (Abst 1660).

81. Gee JM, Hutcheson IR, Knowlden JM et al. The EGFR-selective tyrosine kinase inhibitor ZD 1839 ('Iressa') is an effective inhibitor of tamoxifen-resistant breast cancer growth. *Proc Am Soc Clin Oncol* 2001; **20:** 71a (Abst 282).

13

Effects of aromatase inhibitors on breast cancer

William R Miller

CONTENTS • Introduction • Aromatase • Sites of synthesis • Regulatory factors • Inhibition of aromatase • Aromatase inhibitors • New aromatase inhibitors • Breast endocrinology • Clinical responses • Histopathological changes • Conclusions

INTRODUCTION

About 60% of breast cancers possess estrogen receptors, and many of these tumours will regress if deprived of estrogen.[1] This forms the basis for ablative endocrine therapies, which seek to remove the source of estrogen production. In premenopausal women, this usually takes the form of ovarian irradiation, surgical removal of the ovaries,[2] or the use of gonadotrophin-releasing hormone (GnRH) analogues.[1,2] However, the problem in postmenopausal women is that there are multiple sites of estrogen biosynthesis, most of which are not amenable to ablative procedures.[3,4] Alternative approaches therefore have to be used whereby the trophic effects of estrogens may be suppressed irrespective of the hormone source.[5,6] Amongst these strategies, the use of drugs that inhibit estrogen biosynthesis is particularly attractive.[6,7] Effects can be reversible or self-limiting, so that if therapy proves ineffective, withdrawal of the inhibitor will allow estrogens to return to normal levels. Specific inhibition should affect only estrogens and

minimize side-effects not associated with estrogen deprivation. Furthermore, as the aromatase enzyme appears to be similar irrespective of tissue source,[8] therapy should reduce estrogen synthesis at all sites, reducing both local and circulating hormone levels.[9,10] Consequently, inhibitors should have the potential to suppress trophic effects of estrogen beyond those achievable by ablation of any individual endocrine organ. This accounts for the interest of the pharmaceutical industry in producing drugs that will inhibit estrogen biosynthesis both specifically and potently.

AROMATASE

The classical pathway of estrogen biosynthesis (Figure 13.1) starts with cholesterol and comprises a series of degradative steps whereby cholesterol, a C_{27} sterol, is successively converted by (i) partial removal of the side-chain of the D ring into C_{21} steroids (progestogens and corticoids), (ii) completion of removal of the D-ring side-chain into C_{19} steroids (androgens),

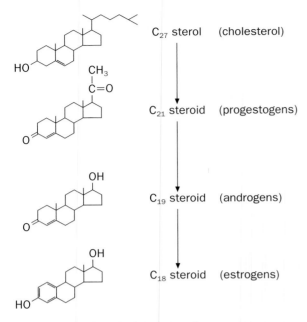

C_{27} sterol   (cholesterol)

C_{21} steroid   (progestogens)

C_{19} steroid   (androgens)

C_{18} steroid   (estrogens)

Figure 13.1 Classical pathway of estrogen biosynthesis from cholesterol.

and finally (iii) removal of the methyl group between the A and B rings into C_{18} steroids (estrogens). These transformations have in common hydroxylation by mixed-function oxidases, but each step is catalysed by a different enzyme. The first step of cholesterol side-chain cleavage is rate-limiting, but the last step in the sequence, catalysed by the aromatase enzyme, is unique to estrogen biosynthesis and is potentially the most interesting. The methyl group between the A and B rings is removed and the A ring becomes aromatic (hence the name aromatase for the enzyme). The reaction requires three hydroxylations, all of which utilize molecular oxygen and the reduced cofactor NADPH. Generation of the latter involves an NADP reductase and a transfer of electrons to a specific cytochrome P450 AROM.[11] The aromatase reaction may utilize several androgen substrates for estrogen production; thus Δ^4-androstenedione is converted to estrone and testosterone to estradiol. Both transformations

are thought to be catalysed by the same enzyme molecule – indeed, there seems to be a single human gene for aromatase,[12] its product being responsible for all estrogen synthesis irrespective of androgen substrate or site of synthesis. In many tissues, androstenedione seems to be the preferred substrate for aromatization, and, under these conditions, full estrogenic activity requires the resulting estrone to be converted into estradiol by the enzyme estrogen 17β-dehydrogenase.

SITES OF SYNTHESIS

Major sites of estrogen biosynthesis differ in pre- and postmenopausal women. Before the menopause, the ovary is mainly responsible for circulating levels of estrogen, which vary through the menstrual cycle. However, in the follicular phase, in the absence of a functioning corpus luteum, non-ovarian sources can account for as much as 50% of estrogens.[13] Peripheral synthesis of estrogen assumes greater importance in women after the menopause, when ovarian estrogen biosynthesis virtually ceases. The postmenopausal ovary still produces substantial amounts of androgen,[14] which can be used as substrate for synthesis of estrogen at peripheral sites. These sites include fat,[15] skin,[16] muscle,[17] liver,[18] and breast cancer.[19] (The adrenal cortex may also synthesize small amounts of estrogen, but – like the postmenopausal ovary – its major contribution appears to be production of androgen precursors.[20]) Consistent with these findings, aromatase activity has been demonstrated by in vitro techniques in all of these peripheral tissues, but levels are small in comparison with classical endocrine organs such as placenta and ovary. Although adipose tissue and muscle display only low levels of estrogen synthesis, their large mass within the body means that potentially they can produce micrograms of estrogen per day.[21,22] In vivo perfusion studies suggest that muscle accounts for up to 30% and adipose tissue for up to 15% of peripheral aromatization of androgen to estrogen.[21] Thus, positive correlations have been found between body weight indices and plasma estrogen levels in post-menopausal women.[22–24] Aromatase activity may also vary between different body sites of the same tissue. For example, adipose tissue from the buttocks possesses much higher activity than that from the thighs.[25]

In women with breast cancer, local production of estrogen within the breast may assume particular importance in maintaining the growth of hormone-dependent tumours. In this respect, it has been shown that both mammary adipose tissue[15,19] and about 70% of breast cancers display aromatase activity[19] and have the potential for estrogen biosynthesis. Estrogen production has also been detected in axillary lymph nodes invaded with breast cancer and metastatic skin nodules. Indeed, on a gram per gram basis, breast cancers may display amongst the highest activities seen in peripheral tissues.[26,27] This may represent picomolar amounts of estrogen being produced in situ within the tumour – sufficient to maintain estrogen-mediated events.[27]

If intratumoral aromatase activity is the source of estrogen that maintains malignant growth, then treatment with drugs that inhibit that activity might be particularly effective in those tumours. There are three studies that have addressed this issue. Bezwoda et al[28] showed that the majority of patients with tumours having high aromatase activity responded to treatment whereas none with low-activity tumours benefited. A similar investigation performed by Miller and O'Neill[29] that only recruited estrogen-receptor-positive tumours yielded identical results, in that most aromatase-positive cancers responded to the inhibitor aminoglutethimide whereas none of the tumours without evidence of in vitro aromatase did so. Finally, tumour aromatase was measured in small groups of patients given neoadjuvant treatment with aminoglutethimide or formestane (4-hydroxyandrostenedione).[30] Whilst tumours with high aromatase had better response rates than those with low activity, the difference failed to reach statistical significance. Nevertheless, these results suggest that tumours with low or no aromatase are unlikely

to respond whereas those with high activity are likely to be sensitive to aromatase inhibitors, although the presence of activity does not guarantee clinical benefits to the drugs.

REGULATORY FACTORS

Control of estrogen production and aromatase activity differs between pre- and post-menopausal women. In premenopausal women, gonadotrophins are the major regulators,[31] but they do not appear to be influential in peripheral tissues.[32] Factors that control the latter are largely undefined, but may include cytokines[33] and prostaglandins.[34] Some clues have been obtained from cultures of established cell lines of both breast cancers and mammary adipose tissue. In terms of the latter, there are preliminary data suggesting that agents that signal through cyclic AMP (cAMP),[35] prostaglandin E_2,[8,34] or Jak–STAT transduction[36,37] may be involved. In terms of the latter, interleukin-6 (IL-6)[38] and tumour necrosis factor α (TNF-α)[39] are prime suspects. Additionally, observations on the nature of mRNA transcripts for aromatase in breast cancers are informative. Thus, whilst there is a single protein for aromatase, there are multiple variants of RNA transcripts, which differ according to the nature of the untranslated exon 1.[40] These variants appear to be tissue-specific,[41] but their preponderance differs in individual breast cancers. This may be of prognostic significance[42] – although this is contested by others.[43] Analysis of the promoter region indicates that there are elements responsive to cAMP, glucocorticoids, and cytokines.[44] The suggestion has been made that transcription of aromatase switches from a glucocorticoid-dependent promoter in normal breast tissue to cAMP-stimulated promoters in breast cancers.[45] The hypothesis is that, in normal breast, aromatase expression is primarily driven by glucocorticoid-dependent promoters because cAMP promoters are suppressed by a silencer element. In breast cancers, the silencer is not detectable, so transcription can occur from the cAMP-dependent promoters.

INHIBITION OF AROMATASE

As estrogens lie at the end of a sequence of steroid transformations, inhibition of any of these conversions will potentially cause a decrease in estrogen levels, but more specific effects result from blockade of the final step in the pathway, the aromatization of androgens into estrogen. Because of this, considerable endeavours have been invested in the development of aromatase inhibitors.

AROMATASE INHIBITORS

The aromatase reaction is complex and requires multiple hydroxylations of the androgen precursor, which utilizes NADPH as an electron donor and employs a specific cytochrome P450.[46] There are therefore several mechanisms by which inhibition may be achieved – but most notably either by blocking electron transfer through the cytochrome P450 system or by competing directly with the androgen substrate binding site within the active site of the enzyme. As a result, two major types of agents have been developed: type I inhibitors, which are invariably androgen

analogues (i.e. steroidal) and compete with the natural substrate at its catalytic site, and type II inhibitors, which are non-steroidal (usually azoles) and interfere with the cytochrome P450 moiety of the enzyme (Figure 13.2).

Given that most type I inhibitors are androgens in structure, it is important that they neither have androgenic activity nor be aromatized into estrogens. The actions of some type I agents are mechanism-based in that for inhibitory activity, the drug requires metabolism by the aromatase enzyme into an active intermediate, which connects itself covalently and irreversibly to the catalytic site of the enzyme;[47] since the enzyme is only inhibited as a consequence of its own mechanism of action, these agents have been termed 'suicide' inhibitors. An inhibitor of this type might be expected to be particularly specific, being only activated by the target enzyme. Additionally, more prolonged in vivo effects might be predicted if the aromatase is irreversibly inhibited, because estrogen biosynthesis will be dependent upon de novo synthesis of aromatase. Consequently steroid inhibitors such as formestane and exemestane are currently being marketed as aromatase inactivators[48] (although in practice the drugs are

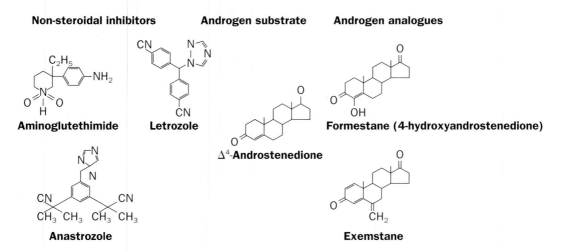

Figure 13.2 Different classes of aromatase inhibitors: non-steroidal inhibitors such as aminoglutethimide, letrozole, and anastrozole are azoles; steroidal inhibitors are androgen analogues.

prescribed to be taken daily and resumption of estrogen production is probably determined more by the half-life of the drug than the time for enzyme biosynthesis).

The properties of type I inactivators may be compared with non-steroidal type II inhibitors, whose action is usually reversible and targeted to cytochrome P450 prosthetic groups and is therefore dependent upon the continued presence of the drug. Furthermore, since many steroid hydroxylases have cytochrome P450 prosthetic groups, type II inhibitors may potentially lack specificity. Indeed, this was the case with early drugs such as aminoglutethimide, which inhibit corticoid production in addition to estrogen biosynthesis.[49] However, more recently developed drugs such as letrozole and anastrozole have a remarkable specificity and possess a differential affinity for the cytochrome P450 and aromatase and can selectively inhibit the enzyme.[50,51]

NEW AROMATASE INHIBITORS

Although drugs such as aminoglutethimide have been available for almost 30 years,[52] they have failed to make a major impact because of their lack of potency and specificity. This has meant that estrogen biosynthesis has not been completely inhibited and toxicities have occurred as other enzymes have been inhibited. Recently developed drugs such as formestane, exemestane, letrozole and anastrozole are more potent and specific, and are currently being used to treat patients with breast cancer.[48,50,51,53–56] It is therefore appropriate to describe the general endocrinology of these agents before considering their effects within the breast.

As shown in Table 13.1, all of these new agents can be shown to inhibit aromatase activity in model systems, such as placental microsomes, with great efficacy and with magnitudes of power greater than aminoglutethimide. Thus values of IC_{50} (50% inhibitory concentration) for exemestane, formestane, letrozole and anastrozole are in the nanomolar range – compared with the micromolar range for aminoglutethimide). These inhibitory influences are translated into effects on circulating estrogens when the drugs are given to postmenopausal women. Thus, in milligram oral daily doses, anastrozole (1 mg), letrozole (2.5 mg), and exemestane (25 mg) almost totally inhibit peripheral aromatase,[57] and circulating levels of estrogen fall to undectectable levels in many individuals.[48,51,58]

Table 13.1 Inhibition of aromatase activity in whole-cell and disrupted-cell preparations: IC_{50} (50% inhibitory concentration) values and relative potency of antiaromatase agents in placental microsomes, breast cancer homogenates, and mammary fibroblast cultures

	Placental microsomes		Breast cancer homogenates		Mammary fibroblast cultures	
	IC_{50} (nM)	Relative	IC_{50} (nM)	Relative	IC_{50} (nM)	Relative
Aminoglutethimide	3000	1	4500	1	8000	1
Anastrozole	12	250	10	450	14	570
Letrozole	12	250	2.5	1800	0.8	10 000
Formestane	50	60	30	150	45	180
Exemestane	50	60	15	300	5	1600

BREAST ENDOCRINOLOGY

The endocrinology within the postmenopausal breast is unusual in that (i) steroid hormone levels (most notably those of estradiol) may be substantially higher than in the circulation,[59] (ii) the breast is able to concentrate estrogen from the circulation against a gradient,[60] and (iii) both mammary adipose tissue[15] and breast cancers[19] are capable of local estrogen biosynthesis. These phenomena may be associated with the enhanced growth of breast cancers, and it is therefore important to determine the effect of novel aromatase inhibitors on the process involved.

Incubations of breast cancers with varying concentrations of inhibitors may be used as in vitro screening to determine the relative potency of newly developed drugs. These have shown that formestane, exemestane, anastrozole, and letrozole are all active agents against breast cancer aromatase, with IC_{50} values in the nanomolar range (Table 13.1). Interestingly, both type I inhibitors and letrozole seem to be more potent in this system than with placental microsomes. Whether this reflects differences between tissues or is a reflection of assay systems (breast cancers are incubated for hours and placenta for minutes) remains to be clarified. Another interesting phenomenon is that aromatase in a proportion of breast cancers appears to be selectively resistant to formestane.[61] A similar phenotype has been artificially created in site-mutagenesis studies.[62] However, the particular mutation producing formestane resistance has not been demonstrated to be present in breast tumours.[63] It is also unclear as to whether this has any clinical significance, although in vivo perfusion studies have also revealed breast tumours in which aromatase activity may be enhanced rather than inhibited by formestane.[61,64]

Whilst assays with disrupted cell preparations such as cancer homogenates demonstrate potential for aromatase inhibition, they are not as physiological as methods that employ whole cells. Similar experiments have therefore been carried out with cultured cells. Because breast cancer cells from primary tumours are notori-

ously difficult to establish and maintain, the most commonly used system is that employing fibroblasts derived from mammary adipose tissue. These display aromatase activity, particularly after pre-incubation with dexamethasone. Using these cultures, it can be shown that aromatase activity may be inhibited by nanomolar concentrations of exemestane, formestane, anastrozole, and letrozole, although aminoglutethimide is only effective at micromolar levels (Table 13.1). Interestingly, once again letrozole seems particularly potent, being 10 000-fold more so than aminoglutethimide. Similarly enhanced potency has been observed for letrozole in other whole-cell systems,[65] and it has been suggested that this results from improved pharmokinetic properties and higher intracellular concentrations of the drug.[66] In order to determine the effects of inhibitors on breast cancers in patients treated with the drugs, studies have been performed in postmenopausal women with large primary tumours who have been offered neoadjuvant therapy. Such protocols often allow sequential biopsies of tumours to be taken before and during treatment. Interestingly, when such biopsies have been assayed for aromatase activity in vitro, paradoxical results have been obtained. For example, treatment with aminoglutethimide–hydrocortisone is frequently associated with markedly raised aromatase activity as assessed in vitro (although this activity is still sensitive to aminoglutethimide, as shown by including the drug within the assay systems).[67] Although in vitro activity in tumour biopsies taken after letrozole treatment was lower than that in assays before treatment, the degree of inhibition was incomplete and paradoxical increases were observed in specimens of nonmalignant breast.[10,68] In contrast, biopsies taken before and after therapy with formestane show the expected fall with treatment.[60] These results probably reflect differences between type I and type II inhibitors that may be revealed when drug-treated tissues are assayed in vitro. Similar results may be obtained in fibroblast cultures, such that preincubation with type II reversible inhibitors causes an apparent induction of aromatase activity, whereas type I inactivators are clearly inhibitory.[69]

In this respect, it is relevant that induction of aromatase in other systems may occur as a result of either increased transcriptional activity[70] or stabilization of enzyme protein.[71,72] The practical implication of these observations is that in vitro measurements of aromatase activity in tissues exposed to reversible inhibitors may not accurately reflect in situ inhibition. Because of this, it is necessary to undertake in vivo studies in order to estimate the true potential of aromatase inhibitors given to patients. A particularly informative protocol involved infusing women with breast cancer with [^{3}H]androgen and [^{14}C]estrogen before surgically removing breast tissue and sampling peripheral blood. By purifying estrogen fractions, it is possible to estimate tumour uptake of estrogen, in situ breast aromatase activity, and endogenous levels of estrogens.[73] These studies have shown that both letrozole[74] and anastrozole,[75] whilst having no consistent effects on tumour uptake of estrogen, markedly inhibit in situ aromatase activity and significantly reduce levels of estrogen within breast tissue (Figures 13.3 and 13.4 depict examples following the use of letrozole).

CLINICAL RESPONSES

The use of neoadjuvant protocols allows tumour responses to be assessed in individual patients by monitoring changes in tumour volume occurring during treatment with aromatase inhibitors (Figure 13.5). In selected groups of patients with estrogen-receptor-rich tumours, such studies have yielded impressive antitumour effects. For example, in a series of 24 tumours treated with either 2.5 or 10 mg daily letrozole, 23 displayed a reduction in volume as assessed by serial ultrasound measurements at 1, 2, and 3 months. Similarly, in another group of patients treated with anastrozole, 18 of 23 tumours showed a greater than 50% reduction in tumour volume at 3 months. These dramatic reductions in tumour size mean that many patients who initially required mastectomy or were technically inoperable could be treated by more conservative surgery to the breast.

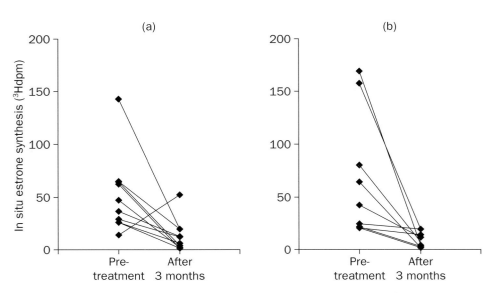

Figure 13.3   In situ synthesis of estrone by breast cancers before and after 3 months' treatment with letrozole at 2.5 mg (a) or 10 mg (b) daily.

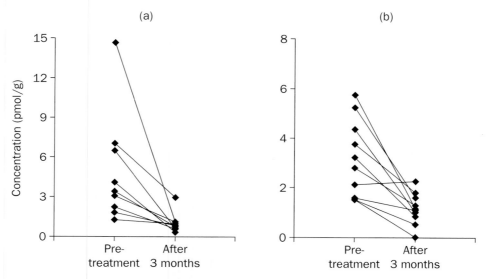

Figure 13.4 Endogenous levels of estrogens (expressed as a combination of estrone and estradiol) in breast cancers before and after 3 months' treatment with letrozole 2.5 mg (a) and 10 mg (b) daily.

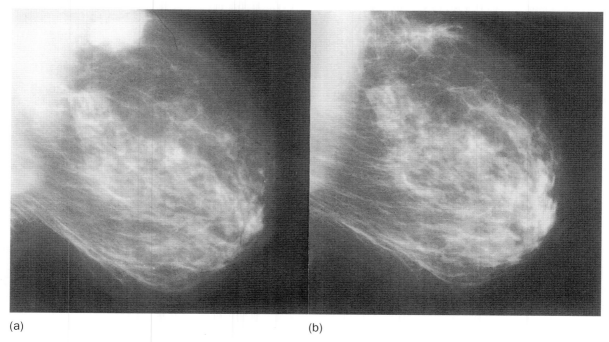

(a) (b)

Figure 13.5 Mammograms of the same breast (a) before and (b) after 3 months' treatment with letrozole. Note the resolution of a large cancer in the upper quadrant with treatment.

HISTOPATHOLOGICAL CHANGES

The ability to study sequential biopsies from the same tumour before and after primary systemic therapy with aromatase inhibitors provides the opportunity to determine the effects of treatment on both tumour morphology and the histopathological expression of important markers.[76] Both letrozole and anastrozole are capable of producing marked changes in tumour morphology. Thus, in the two small studies referred to in the previous section, pathological responses were detected in 75% of tumours treated with letrozole and in 61% of those treated with anastrozole. Although in

most cases these responses comprised decreased cellularity/increased fibrosis, in several tumours only microscopic loci of residual disease were evident after three months' treatment and there was one instance of a complete pathological response to letrozole. Histochemical staining of tumour sections also provides evidence of profound effects of treatment. Thus staining with the Mib1 antibody (which is recognized as a useful surrogate marker for proliferative activity) shows that the proportion of positive cells was consistently reduced following treatment with either letrozole[77] or anastrozole[78] (Figure 13.6). Similarly, staining for progesterone receptors was significantly

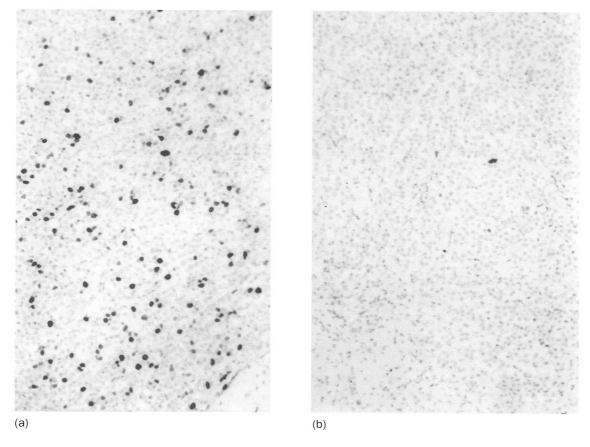

(a)　　　　　　　　　　　　　　　　　　(b)

Figure 13.6　Immunohistochemical staining for Mib1 (a) before and (b) after 3 months' treatment with letrozole. Note the marked decrease in staining with treatment.

reduced in terms of both intensity and the proportion of positive cells in the majority of tumours. These results are consistent with antiestrogenic and antitumour effects of these aromatase inhibitors.

CONCLUSIONS

The new generation of aromatase inhibitors are potent and specific drugs that are capable of almost totally inhibiting aromatase activity in the breasts of postmenopausal women. The consequence of this is that local endogenous estrogens fall profoundly. These endocrine changes are reflected in antitumour effects within hormone-sensitive breast cancers. Thus, in most cases, there is a rapid sustained shrinkage in tumour volume and a marked decrease in markers of proliferation and estrogen action. Such observations suggest that these drugs have an immense potential not only in the treatment of established breast cancers but also in the chemoprevention of the disease.

REFERENCES

1. Miller WR. Estrogens and endocrine therapy for breast cancer. In: *Estrogen and Breast Cancer* (Miller WR, ed). Austin, TX: RH Landes, 1996: 125–50.

2. Nissen-Meyer R. Castration as part of the primary treatment for operable female breast cancer. *Acta Radiol Suppl* 1965; 249: 1–133.

3. Miller WR. Sources of estrogen and sites of biosynthesis. In: *Estrogen and Breast Cancer* (Miller WR, ed). Austin, TX: RH Landes, 1996: 75–94.

4. Simpson E, Rubin G, Clyne C et al. Local estrogen biosynthesis in males and females. *Endocr Rel Cancer* 1999; **6:** 131–7.

5. Jordan VC, Parker CJ, Morrow M. Update: breast cancer treatment and prevention with antioestrogens in the 1900s. *Endocr Rev* 1993; **1:** 82–5.

6. Miller WR. Aromatase inhibitors and breast cancer. *Cancer Treat Rev* 1997; **23:** 171–87.

7. Miller WR. Aromatase inhibitors in the treatment of advanced breast cancer. *Cancer Treat Rev* 1989; **16:** 83–93.

8. Simpson ER, Mendelson CR. The regulation of

oestrogen biosynthesis in human adipose tissue. *Proc R Soc Edin* 1989; **95B:** 153–9.

9. Samojlik E, Santen RJ, Worgul TJ. Suppression of residual oestrogen production with aminoglutethimide in women following surgical hypophysectomy or adrenalectomy. *Clin Endocrinol* 1984; **20:** 43–51.

10. Miller WR. Biology of aromatase inhibitors: pharmacology/endocrinology within the breast. *Endocr Rel Cancer* 1999; **6:** 187–95.

11. Bulun SE, Simpson ER. Regulation of aromatase expression in human tissues. *Breast Cancer Res Treat* 1994; **30:** 19–29.

12. Means GD, Mahendroo M, Corbin CJ et al. Structural analysis of the gene encoding human aromatase cytochrome P-450, the enzyme responsible for estrogen biosynthesis. *J Biol Chem* 1989; **264:** 19385–91.

13. Kirschner MA, Schneider G, Ertel NH et al. Obesity, androgens, estrogens and cancer risk. *Cancer Res* 1982; **42**(Suppl): 3281S–5S.

14. Judd HL, Judd GE, Lucas WE, Yen SS. Endocrine function of the postmenopausal ovary: concentration of androgens and estrogens in ovarian and peripheral vein blood. *J Clin Endocrinol Metab* 1974; **39:** 1020–4.

15. Perel E, Killinger DW. The interconversion and aromatization of androgens by human adipose tissue. *J Steroid Biochem* 1979; **10:** 623–7.

16. Schweikert HU, Milewich L, Wilson JD. Aromatization of androstenedione by cultured human fibroblasts. *J Clin Endocrinol Metab* 1976; **43:** 785–95.

17. Longcope C. Methods and results of aromatization studies in vivo. *Cancer Res* 1982; **42**(Suppl): 3307S–11S.

18. Smuk M, Schwers J. Aromatization of androstenedione by human adult liver in vitro. *J Clin Endocrinol Metab* 1977; **45:** 1009–12.

19. Miller WR, Mullen P, Sourdaine P et al. Regulation of aromatase activity within the breast. *J Steroid Biochem* 1997; **61:** 193–202.

20. Baird DT, Uno A, Melby JC. Adrenal secretion of androgens and oestrogens. *J Endocrinol* 1969; **45:** 135–6.

21. Longcope C, Pratt JH, Schneider SH et al. In vivo studies on the metabolism of estrogens by muscle and adipose tissue of normal males. *J Clinical Endocrinol Metab* 1976; **43:** 1134–45.

22. James VHT, Reed MJ, Folkard EJ. Studies of estrogen metabolism in postmenopausal women with cancer. *J Steroid Biochem* 1981; **15:** 235–45.

23. MacDonald PC, Edman CD, Hemsell DL et al. Effect of obesity on conversion of plasma androstenedione to estrone in postmenopausal women with and without endometrial cancer. *Am J Obstet Gynecol* 1978; **130:** 19–26.

24. Vermeulen A, Verdonck L. Sex hormone concentrations in postmenopausal women. *Clin Endocrinol* 1978; **9:** 59–66.

25. Killinger DW, Perel E, Daniilescu D et al. The relationship between aromatase activity and body fat distribution. *Steroids* 1987; **50:** 61–72.

26. Abul-Hajj YJ, Iverson R, Kiang DT. Aromatization of androgens by human breast cancer. *Steroids* 1979; **33:** 205–22.

27. Miller WR. Steroid metabolism in breast cancer. In: *Breast Cancer: Treatment and Progress* (Stoll BA, ed). Oxford: Blackwell Science, 1986: 156–72.

28. Bezwoda WR, Mansoor N, Dansey R. Correlation of breast tumour aromatase activity and response to aromatase inhibition with aminoglutethimide. *Oncology* 1987; **44:** 345–9.

29. Miller WR, O'Neill JS. The importance of local synthesis of estrogen within the breast. *Steroids* 1987; **50:** 345–9.

30. Miller WR, Anderson EC. The biological relevance of aromatase activity in breast tumours. In: *Clinical Use of Aromatase Inhibitors, Current Data and Future Perspectives* (Robustelli Della Cuna G, Manni A, Pannutti F, eds). Pavia: Edizioni Medico Scientifiche, 1995: 89–93.

31. Hillier SG, Whitelaw PF, Smyth CD. Follicular oestrogen synthesis: the 'two-cell, two-gonadotrophin' model revisited. *Mol Cell Endocrinol* 1994; **100:** 51–4.

32. Folkerd EJ, Jacob HS, van der Spuy et al. Failure of FSH to influence aromatization in human adipose tissue. *Clin Endocrinol* 1982; **16:** 621–5.

33. Reed MJ, Purohit A. Breast cancer and the role of cytokines in regulating estrogen synthesis: an emerging hypothesis. *Endocr Rev* 1997; **18:** 701–15.

34. Singh A. Purohit A, Ghilchik MW, Reed MJ. The regulation of aromatase activity in breast fibroblasts: the role of interleukin-6 and prostaglandin E$_2$. *Endocr Rel Cancer* 1999; **6:** 139–47.

35. Miller WR, Mullen P. Factors influencing aromatase activity in the breast. *J Steroid Biochem Mol Biol* 1993; **44:** 597–604.

36. Zhao Y, Nichols JE, Bulun SE et al. Aromatase P450 gene expression in human adipose tissue. Role of a Jak/STAT pathway in regulation of the adipose-specific promoter. *J Biol Chem* 1995; **270:** 16449–57.

37. Miller WR, Mullen P, Sourdaine P et al. Regulation of aromatase activity within the breast. *J Steroid Biochem Mol Biol* 1997; **61:** 193–202.

38. Purohit A, Ghilchik MW, Duncan LJ et al. Aromatase activity and interleukin-6 production by normal and malignant breast tissues. *J Clin Endocrin Metab* 1995; **80:** 3052–8.

39. Macdiarmid F, Wang DY, Duncan LJ et al. Stimulation of aromatase activity in breast fibroblasts by tumour necrosis factor alpha. *Mol Cell Endocrinol* 1995; **106:** 17–21.

40. Means GD, Kilgore MW, Mahendroo MS et al. Tissue-specific promoters regulate aromatase cytochrome P450 gene expression in human ovary and fetal tissues. *Mol Endocrinol* 1991; **5:** 2005–13.

41. Harada N, Utsumi T, Takagi Y. Tissue specific expression of the human aromatase cytochrome P-450 gene by alternative use of multiple exons 1 and promoters and switching of tissue specific exons 1 in carcinogenesis. *Proc Natl Acad Sci USA* 1993; **90:** 11312–16.

42. Harada N, Yamada K. Ontogeny of aromatase messenger-ribonucleic-acid in mouse brain – fluorometrical quantitation by polymerase chain-reaction. *Endocrinology* 1992; **131:** 2306–12.

43. Howie AF, Morley SD, Miller WR, Mason JI. Aromatase transcripts in breast cancer. In: *Proceedings of 'Aromatase and its Inhibitors', Prague*, 1998: Abst 11.

44. Harada N, Honda S. Molecular analysis of aberrant expression of aromatase in breast cancer. *Breast Cancer Res Treat* 1998; **49:** S15–21.

45. Chen S, Zhou D, Okubo T et al. Breast tumor aromatase: functional role and transcriptional regulation. *Endocr Rel Cancer* 1999; **6:** 149–56.

46. Simpson ER, Mahendroo MS, Means GD et al. Aromatase cytochrome P450, the enzyme responsible for estrogen biosynthesis. *Endocr Rev* 1994; **15:** 342–55.

47. Johnston JO, Metcalf BW. Aromatase: a target enzyme in breast cancer. In: *Novel Approaches to Cancer Chemotherapy*. London: Academic Press, 1984: 307–328.

48. Clemett D, Lamb HM. Exemestane: a review. *Drugs* 2000; **59:** 1279–96.

49. Santen RJ, Misbin RI. Aminoglutethimide: review of pharmacology and clinical use. *Pharmacotherapy* 1981; **1:** 95–120.

50. Bhatnagar AS, Hausler A, Schieweck KL et al. Highly selective inhibition of estrogen biosynthesis by CGS 20267, a new non-steroidal aromatase inhibitor. *J Steroid Biochem Mol Biol* 1990; **37:** 1021–7.

51. Yates RA, Dowsett M, Fisher GV et al. Arimidex (ZD1033): a selective, potent inhibitor of aromatase in postmenopausal female volunteers. *Br J Cancer* 1996; 73: 543–8.

52. Griffiths CT, Hall TC, Saba Z et al. Preliminary trial of aminoglutethimide in breast cancer. *Cancer* 1973; **32:** 31–7.

53. Perez-Carrion R, Alberola CV, Calabresi F et al. Comparison of the selective aromatase inhibitor formestane with tamoxifen as first-line hormonal therapy in postmenopausal women with advanced breast cancer. *Ann Oncol* 1994; **5:** S19–24.

54. Buzdar AU. Role of aromatase inhibitors in advanced breast cancer. *Endocr Rel Cancer* 1999; **6:** 219–25.

55. Ragaz J. Status of aromatase inhibitors in relation to other breast cancer treatment modalities. *Endocr Rel Cancer* 1999; **6:** 277–91.

56. Jones S, Vogel C, Arkhipov A et al. Multicenter phase II trial of exemestane as third-line hormonal therapy of postmenopausal women with metastatic breast cancer. *J Clin Oncol* 1999; **17:** 3418–25.

57. Lonning PE. Pharmacology of new aromatase inhibitors. *Breast* 1996; **5:** 202–8.

58. Demers LM, Lipton A, Harvey HA et al. The efficacy of CGS20267 in suppressing estrogen biosynthesis in patients with advanced stage breast cancer. *J Steroid Biochem* 1993; **44:** 687–91.

59. Vermeulen A. Human mammary cancer as a site of sex steroid metabolism. *Cancer Surv* 1986; **5:** 585–95.

60. Miller WR. Uptake and synthesis of steroid hormones by the breast. *Endocr Rel Cancer* 1997; **4:** 307–11.

61. Miller WR. In vitro and in vivo effects of 4-hydroxyandrostenedione on steroid and tumour metabolism. In: *4-Hydroxyandrostenedione – A New Approach to Hormone-Dependent Cancer* (Coombes RC, Dowsett M, eds). London: Royal Society of Medicine International Congress and Symposium Series, 1992: 45–50.

62. Kadohama N, Yarborough C, Zhou D et al. Kinetic properties of aromatase mutants Pro308Phe, Asp309Asn and Asp309Ala and their interactions with aromatase inhibitors. *J Steroid Biochem Mol Biol* 1992; **43:** 693–701.

63. Sourdaine P, Parker MG, Telford J, Miller WR. Analysis of the aromatase cytochrome P450 gene in human breast cancers. *J Mol Endocrinol* 1993; **13:** 331–7.

64. James VHT, Reed MJ, Adams EF et al. Oestrogen uptake and metabolism in vivo. *Proc R Soc Edin* 1989; **95B:** 185–93.

65. Long BJ, Tighman S, Yue W et al. The steroidal antiestrogen ICI 182,780 is an inhibitor of cellular aromatase activity. *J Steroid Biochem Mol Biol* 1998; **67:** 293–304.

66. Bhatnagar A, Miller WR. Pharmacology of inhibitors of estrogen biosynthesis. In: *Handbook of Experimental Pharmacology: Estrogens and Antiestrogens* (Oertel M, Schillinger E, eds). Berlin: Springer-Verlag, 1999: 223–30.

67. Miller WR, O'Neill J. The importance of local synthesis of estrogen within the breast. *Steroids* 1987; **50:** 537–40.

68. Miller WR, Mullen P, Telford J, Dixon JM. Clinical importance of intratumoral aromatase. *Breast Cancer Res Treat* 1998; **49:** S27–32.

69. Miller WR, Raghavan V, Mullen P, Dixon JM. Induction and suppression of aromatase by inhibitors. In: *Aromatase and Breast Cancer* (Miller WR, Santen RJ, eds). New York: Marcel Dekker, 2000: 213–25.

70. Kao Y-C, Okubo T, Sun X-Z, Chen S. Induction of aromatase expression by aminoglutethimide, an aromatase inhibitor that is used to treat breast cancer in postmenopausal women. *Anticancer Res* 1999; **19:** 2049–56.

71. Harada N, Hatano O. Inhibitors of aromatase prevent degradation of the enzyme in cultured human tumour cells. *Br J Cancer* 1998; **77:** 567–72.

72. Harada N, Honda S-I, Hatano O. Aromatase inhibitors and enzyme stability. *Endocr Rel Cancer* 1999; **6:** 211–18.

73. Reed MJ, Owen AM, Lai C et al. In situ oestrone synthesis in normal breast and breast tumour tissues: effect of treatment with 4-hydroxyandrostenedione. *Int J Cancer* 1989; **44:** 233–7.

74. Miller WR, Telford J, Love C et al. Effects of letrozole as primary medical therapy on in situ oestrogen synthesis and endogenous oestrogen levels within the breast. *Breast* 1998; **7:** 273–6.

75. Miller WR, Dixon JM, Grattage L et al. Effects of neoadjuvant treatment with the aromatase inhibitor, anastrozole ('Arimidex'), on peripheral and in situ estrogen synthesis and uptake by breast tissue in postmenopausal women. *Breast Cancer Res Treat* 1999; **57:** 32.

76. Dixon JM, Love CDB, Renshaw L et al. Lessons from the use of aromatase inhibitors in the neoadjuvant setting. *Endocr Rel Cancer* 1999; **6:** 227–30.

77. Miller WR, Anderson TJ, Marson L et al. Histological changes in breast cancers following primary systemic treatment with either letrozole or tamoxifen. *Breast* 1999; **8:** 216.

78. Anderson TJ, Dixon JM, Stuart M et al. Effect of neoadjuvant treatment with anastrozole (Arimidex) on pathological markers in tumors in postmenopausal women with large (>3 cm) operable breast cancer. *Proc Am Assoc Cancer Res* 2000: Abst 4708.

14

Effects of progesterone receptor antagonists on breast cancer

Jens Hoffmann, Rosemarie B Lichtner, Ulrike Fuhrmann, Horst Michna, Karsten Parczyk, Günter Neef, Kristof Chwalisz, Martin R Schneider

CONTENTS • Introduction • Biological mechanisms of action of progesterone antagonists • Preclinical models for assessing antiprogestogenic activity • Comparison with standard hormonal therapy

INTRODUCTION

Endocrine therapy of breast cancer has been established for decades. The therapies available to block steroid-hormone-receptor-mediated tumour growth are based on two principles: ligand depletion or receptor blockade. Ligand depletion can be achieved either by removal of steroid-producing glands or by inhibition of steroid biosynthesis. The latter can be done through inhibition of enzymes (e.g. aromatase) or through the induction of negative-feedback mechanisms (e.g. with the use of gonadotropin-releasing hormone (GnRH) agonists). Estrogen receptors can be blocked either with selective estrogen receptor modulators (SERMs), which are partial agonists (and of which the antiestrogen tamoxifen is presently the compound of choice for the endocrine treatment of breast cancer) or with a new class of compounds, the pure antiestrogens.

In addition to estradiol, it is well known that progesterone in physiological concentrations participates in the proliferation of mammary carcinomas. Therefore it is to be expected that antiprogestins can block the growth of breast tumours functionally expressing the progesterone receptor (PgR) and might be promising new tools for breast cancer therapy. These compounds clearly need a functionally expressed PgR to block tumour growth, but there is strong experimental evidence that their tumour inhibition is based on more than just progesterone antagonism. The ability of these compounds to induce tumour cell differentiation that leads to apoptosis is unique among all other endocrine therapeutics.

Different classes of antiprogestins have been identified, but a broad spectrum of either agonistic or antagonistic activity on other steroid receptors (i.e. glucocorticoid, estrogen, and androgen receptors) has also been observed for some compounds.

This chapter focuses on the preclinical and clinical development of new antiprogestins with high receptor specificity for breast cancer treatment.

Considerable progress has been made in elucidating the mechanism of action of antiprogestins. The antagonists bind to the hormone receptors, which are ligand-inducible transcription factors, and modulate their gene-regulatory activities. In most instances, a steroid receptor such as PgR is transcriptionally inactive when complexed with an antagonist and competitively inhibits transactivation of a target steroid-responsive gene by the cognate hormone-occupied receptor. Recent results, however, have revealed that the biological response to a progesterone antagonist depends on further factors and does not seem to be simply the result of competition with progesterone.

BIOLOGICAL MECHANISMS OF ACTION OF PROGESTERONE ANTAGONISTS

The physiological effects of progesterone are mediated by two receptor proteins (members of the nuclear receptor superfamily of transcription factors), termed PgR-A and PgR-B, that arise from a single gene and act as ligand-activated transcription factors to regulate the expression of reproductive target genes. The structure and functional properties of the PgR isoforms and how functional differences between these proteins are likely to impact on the overall physiologic role of the receptor in reproductive systems are discussed in detail by Conneely et al.[1]

In most cases, PgR expression is induced by estrogen, implying that many of the in vivo effects attributed to progesterone could also be the result of concomitantly administered estrogen. Therefore, to clearly define those physiological events that are specifically attributable to progesterone in vivo, a mouse model carrying a null mutation of the *PgR* gene has been generated using embryonic stem cell/gene targeting techniques.[2,3]

Null mutation of both PgR proteins in mice leads to pleiotropic reproductive abnormalities.[4] Male and female embryos homozygous for the *PgR* mutation (PRKO) developed normally to adulthood; however, they displayed significant defects in all reproductive organs. These included an inability to ovulate, uterine hyperplasia and inflammation, severely limited mammary gland development, and an inability to exhibit sexual behaviour.

The PRKO model was also used to study the effects of the stromal and epithelial PgRs on ductal and lobuloalveolar development in the mouse mammary gland.[5] In reciprocal transplantation experiments, it was found that in the absence of PgR in transplanted donor epithelium, but not in recipient stroma, normal lobuloalveolar development in response to estrogen and progesterone treatment was prevented. Conversely, the presence of PgR in the transplanted donor epithelium, but not in the recipient stroma, revealed that PgR in the stroma may be necessary for ductal development. These mammary gland transplantation experiments have shown that the luminal epithelial compartment of the mammary gland is responsive to the progesterone-induced signal.

There is strong evidence that the PgR may extend its proliferative effects to induce side-branching to neighbouring mammary epithelial cells that lack the receptor, probably through as-yet unidentified paracrine factors.[6,7]

Wnt proteins might function as the paracrine factors that operate downstream of progesterone and the PgR to mediate the process of side-branching. These factors are secreted glycoproteins that bind to members of the Frizzled family of seven-transmembrane-domain receptors and can function as oncogenes. Wnt proteins play important roles in the development of various vertebrate and invertebrate tissues.[8,9]

A member of the Wnt growth factor family, Wnt-4, was employed as a molecular marker of steroid hormone action in the mammary gland stroma and epithelium, respectively, to investigate the systemic effects of progesterone.[10] Progesterone induces Wnt-4 in mammary epithelial cells and is required for increased Wnt-4 expression during pregnancy. In the absence of the PgR from the mammary epithelium, ductal side-branching fails to occur. Transplantation studies with mammary epithelia from *wnt-4*[-/-] mice showed that Wnt-4 plays an essential role in side-branching early in pregnancy. Although *wnt-4* is the only *wnt* gene directly induced by progesterone, and Wnt signalling seems to be essential in mediating progesterone function during early mammary gland morphogenesis, it is not unique in its ability to trigger side-branching, since late in pregnancy, the ductal epithelium of *wnt-4*$^{-/-}$ mice shows normal side-branching. It could be speculated that this compensation is due to the expression of other Wnt proteins later in pregnancy.[11,12]

The PRKO model was also used to define the controversial role of progesterone-initiated intracellular signalling in mammary gland tumorigenesis.[13] In combination studies with tissue transplantation and an established carcinogen-induced (using 7,12-dimethylbenz[a]-anthracene, DMBA) mammary tumorigenesis system, it was shown that there was a marked reduction in mammary tumour incidence in PRKO mice as compared with isogenic wild types.

This observation demonstrates that in the absence of PgR function, prolactin alone is not sufficient to induce the neoplastic transformation and that progesterone may activate mitogenic mediators of the prolactin pathway. Under these conditions, the epithelial cells might exhibit a low proliferative index and at the time of carcinogen administration be a poor candidate for malignant transformation.

Not only has the luminal epithelial compartment been considered to be primarily responsive to the progesterone induced proliferative signals and to be the primary site for the initial carcinogenic insult, but additionally PgR expression has been localized predominantly to these cells. One interpretation for the reduction of mammary tumorigenesis could be that the progenitor cells for alveologenesis – the PgR-expressing epithelial cells – are absent in the PRKO mice. Because the majority of mammary tumours are of alveolar origin, the absence of these progenitor cells might reduce the number of target cells for neoplastic transformation.

These results give strong support for the use of antiprogestins in breast cancer, because they might inhibit the prolactin mitogenic action on the luminal epithelium.

Interactions between progestins, PgR, and growth factor receptors

Depending on the tissue, progesterone is classified as a proliferative or a differentiative hormone. This has been extensively studied in cultured human T47D breast cancer cells. Treatment of PgR-positive T47D cells with progestin produces biphasic effects. Studies focusing on the initial growth-stimulatory components show that progestin-induced entry of cells into S phase is accompanied by transient increases in the activity of cyclin D1 and cyclin-dependent kinase (cdk) 4.[14] Growth stimulation by progestins is restricted to one cycle, however, and is followed by growth arrest at the G_1/S boundary of the second cycle.[14,15] Cells then enter a period of resistance to growth-regulatory effects of additional progesterone, accompanied by hypophosphorylation and profound downregulation of retinoblastoma protein (pRb), loss of cyclins D, A, and B, and subsequential increases first in the levels of the cdk inhibitor p21 followed by increases in the cdk inhibitor p27.[14]

During the progesterone-arrested state, cells upregulate epidermal growth factor (EGF) receptor (EGFR) three- to fivefold and acquire sensitivity to the proliferative effects of EGF.[14] It has been shown that progestin potentiates the effects of EGF on T47D cells by upregulation of EGFR, ErbB2, and ErbB3, and enhances tyrosine phosphorylation of signalling molecules known to associate with activated type I receptors.[16,17] This led to the model proposed by Horwitz and co-workers, in which progesterone is a competence factor that switches breast cancer growth from steroid hormone to growth factor dependence.

Growth arrest accompanied by upregulation of p21 has been implicated not only in inhibiting proliferation but also in promoting differentiation.[18] Furthermore, this cdk inhibitor has been postulated to be a key intermediary protein in the pathway that determines whether cells proliferate or differentiate.[19] The promoter of p21 lacks a canonical progesterone element, and thus is activated by progesterone through a novel mechanism that involves interactions between PgRs and CPB/p300, similarly to other agents such as phorbol esters, butyrate, BRCA1, and transforming growth factor β (TGF-β).[20]

There is considerable evidence linking the EGF and progesterone signalling pathways in breast cancer. This includes attenuation of progestin responsiveness and decreases in PgR levels in cells treated with EGF,[21] as well as progestin-specific regulation of EGF and EGFR levels.[21,22]

Induction of differentiation and apoptosis

The progesterone antagonists onapristone (ZK 98299) and ZK 112993 (Figure 14.1) exert a strong tumour inhibiting effect in a panel of

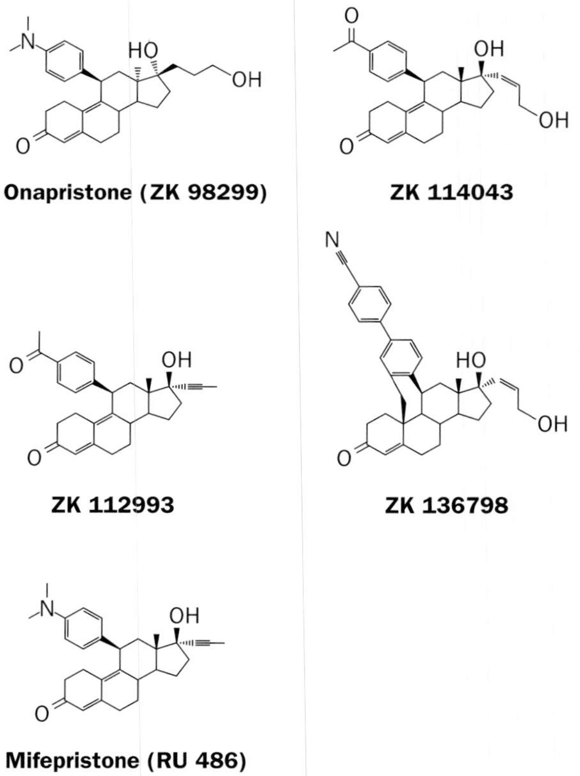

Onapristone (ZK 98299)

ZK 114043

ZK 112993

ZK 136798

Mifepristone (RU 486)

Figure 14.1 Structure of the antiprogestins onapristone, ZK 114043, ZK 112993, ZK 136798 and mifepristone.

hormone-dependent rodent mammary tumour models.[23] Quantitative light and electron microscopic data from these experiments indicate that the antitumour action of antiprogestins is accompanied by the initiation of terminal differentiation, leading to apoptotic cell death.[23] Flow cytometry studies revealed an accumulation of the tumour cells in the G_0–G_1 phase of the cell cycle, which may result from induction of differentiation, since a differentiation-specific G_1 arrest has already been proposed for other stem cell systems.

Further experiments to characterize the antitumour mechanism of progesterone antagonists have been described.[24] In these experiments, the effects of onapristone and ZK 112993 on DMBA-induced and N-methyl-N-nitrosourea (MNU)-induced-mammary tumours of the rat and on syngenic mouse mammary tumours (MXT) with different therapy intervals were investigated. Hormone-dependent mammary tumours normally display intraductal growth in papillary, cribriform, or solid formation. After treatment periods of 2–6 weeks with progesterone antagonists, these tumours displayed dysplastic ductal and acinous formations, usually filled with secretory material. Whereas tumour size, mitotic index, and grade of tumour malignancy decreased distinctly, the volume fraction of glandular structures in the tumours as well as the appearance of apoptosis increased threefold compared with controls. In addition, the mammary glands of antiprogestin-treated animals showed the morphological features of differentiation, with the appearance of secretory activity. Interestingly, the staining pattern of some of the lectins used, especially the UEA 1 binding pattern, fits the concept of differentiation, since recent studies have revealed a higher degree of fucosylation only in benign lesions of human breast cancers.

Differential gene expression in response to antiprogestin treatment

Antiprogestins can only exert their antitumour activity in cells expressing PgR,[25] and therefore it is speculated that the antiprogestins exert their antiproliferative effect via binding to PgR. The molecular mechanism responsible for this antiproliferative effect is unclear. According to the commonly accepted hypothesis, in the absence of an agonistic ligand, a receptor antagonist should not induce any pronounced effects. It could be that these compounds act as inverse agonists by directly regulating PgR transcription factor activities. Further, it is possible that the antiprogestin-liganded PgR sequestrates co-regulatory proteins, thereby limiting the activity of other transcription factors (this phenomenon has also been called 'squelching'). In this respect, it could be that the transcriptional activity of the PgR is impaired by a 'squelching' phenomenon.

One possible way in which to elucidate this phenomenon is to study the effects of estrogens, antiestrogens, and antiprogestins on the expression of a larger number of genes. When T47D breast cancer cells were cultivated in a medium containing 5% charcoal-treated fetal calf serum, proliferation could be significantly stimulated with 0.1 nM estradiol. The PgR was expressed at relatively high levels (around 900 fmol/mg protein), and these cells are highly susceptible to growth inhibition by antiprogestins. Since these experiments were performed in the absence of any relevant levels of a progestin, it was surprising to find that the antiprogestin was able to inhibit cell proliferation in a very prominent manner. A similar observation has been made in animal experiments where tumour growth induced by estrogens could also be efficiently blocked by antiprogestins.[25] A thorough analysis of gene expression is possible using chip-driven technologies such as Affymetrix Genechip Assays. By comparing the effects of these hormones and antihormones, it is possible to determine whether or not the gene expression patterns induced by antiprogestins and antiestrogens are comparable (i.e. whether or not antiprogestins act functionally like antiestrogens). The appropriate experiments are ongoing. The antiprogestin-mediated induction of terminal differentiation, resulting in apoptosis, already described in in vivo

tumour model systems, might also be reflected at the level of gene expression.

PRECLINICAL MODELS FOR ASSESSING ANTIPROGESTOGENIC ACTIVITY

In vitro models for antiprogestin characterization

Transactivation assay
The transactivation assay is based on the observation that steroid receptors act as ligand-regulated transcriptional activators. After binding of hormone, the steroid receptor interacts with hormone response elements (HREs) of hormone-regulated genes, thereby inducing a cascade of transcriptional events. This hormone-dependent transcriptional activation can be determined in tissue culture by transfection into cells of the steroid receptor under investigation and a reporter gene linked to a hormone-responsive promoter. The transactivation assay allows determination of both the agonistic and the antagonistic potency of a given compound. In order to determine the antiprogestogenic and progestogenic potency of antiprogestins, cells stably transfected with either human PgR-A or PgR-B together with the luciferase reporter gene linked to the mouse mammary tumour virus promoter (MMTV-LUC) are used. For the determination of antagonistic activity, cells are treated with 0.1 nmol/l of the synthetic progestin R5020 and, in addition, with increasing amounts of the test compound. As a positive control for reporter gene inhibition, cells are treated with the antiprogestin mifepristone (Figure 14.1).

To determine agonistic activity, cells are cultured only in the presence of the test compound. As a positive control for reporter gene induction, cells are incubated with increasing amounts of R5020. As a negative control for reporter gene induction, cells are cultured in 1% ethanol. After 24 hours, a luciferase assay is carried out. Figure 14.2(a) shows an example of a transactivation assay carried out with the antiprogestin ZK 136798 (Figure 14.1), which is

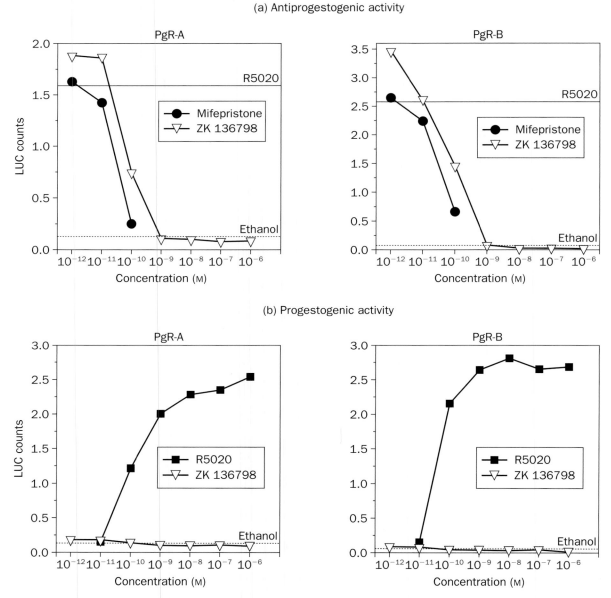

Figure 14.2 Progesterone-stimulated transactivation of the PgR-A and PgR-B isoforms is inhibited by the antiprogestin ZK 136798. In order to determine the antiprogestogenic and progestogenic potency of ZK 136798, in vitro transactivation assays were carried out with cells stably transfected with either human PgR-A or PgR-B. ZK 136798 showed strong antiprogestogenic activity on both PgR isoforms comparable to that of mifepristone. ZK 136798 did not show any progestogenic activity. LUC, luciferase.

a strong antagonist on both PgR isoforms, with IC$_{50}$ values of 7.7×10^{-11} M (PgR-A) and 1.2×10^{-10} M (PgR-B). Furthermore, ZK 136798 did not show any progestogenic activity (Figure 14.2b).

Inhibition of breast cancer cell proliferation

Growth inhibition studies in breast cancer cell lines can be used to screen antiprogestins for antiproliferative activity. Principally, cells were grown in charcoal-treated serum supplemented with 0.1 nM estradiol plus the indicated compounds for 6 days with one change of medium. Following fixation and subsequent staining with crystal violet, the absorbance was recorded and values normalized to the absorbance of untreated controls as described elsewhere.[26] Figure 14.3(a) demonstrates inhibition of estradiol-stimulated growth in T47D cells by 4-hydroxytamoxifen, while onapristone was ineffective. In contrast, the antiprogestin ZK 136798 was able to inhibit estradiol-stimulated cell proliferation in a dose-dependent manner (Figure 14.3b).

In vivo models for antiprogestin characterization

The standard model for screening of progestogenic and antiprogestogenic activity is the estradiol-primed rabbit. However, further models in rat and mice have been developed to characterize the antiproliferative and differentiation-promoting activities of antiprogestins. This chapter will focus on the two antiprogestins that have entered a clinical development programme, namely mifepristone (RU 486) and onapristone (ZK 98299), and two experimental drugs, namely ZK 112993 and ZK 136798 (Figure 14.1).

Antiprogestogenic effects on mouse mammary glands

To test directly the antiproliferative and differentiation-promoting activities of antiprogestins on the normal mammary gland, whole-organ cultures of mammary glands from estradiol/

(a)

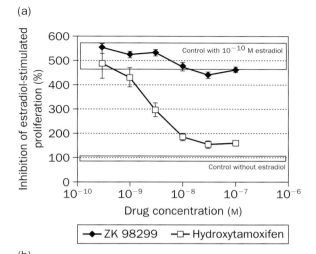

(b)

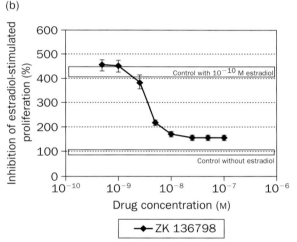

Figure 14.3 Estradiol-stimulated growth of the T47D breast cancer cell line is inhibited by the antiprogestin ZK 136798. T47D cells were grown in medium with 10% charcol-stripped serum. Upper and lower shaded bars represent cells grown in the presence or absence respectively of 10^{-10} M estradiol, while the graphs indicate the proliferation in the presence of 10^{-10} M estradiol plus increasing concentrations of ZK 98299, 4-hydroxytamoxifen, and ZK 136798.

progesterone-primed virgin mice maintained in a serum-free medium with aldosterone, prolactin, insulin, and hydrocortisone were used.[27] In this model, it was shown that a 4-day treatment of organ cultures with investigational antiprogestins led to a strong inhibition of epithelial DNA synthesis. In parallel, it was shown that antiprogestins cause alveolar cells to acquire a more differentiated phenotype distinguished by secretory active alveoli composed of single cell layers with increased fat droplet accumulation and enhanced expression of the milk proteins β-casein and whey acidic protein.[27]

In addition, this model allowed investigations of the mechanism of action of antiprogestins,[27] since particularly strong effects were found on the expression of mammary-derived growth inhibitor (MDGI). Both half-maximal inhibition of epithelial DNA synthesis and stimulation of MDGI mRNA expression were found at about 5 ng/ml of ZK 114043. This was not due to the antiglucocorticoid effects of ZK 114043, since the medium was supplemented with 5 μg/ml hydrocortisone. Furthermore, the prevention of action of ZK 114043 by the progesterone agonist R5020 and the ZK 114043-stimulated expression of β-casein and MDGI mRNA in cultured glands of 10-week-old unprimed virgin mice suggested a PgR-mediated mechanism of antiprogestin action. The other antiprogestins, mifepristone and onapristone, likewise stimulated MDGI expression. These data provide direct evidence that antiprogestins act like a differentiation factor in the normal mammary gland. Although the underlying mechanism is not clear, induction of functional differentiation of mammary glands appears to be a major event.

Antiprogestogenic effects on rat mammary glands

A similar bioassay that allows quantification of the antiproliferative potency of antiprogestins on the mammary gland in the rat was developed by Michna et al.[27] For this purpose, ovariectomized rats were substituted with estrone and progesterone and a further group was simultaneously treated with mifepristone, onapristone, ZK 112993, and ZK136798. A morphometric analysis of the tubulo-alveolar buds in the inguinal mammary glands revealed a dramatic antiproliferative effect of mifepristone and onapristone after only 3 days of treatment.[28] This bioassay measures the potency of

antiprogestins to competitively antagonize the specific effects of progesterone on the target organ mammary gland. Further advantages of this bioassay are the use of a hormonally standardized biological system, the quantitative results, and the small amount of test compound necessary, as well as the substitution with progesterone and estrone since the antiproliferative potency of antiprogestins on experimental hormone-dependent mammary carcinomas is most potently displayed in ovariectomized animals substituted with both sex hormones.

ZK 112993 and ZK 136798 given in a daily dose of 0.1 mg subcutaneously significantly reduced the dry weights of the inguinal mammary glands as well as the weights of 'wholemount' preparations of mammary glands. As a more sensitive and valid parameter of antiproliferative effects, the inhibition of the development of tubulo-alveolar buds was quantified with morphometrical methods on 'wholemount' preparations of mammary glands. ZK 136798 strongly reduced the development of tubulo-alveolar buds after only 3 days' treatment (Table 14.1).

Profiling activity against other steroid receptors

For the first antiprogestin described, mifepristone, the antiglucocorticoid effect is the main side-effect that might be a problem for its development in oncological indications. Therefore, screening on antiglucocorticoid activity has to be implemented early into the drug screening process. Antiglucocorticoid activity has to be compared with dexamethasone and mifepristone. Most compounds (e.g. ZK 136798) have been found not to be glucocorticoid in comparison with dexamethasone.

Androgenicity/antiandrogenicity

The growth and function of the prostate and the seminal vesicles are dependent on the presence of androgens. Orchiectomy results in a decrease in endogenous androgens, leading to growth inhibition of these organs. Treatment with compounds showing androgenic activity stimulates growth in a dose-dependent manner. This assay

Table 14.1 Antiproliferative potency of antiprogestins on the development of tubulo-alveolar buds in rats

	Antiprogestin (s.c. mg/rat)	Estrone (μg/rat)	Progesterone (mg/rat)	Development of tubulo-alveolar buds (mm^3)
Control	—	10	3	3760 ± 358
ZK 112993	0.1	10	3	2123 ± 321[a]
ZK 136798	0.1	10	3	2480 ± 259[a]

[a]Statistically significant difference from control.

Table 14.2 Androgenic effect of ZK 136798 in the orchiectomized rat and antiandrogenic effect in the testosterone propionate (TP)-primed orchiectomized rat

	TP (mg/rat)	Antiprogestin (mg/rat)	Seminal vesicle (mg/100 g bw)	Prostate (mg/100 g bw)
Androgen assay				
Control	—	—	6 (±1)	4 (±1)
Control	0.1	—	77 (±11)	45 (±7)
ZK 136798	—	1.0[a]	9 (±1)	8 (±2)
ZK 136798	—	3.0[a]	15 (±2)	10 (±3)
ZK 136798	—	10.0[a]	27 (±7)	18 (±2)
Antiandrogen assay				
Control	—	—	20 (±3)	10 (±3)
Control	0.1	—	116 (±23)	49 (±17)
ZK 136798	0.1	3.0[b]	143 (±26)	49 (±17)
Cyproterone acetate	0.1	3.0[b]	22 (±3)	17 (±4)

[a]Daily for 12 days s.c. [b]Daily for 7 days s.c.

can also be used to determine the antiandrogenic activity of a given substance.

Additionally, the musculus levator ani is rich in androgen receptors. Thus an increase in its weight is a good parameter for the anabolic activity of a compound.

In the classical orchiectomized rat model, ZK 136798 induced a dose-dependent but weak androgenic activity after a treatment period of 12 days (Table 14.2). However, this weak androgenic effect observed at a dose of 10 mg/animal/day was not statistically significant. Mifepristone did not reveal any androgenic potential on prostate and seminal vesicles at various doses (1, 3, and 10 mg/animal/day subcutaneously) either.

ZK 136798 showed no antiandrogenic activity at a dose of 3 mg/animal/day (Table 14.2), in contrast to mifepristone, which showed antiandrogenic activity in previously performed experiments. In conclusion, ZK 136798 is an antiprogestin devoid of antiandrogenic activity in vivo with a marginal androgenic activity at higher doses of 3 and 10 mg/animal/day.

Estrogenicity/antiestrogenicity

In mice, ZK 136798 in doses of 3 and 10 mg/kg exerted no estrogenic effects on the weights of the uterus and vagina of ovariectomized mice after 7 days' treatment. At the highest dose of 30 mg/kg, the weights of these organs were significantly enhanced, although no estrogenic reactions (cornification of the vagina) could be detected. The corresponding histology of the uterus indicated reactions that might rather be related to the androgenic effect of the compound.

In contrast to experiments in mice, no estrogenic reactions at the level of genital organ weights were seen in ovariectomized rats after treatment with ZK 136798 in doses of 3, 10, and 30 mg/kg. Nevertheless, at the highest dose, the myoepithelial cells of the uterus displayed histological characteristics of a marginal activation.

Using ovariectomized rats in which ZK 136798 was administered for 5 consecutive days at doses of 5, 10, and 20 mg/kg, no influence on estradiol-induced growth of the genital organs was observed.

Therapeutic efficacy in preclinical breast cancer models

For the characterization of new mammary tumour-inhibiting compounds, the use of a panel of tumour models is highly recommended. In the case of hormone-sensitive mammary carcinomas, syngeneic mouse mammary tumours (MXT), chemically induced (DMBA and MNU) rat mammary carcinomas, and human breast cancer xenografts implanted into athymic nude mice are all useful models.

Chemically induced tumours in the rat

Experimental mammary tumours induced by chemical carcinogens such as DMBA in female rats have a similarity to human breast cancers. These tumours are estrogen receptor (ER)- and PgR-positive, and their growth is hormone-responsive (i.e. estrogen can stimulate whereas ovariectomy suppresses tumour growth). Known antiestrogens or aromatase inhibitors are effective in this tumour model, indicating that it is useful for testing the antitumour efficacy of new hormonal or antihormonal agents, especially antiprogestins.

In intact control animals, progressive tumour growth was observed, whereas ovariectomy caused complete tumour regression in 90% of the animals. Treatment with ZK 136798 at doses of 0.2, 1, and 5 mg/kg resulted in a significant inhibition of tumour growth compared with control (Figure 14.4a). Treatment with 0.2 mg/kg resulted in a growth inhibition that was improved with 1 mg/kg. At this dose, maximal growth inhibition was observed – a further dose increase did not lead to better control of tumour growth. In these groups, a complete tumour regression was seen in 30–45% of the rats. The effect of the lowest dose of ZK 136798 tested in this experiment (0.2 mg/kg), was comparable to that of onapristone at 5 mg/kg. At equal doses, the newer investigational drug ZK 136798 was distinctly more potent than onapristone.

It was established by morphometric procedures that treatment with onapristone triggers differentiation of the mitotically active polygonal tumour epithelial cell towards secretorily active glandular structures and acini. Quantitative light and electron microscopic data indicate that the antitumour action of antiprogestins is accompanied by the initiation of terminal differentiation, leading to apoptotic cell death.[23,24] Surprisingly, the antitumour activity of antiprogestins is evident in spite of elevated serum levels of ovarian and pituitary hormones.

The MNU-induced, aggressively growing mammary carcinoma of the rat is strongly ovarian hormone-dependent but less prolactin-dependent than the DMBA-induced tumour model. Measurements revealed progressive

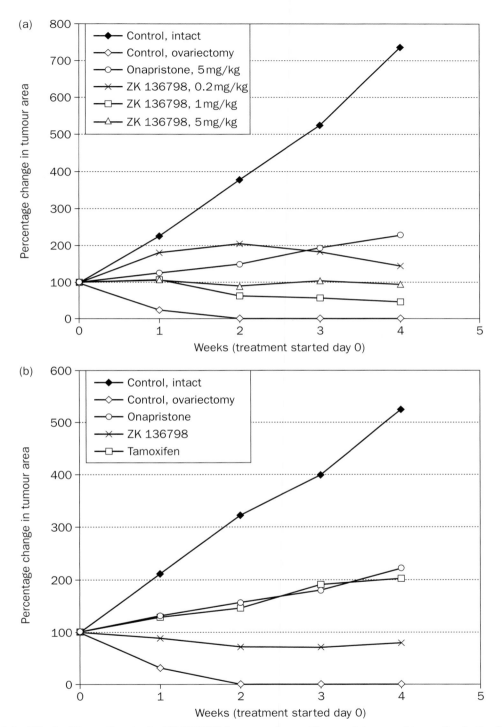

Figure 14.4 Effect of the antiprogestin ZK 136798 in comparison with onapristone and tamoxifen in the DMBA- and MNU-induced mamary carcinoma of the Sprague–Dawley rat. (a) DMBA-model rats were treated subcutaneously once daily for 28 days. (b) MNU-model rats were treated orally once daily with 5mg/kg for 28 days.

growth in intact controls, whereas ovariectomy at day 0 of treatment almost extinguished the tumours, demonstrating the strong hormone dependence of the model.

ZK 136798 was compared with tamoxifen and onapristone (all 5 mg/kg daily orally) over a treatment period of 4 weeks. Whereas tamoxifen and onapristone led to a significant reduction of tumour growth, interestingly ZK 136798 was even more potent, and in the MNU-induced model reached statistically the effect of ovariectomy (Figure 14.4b). No effect on follicle-stimulating hormone and only a marginal stimulation of luteinizing hormone levels were seen after treatment with ZK 136798, and no influences on prolactin and estradiol levels were observed (data not shown).

Syngeneic breast cancer models in mice

The MXT mammary tumour was originally induced by urethane and then kept as in vivo lines existing in various lines with different characteristics. The MXT (+) line exerts pronounced steroid hormone sensitivity in that its growth is strongly inhibited by deprivation of estrogens and progestins.

MXT (+) mammary tumours obtained from donor mice were implanted in fragments of about 2 mm diameter in the inguinal region of female BDF1 mice. Established MXT (+) tumours were treated with ZK 136798 starting 21 days after tumour implantation, with a daily subcutaneous dose of 1 mg/kg. In this model also, ZK 136798 exerted a growth-inhibitory effect comparable to that of ovariectomy (Figure 14.5). Previous reports using the MXT model have shown that tamoxifen causes only relatively weak effects and that megestrol acetate or medroxyprogesterone acetate have no effects on tumour growth in this model.[29] In the MXT model, ZK 136798 is approximately fivefold more active than onapristone.

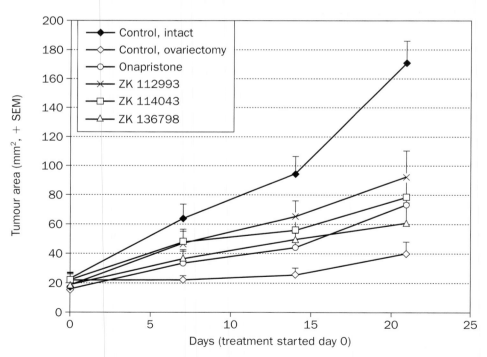

Figure 14.5 Effect of the antiprogestins onapristone, ZK 114043, ZK 112993, and ZK 136798 in comparison with ovariectomy on the growth of established MXT (+) mammary tumours of the mouse. Mice were treated subcutaneously once daily for 21 days with 1 mg/kg.

Xenografted human breast cancer tissue in immunodeficient mice

The human postmenopausal, ER- and PgR-positive T 61 mammary carcinoma (originally provided by Professor Bastert, University Clinic, Homburg, Germany) implanted in castrated male nude mice is a hormone-sensitive tumour that is strongly inhibited by tamoxifen.[30,31] First studies with onapristone using a line with a very high PgR content of almost 200 fmol/mg protein reported a significant growth-inhibitory effect at a dose of 1 mg/mouse (=50 mg/kg).[32]

Using the T 61 model, it was found that, in parallel treatment groups, onapristone when given alone had no effect on tumour growth. When given concomitantly with estradiol benzoate, however, onapristone in the relatively low dose of 10 mg/kg showed strong and significant ($p < 0.05$, Dunnett test) tumour inhibition. Tamoxifen in the same dose of 10 mg/kg again had a pronounced antitumour effect and stimulated the PgR owing to its known estrogenicity in mice.[33] These data on PgR expression were confirmed by immunocytochemical analyses of tumour sections. Whereas in the control tumours no PgRs could be localized, after stimulation with estradiol benzoate as well as in the group receiving estradiol benzoate plus onapristone, an intense staining was found.

El Etreby and colleagues[34] have reported an in vivo antitumour activity of antiprogestins (mifepristone and onapristone) alone and in combination with tamoxifen in the MCF-7 human breast cancer model. The MCF-7 cells produced progressively growing tumours in female nude mice supplemented with estradiol. Tumour regression was observed following either estrogen ablation alone or estrogen ablation in combination with tamoxifen. Monotherapy with tamoxifen or antiprogestins caused a retardation of estrogen-induced tumour progression. Complete inhibition or prevention of tumour growth occurred as a result of simultaneous administration of mifepristone and tamoxifen.

COMPARISON WITH STANDARD HORMONAL THERAPY

It has been shown that the new progesterone antagonists such as onapristone, ZK 112993, and ZK 136798, which are highly selective for the PgR and possess a reduced antiglucocorticoid activity compared with mifepristone, exert a strong tumour inhibiting effect in a panel of hormone-dependent mammary tumour models. Unexpected new experimental observations from these preclinical experiments in different model systems has led to the conclusion that the strong antitumour activity of these 'pure' antiprogestins in breast cancer might not only depend on a primarily classical antihormonal mechanism. For the first time, Michna et al[23,24] showed that the morphological pattern in experimental breast tumours after treatment with antiprogestins differs totally from that after treatment with tamoxifen or high-dose estrogen or ovariectomy. Using quantitative light and electron microscopy, they found that the antitumour action of antiprogestins is accompanied by the initiation of differentiation by induction of secretory active glandular formations, with the disappearance of undifferentiated epithelial tumour cells. Mammary glands and breast tumours of onapristone-treated rats displayed morphometrical features of terminal differentiation, with the appearance of apoptotic cell death.

In addition, flow cytometry studies revealed an accumulation of the tumour cells in G_0–G_1 phase of the cell cycle, together with a significant and biologically relevant reduction in the number of cells in G_2–M and S phases, which may result from induction of differentiation, since a differentiation-specific G_1 arrest has already been proposed for other stem cell systems.[24] In contrast, conventional endocrine therapeutics for breast cancer such as tamoxifen as well as ovariectomy displayed no changes in the distribution of cells within the cell cycle.

It can be concluded from these data that PgR antagonists differ in their mode of action from compounds used in established endocrine treatment strategies for mammary carcinoma. It was shown by morphometric procedures that treatment with onapristone triggers differentiation of the mitotically active polygonal tumour epithelial cell towards secretory active glandular structures and acini. The antiprogestin-related reduction of the number of mammary tumour cells in S phase in experimental tumour models (G_0–G_1 arrest) emphasizes the unique innovative mechanism of action of these new agents in the treatment of human breast cancer.

The ability of progesterone antagonists to reduce the number of cells in S phase may offer a significant clinical advantage, since it has been established that the S phase fraction is a highly significant predictor of disease-free survival among axillary node-negative patients with diploid mammary tumours.

Clinical studies were therefore initiated to investigate the new antiprogestin onapristone as first- and second-line endocrine therapy in patients with breast cancer. In an exploratory phase II clinical trial,[35] 19 patients who either had locally advanced breast cancer (12 patients) or were elderly and unfit with primary breast cancer (7 patients) received onapristone 100 mg/day. Of the 19 tumours, 17 expressed ER whilst 12 of the 18 tumours tested expressed PgR. Tumour remission was categorized according to International Union Against Cancer criteria. One patient was withdrawn after 4.5 months. Of the remaining 18 patients, 10 (56%) showed a partial response and 2 (11%) durable static disease (for 6 months or longer), giving an overall tumour remission rate of 67%, confirming that onapristone can induce tumour responses in human breast cancer. The median duration of remission was 70 weeks. Studies are ongoing to investigate whether the biological effects of onapristone on these human breast cancers were similar to the changes seen in the in vivo models described above.

However, irrespective of the biological changes seen, the clinical results suggest a potential benefit of adding antiprogestins to the panel of endocrine breast cancer therapeutics, especially to extend the therapeutic options in antiestrogen-refractory diseases.

It has been shown that antiprogestins induce cellular differentiation and apoptosis. Besides their use as single treatment of breast cancer, preclinical experiments indicate that combination therapy as well as the extension of endocrine treatments to several other tumour entities are promising approaches for further developments.

El Etreby et al[36] have demonstrated an additive effect of the antiprogestin mifepristone in combination with 4-hydroxytamoxifen on the increase in induction of apoptosis and on downregulation of Bcl-2 in the human breast cancer cell line MCF-7. These results and other published data suggested that antiprogestins and the antiestrogen tamoxifen interact with their respective receptors to initiate an additive effect on cell death. As mechanisms, the downregulation of Bcl-2, changes in the activity of proteinkinase C (PKC), and induction of TGF-β1 have been discussed. These in vitro experimental results were confirmed by demonstrating an in vivo antitumour activity of antiprogestins alone and in combination with tamoxifen in the MCF-7 human breast cancer model.[34] Complete inhibition or prevention of tumour growth occurred as a result of simultaneous administration of mifepristone and tamoxifen. These results suggest a potential clinical benefit of adding an antiprogestin to antiestrogen therapy of breast cancer patients.

The effects of antiprogestins has been investigated in other tumour types – both classical endocrine-sensitive tumours (i.e. prostate cancer) and non-classical endocrine-sensitive tumours (i.e. gastrointestinal cancer).

The effect of onapristone and concomitant estrogen supplements on the growth of human gastrointestinal cancer xenografts was examined by Robertson and colleagues.[37] Estradiol-stimulated RD19 (gastric) tumour growth in female mice was inhibited on treatment with onapristone ($p < 0.05$). Pancreatic tumours (PAN-1) were significantly stimulated by estrogen (by 64% of control; $p = 0.02$), and onapristone treatment inhibited estradiol-stimulated growth (52% reduction of estrogen control; $p > 0.05$). Xenografts of some gastrointestinal tumour cell lines grow at different rates in male and female mice. Estrogen may cause additional growth stimulation, and estrogen-stimulated growth can be reversed by onapristone to basal levels.

In prostate tumours that have relapsed from androgen ablation therapies, the androgen receptor (AR) is still expressed, and, compared with the primary tumours, its level is often even enhanced.[38] Mutated ARs can be activated by other compounds, such as adrenal steroids, estrogens, progestins, and even antiandrogens. Thus, relapse of tumours under the selective pressure of common androgen ablation therapies can be caused by acquired androgen hypersensitivity and AR activation by ligands other than (dihydro)testosterone. There is a clinical need for future compounds that are effective inducers of apoptosis in recurrent tumours. Published data indicate that mifepristone can inhibit prostate cancer cell growth in vitro and in vivo.[39,40] The results from El Etreby's group indicate that mifepristone seems to be an effective inducer of apoptosis, and may represent a novel therapeutic approach, not directed towards the AR, to overcome a potential intrinsic apoptosis resistance of androgen-independent prostate cancer cells. Similar opportunities may be possible in breast cancer too, and should be investigated further.

REFERENCES

1. Conneely OM, Lydon JP, De Mayo F, O'Malley BW. Reproductive functions of the progesterone receptor. *J Soc Gynecol Investig* 2000; **7:** S25–32.
2. Lydon JP, DeMayo FJ, Funk CR et al. Mice lacking progesterone receptor exhibit pleiotropic reproductive abnormalities. *Genes Dev* 1995; **15:** 2266–78.
3. Lydon JP, DeMayo FJ, Conneely OM, O'Malley BW. Reproductive phenotypes of the progesterone receptor null mutant mouse. *J Steroid Biochem Mol Biol* 1996; **56:** 67–77.
4. Chappell PE, Lydon JP, Conneely OM et al. Endocrine defects in mice carrying a null mutation for the progesterone receptor gene. *Endocrinology* 1997; **138:** 4147–52.
5. Humphreys RC, Lydon J, O'Malley BW, Rosen JM. Mammary gland development is mediated by both stromal and epithelial progesterone receptors. *Mol Endocrinol* 1997; **11:** 801–11.
6. Brisken C, Park S, Vass T et al. A paracrine role for the epithelial progesterone receptor in mammary gland development. *Proc Natl Acad Sci USA* 1998; **95:** 5076–81.
7. Kurita T, Young P, Brody JR et al. Stromal progesterone receptors mediate the inhibitory effects of progesterone on estrogen-induced uterine epithelial cell deoxyribonucleic acid synthesis. *Endocrinology* 1998; **139:** 4708–13.
8. Nusse R, Varmus HE. Wnt genes. *Cell* 1992; **69:** 1073–87.
9. Cadigan KM, Nusse R. Wnt signaling: a common theme in animal development. *Genes Dev* 1997; **11:** 3286–305.
10. Brisken C, Heineman A, Chavarria T et al. Essential function of Wnt-4 in mammary gland development downstream of progesterone signaling. *Genes Dev* 2000; **14:** 650–4.
11. Gavin BJ, McMahon AP. Differential regulation of the Wnt gene family during pregnancy and lactation suggests a role in postnatal development of the mammary gland. *Mol Cell Biol* 1992; **12:** 2418–23.
12. Weber-Hall SJ, Phippard DJ, Niemeyer CC, Dale TC. Developmental and hormonal regulation of Wnt gene expression in the mouse mammary gland. *Differentiation* 1994; **57:** 205–14.
13. Lydon JP, Ge G, Kittrell FS et al. Murine mammary gland carcinogenesis is critically dependent on progesterone receptor function. *Cancer Res* 1999; **59:** 4276–84.
14. Groshong SD, Owen GI, Grimison B et al. Biphasic regulation of breast cancer cell growth by progesterone: role of the cyclin-dependent kinase inhibitors, p21 and p27^{Kip1}. *Mol Endocrinol* 1997; **11:** 1593–607.
15. Musgrove EA, Lee CS, Cornish AL et al. Antiprogestin inhibition of cell cycle progression in T-47D breast cancer cells is accompanied by induction of the cyclin-dependent kinase inhibitor p21. *Mol Endocrinol* 1997; **11:** 54–66.
16. Lange CA, Richer JK, Shen T, Horwitz KB. Convergence of progesterone and epidermal growth factor signaling in breast cancer. *J Biol Chem* 1998; **273:** 31308–16.
17. Richer JK, Lange CA, Manning NG et al. Convergence of progesterone with growth factor and cytokine signaling in breast cancer. *J Biol Chem* 1998; **273:** 31317–26.

18. Xiong Y, Hannon GJ, Zhang H et al. *Nature* 1993; **366:** 701–4.

19. Steinman RA, Hoffman B, Iro A et al. *Oncogene* 1994; **9:** 3389–96.

20. Owen GI, Richer JK, Tung L et al. Progesterone regulates transcription of the p21^{WAF1} cyclin-dependent kinase inhibitor gene through Sp1 and CBP/p300. *J Biol Chem* 1998; **273:** 10696–701.

21. Sarup JC, Rao KVS, Fox CF. Decreased progesterone binding and attenuated progesterone action in cultured human breast carcinoma cells treated with epidermal growth factor. *Cancer Res* 1988; **48:** 5071–8.

22. Murphy LC, Dotzlaw H, Johnson Wong MS et al. Mechanisms involved in the evolution of progestin resistance in human breast cancer cells. *Cancer Res* 1991; **51:** 2051–7.

23. Michna H, Gehring S, Kuhnel W et al. The anti-tumor potency of progesterone antagonists is due to their differentiation potential. *J Steroid Biochem Mol Biol* 1992; **43:** 203–10.

24. Michna H, Nishino Y, Neef G et al. Progesterone antagonists: tumor-inhibiting potential and mechanism of action. *J Steroid Biochem Mol Biol* 1992; **41:** 339–48.

25. Michna H, Schneider MR, Nishino Y, el Etreby MF. Antitumor activity of the antiprogestins ZK 98.299 and RU 38.486 in hormone dependent rat and mouse mammary tumors: mechanistic studies. *Breast Cancer Res Treat* 1989; **14:** 275–88.

26. Lichtner RB, Parczyk K, Birchmeier W, Schneider MR. Differential cross-talk of estrogen and growth factor receptors in two human mammary tumor cell lines. *J Steroid Biochem Mol Biol* 1999; **71:** 181–9.

27. Li M, Spitzer E, Zschiesche W et al. Antiprogestins inhibit growth and stimulate differentiation in the normal mammary gland. *J Cell Physiol* 1995; **164:** 1–8.

28. Michna H, Nishino Y, Schneider MR et al. A bioassay for the evaluation of antiproliferative potencies of progesterone antagonists. *J Steroid Biochem Mol Biol* 1991; **38:** 359–65.

29. Schneider MR, Michna H, Nishino Y, el Etreby MF. Antitumor activity of the progesterone antagonists ZK 98.299 and RU 38.486 in the hormone-dependent MXT mammary tumor model of the mouse and the DMBA- and the MNU-induced mammary tumor models of the rat. *Eur J Cancer Clin Oncol* 1989; **25:** 691–701.

30. Brunner N, Spang-Thomsen M, Vindelov L et al. Effect of tamoxifen on the receptor-positive T61 and the receptor-negative T60 human breast carcinomas grown in nude mice. *Eur J Cancer Clin Oncol* 1985; **21:** 1349–54.

31. Brunner N, Spang-Thomsen M, Skovgaard Poulsen H et al. Endocrine sensitivity of the receptor-positive T61 human breast carcinoma serially grown in nude mice. *Int J Cancer* 1985; **35:** 59–64.

32. Brunner N, Bastert GB, Poulsen HS et al. Characterization of the T61 human breast carcinoma established in nude mice. *Eur J Cancer Clin Oncol* 1985; **21:** 833–43.

33. Schneider MR, Michna H, Habenicht UF et al. The tumour-inhibiting potential of the progesterone antagonist onapristone in the human mammary carcinoma T61 in nude mice. *J Cancer Res Clin Oncol* 1992; **118:** 187–9.

34. El Etreby MF, Liang Y. Effect of antiprogestins and tamoxifen on growth inhibition of MCF-7 human breast cancer cells in nude mice. *Breast Cancer Res Treat* 1998; **49:** 109–17.

35. Robertson JFR, Willsher PC, Winterbottom L et al. Onapristone, a progesterone receptor antagonist, as first-line therapy in primary breast cancer. *Eur J Cancer* 1999; **35:** 214–18.

36. El Etreby MF, Liang Y, Wrenn RW, Schoenlein PV. Additive effect of mifepristone and tamoxifen on apoptotic pathways in MCF-7 human breast cancer cells. *Breast Cancer Res Treat* 1998; **51:** 149–68.

37. Jacobs E, Watson SA, Ellis IO et al. The effect of onapristone, a progesterone antagonist, on the growth of human gastrointestinal cancer xenografts. *Eur J Cancer* 1997; **33:** 1130–5.

38. Culig Z, Hoffmann J, Erdel M et al. Switch from antagonist to agonist of the androgen receptor bicalutamide is associated with prostate tumour progression in a new model system. *Br J Cancer* 1999; **81:** 242–51.

39. El Etreby MF, Liang Y, Lewis RW. Induction of apoptosis by mifepristone and tamoxifen in human LNCaP prostate cancer cells in culture. *Prostate* 2000; **43:** 31–42.

40. El Etreby MF, Liang Y, Johnson MH, Lewis RW. Antitumor activity of mifepristone in the human LNCaP, LNCaP-C4, and LNCaP-C4-2 prostate cancer models in nude mice. *Prostate* 2000; **42:** 99–106.

Part III
Future Strategies

15

Future prospects for the endocrine management of breast cancer

Robert I Nicholson, Julia MW Gee

CONTENTS • **Introduction** • **New therapeutic targets for candidate pathways** • **New therapeutic targets for non-candidate pathways** • **Conclusions**

INTRODUCTION

Increasing knowledge of the molecular biology of steroid hormone and growth factor signalling is providing new ideas regarding the mechanisms of action of estrogens, progestins, and antihormones (Chapters 9 and 11–14), and moreover possible explanatory hypotheses for the tumour growth associated with the phenomena of de novo and acquired endocrine resistance (Chapter 10). Thus, in hormone-sensitive breast cancer cells, it is likely that input signals generated both by steroid hormones and by a pattern of preferred growth factors are processed by the steroid hormone receptor-positive cells comprising endocrine-responsive tumours to ultimately induce/activate a profile of nuclear transcription factors, for example steroid hormone receptors, Fos and Jun (AP-1), Myc, and Elk-1. Such inductive events are not autonomous: they are markedly strengthened by the interplay of the steroid hormone receptor and growth factor signalling pathways. The net effect of such concerted activation is to markedly influence patterns of gene expression, leading to the gain of positive influ-

ences on cell cycle regulation (e.g. cyclin D1) and cell survival, with a parallel suppression of negative influences (e.g. transforming growth factor β, TGF-β). In the presence of adequate steroid hormone and growth factor input signals, cells are recruited into, and successfully proceed through, the cell cycle, resulting in tumour growth. Importantly, although it is likely that crosstalk between steroid and growth factor pathways enables efficient growth signalling, reductions in the input signals originating from steroid hormones alone (e.g. via antihormones or depletion of the estrogenic environment) appear sufficient to reduce proliferation and induce programmed cell death, thereby leading to excellent initial tumour remissions in endocrine-responsive patients. In this model, differences between endocrine responses exhibited by normal and cancerous cells would be expected to be minimal if oncogenic events occurred in those cellular pathways that either act to limit the extent of growth, but still require an input signal for growth (i.e. that normally maintain tissue size and architecture through negative-feedback and homeostasis mechanisms), or facilitate a more efficient use of input signals from steroid hormones.

In cancers unresponsive to current endocrine measures, it is likely that further alterations have occurred in those elements of growth factor signalling pathways that have the following effects:

1. *Have a positive influence on steroid hormone receptor signalling and facilitate the biological functions of the receptor in a lowered endocrine environment (or indeed in the presence of anti-hormones).* Retention of the estrogen receptor (ER) protein in such cells (as a continued orchestrator of growth responses) would facilitate additional responses to endocrine measures that act by different mechanisms (i.e. aromatase inhibitor/pure antiestrogen substituting for tamoxifen). Such second-line responses certainly occur in over 50% of women with acquired resistant disease who have benefited from a first-line endocrine response.

2. *Circumvent the cellular requirement for steroid hormones via bypassing those elements of their response pathways that impinge upon cell proliferation and survival (i.e. post-receptor mechanisms).* Such phenotypic/genotypic changes may be severe enough to override the importance of crosstalk and hence effectively dislocate growth from a reliance on the steroid hormone receptor. Additional influences may arise from changes in cell cycle components or tumour suppressor genes. Importantly, the majority of patients who fail to respond to one form of endocrine therapy de novo rarely respond to another, suggesting that the influence of the ER in their tumour cells is entirely nullified or circumvented at the time of presentation. This mechanism may also account for the eventual development of acquired resistance to multiple endocrine measures.

3. *Provide a mitogenic input in tumours lacking ER.* ER negativity is predictably associated with de novo endocrine resistance, comprising some 20–30% of breast tumours at presentation. Although it is as yet unknown if such a phenotype arises from aberrant loss of the steroid hormone receptor or from selective outgrowth of steroid hormone receptor-negative cells, the regulation of such tumours is severed from the steroid hormone environment, and they appear to be wholly dependent on elements of growth factor signalling. In addition, perturbed regulation of the cell cycle (e.g. via p53 mutation or loss of BRCA1 expression) may also contribute to the considerable proliferation and aggressive tumour growth associated with steroid hormone receptor-negative, endocrine-unresponsive disease.

NEW THERAPEUTIC TARGETS FOR CANDIDATE PATHWAYS

It is hoped that the above model for endocrine response and failure will ultimately aid progress in many aspects of the clinical management of breast cancer. For example, more accurate stratification of patients for appropriate therapy should be feasible – a feature that will be essential if endocrine therapies are to be directed towards earlier stages of the disease where treatment responses are not readily monitorable. In particular, however, since we believe that such knowledge contributes significantly towards the precise delineation of those molecular pathways involved in the development of de novo and acquired resistance, elucidation of potential targets for novel treatment strategies should also be possible. Based on the above model for loss of endocrine response in breast cancer, therefore, several therapeutic approaches can be envisaged that would be predicted to delay the appearance of, or even treat, endocrine insensitivity/resistance, hence severely compromising the disease process. These include the targeting of ER, growth factor receptors, signal transduction pathways, and nuclear transcription factors.

ER: pure antiestrogens and anti-steroid-hormone-receptor regimes

The most efficient theoretical means of eliminating the influences of pathway crosstalk occurring via ER would be to reduce cellular levels of this receptor. We have recognized ER downregulation as a property of pure antiestrogens that is not shared by other antihormonal drugs[1,2] – a feature that is believed to reside in the ability of these compounds to increase the susceptibility of ER to protolytic degradation.[3] Indeed, these agents are certainly more potent promoters of tumour remission than tamoxifen in several models of human breast cancer, additionally inhibiting growth-factor-induced cell proliferation in both estrogen-sensitive and -resistant ER-positive breast cancer cells.[1,2] Similarly, pure antiestrogens appear to be highly effective in diminishing the cellular ER level and associated expression of estrogen-regulated mRNAs and proteins in clinical breast cancer specimens,[4–6] and furthermore can promote long-lasting tumour remissions in patients who have developed tamoxifen resistance.[7,8]

Importantly, however, even in pure antiestrogen-treated cells, we have noted that ER mRNA expression is maintained on therapy, at least in the short term.[5] Moreover, the ER protein is eventually re-expressed at significant levels within pure antiestrogen-treated cells – an event that coincides with enhanced estrogen-regulated gene expression and the development of a pure-antiestrogen-resistant state.[9] Although the mechanisms associated with the regain of these cellular functions are as-yet unknown, ER re-expression coincident with the development of resistance may again imply that additional therapeutic benefit may accrue from re-instigating receptor loss. In this light, the major thrust of drug design in the pharmaceutical industry targeting endocrine-responsive breast cancers has to date focused on the use of ER-ligand derivatives. However, we believe that ER downregulation through gene inhibition may confer significant advantages on both target cell and hormone receptor specificity. In this light, we are currently evaluating *ER* gene inhibition strategies for their efficacy in reducing the intracellular activity of the ER.[10] These strategies employ antisense technologies (to inhibit *ER* expression) and *ER* dominant-negative mutants (to interfere with ER protein function). Certainly, the transient expression of our truncated version of the ER protein (DNER-1), which notably lacks the C-terminal hormone-binding and AF-2 domains of the receptor, efficiently reduces the ability of the wild-type ER protein to transactivate estrogen response element (ERE) reporter gene constructs in co-transfected ER-positive breast cancer cell lines with parallel growth-inhibitory effects.

Growth factor receptors: anti-ligand and receptor regimes

Given the role established for ErbB tyrosine kinase receptors in the regulation of cellular growth responses, a number of approaches have been used to reduce the signalling primed by the epidermal growth factor receptor (EGFR) and c-ErbB2 receptor within cancer cells.

Several groups have successfully employed immunotherapy with monoclonal antibodies specifically targeting the EGFR or ErbB2 proteins to disrupt their subsequent signalling and inhibit autocrine loops.[11–17] Growth inhibition of EGFR- and c-ErbB2-overexpressing tumours can thereby be enabled both in vitro and in vivo.[13,18,19]

Indeed, phase II clinical trials with a recombinant humanized anti-ErbB2 antibody (trastuzumab, Herceptin) performed on node-positive breast cancer patients showed an overall response rate of 12%.[16] Preliminary data from a phase III trial indicate a 16% response rate to Herceptin and a mean duration of remission of 9 months in metastatic breast cancer, with additive benefits with chemotherapy.[17,20–24] Additionally, such receptor antibodies (or antibody fragments) have also been used to deliver drugs, radiation, or prodrug-activating enzymes,[25] in each instance with some evidence of therapeutic benefit. Finally, toxin conjugates of relevant ligands that damage ErbB-expressing cells have also been described,[11,26–29] as have appropriate antisense mRNA strategies.[30]

Other ways to exploit tumour dependence on growth factor signalling have been (i) to block ligand binding to receptors, using agents such as the trypanocidal drug suramin[31] or its derivatives[32] and (ii) to use cell-permeable low-molecular-weight inhibitors specific to a particular protein tyrosine kinase.[33] Potential inhibitors of protein kinases include ATP analogues and peptide-based inhibitors, including those competing for the SH2 domain (reviewed by Lawrence and Niu[34]). Of particular promise are the tyrosine-specific protein kinase inhibitors, notably tyrphostins[34] and, more recently, quinazoline derivatives,[35–37] while several naturally occurring compounds may also be relevant (e.g. erbstatin,[38,39] lavendustin A,[40] and genistein[41]). Encouragingly, quinazolines not only specifically block the growth-promoting effects of EGFR ligands applied exogenously in culture,[36,42,43] but have also been shown in a number of cases to reduce basal growth under serum-free conditions[43] and to effectively instigate programmed cell death and inhibit tumour cell invasion.[36,43–45] Therefore, while it appears that many such cells are certainly capable of synthesizing and secreting ligands that can activate the EGFR in an autocrine manner, it is nevertheless likely that such pathways may be equally susceptible to the inhibitory properties of these new compounds, where they may also fortuitously instigate programmed cell death. Additionally, EGFR-selective tyrosine kinase inhibitors when in vitro can (i) block the cellular actions of estrogens on breast cancer cells,[36] (ii) reduce the growth of ER-positive estrogen-growth-independent[1,2] and fulvestrant-resistant[45] cells, and (iii) show additive inhibitory properties when combined with antiestrogens.[46]

Signal transduction pathways

An extensive biological evaluation of the cellular effects of various inhibitors of individual downstream elements in growth factor signalling pathways is being undertaken by numerous groups.[47] However, of particular interest are Ras protein inhibitors,[48] which either inactivate the enzymes that catalyse the post-translational modification of Ras by farnesylation (farnesyl protein transferase[49,50]) or act to lower *ras* mRNA levels through the use of antisense oligonucleotides and ribozymes.[51–53] Many naturally occurring compounds also inhibit Ras function, often by preventing association with the membrane, including a vinca alkaloid,[54] squalene (found in olive oil),[55] diallyl disulfide (found in garlic),[56] and damnacanthal.[57]

Ras-inhibitory compounds, like EGFR-selective tyrosine kinase inhibitors, might be expected to influence both steroid hormone and growth factor signalling, as would pharmacological and antisense inhibitors of protein kinase C (PKC),[58–62] Grb2,[63] Raf,[64] mitogen-activated protein (MAP) kinase[65,66] and c-Src.[67,68] Indeed, several clinical trials (phase I or II) employing antisense inhibitory strategies to target genes encoding signal transduction and subsequent cell cycle molecules are currently ongoing (e.g. for PKC,[61] Raf,[64] Ras,[51] and p53.[69] In our own hands, inhibition of MAP kinase activity by the compound PD098059 is effective not only as a means of reducing growth-factor-driven proliferative responses within ER-positive breast cancer cells, but also as an inhibitor of ER activation of ERE reporter gene constructs following transient transfection. Equally, PD098059 blocks (i) MAP kinase-induced expression of the early intermediate response gene Fos, (ii) the subsequent activation of AP-1-mediated signalling (see below), (iii) productive associations between steroid hormone and growth factor signalling pathways in driving gene responses, and (iv) estrogen- and growth-factor-promoted proliferation of the cells.

Nuclear transcription factors

Potentially useful antitumour effects can be generated in breast cancer cells in vitro through the inhibition of AP-1 signalling.[70] Relevant inhibitory agents include glucocorticoids.[71–79] and retinoids, as well as AP-1 dominant-negative[76] and antisense strategies.[72] In a number of instances, it has been shown that compounds such as all-*trans*-retinoic acid not only have antiproliferative activity, as mediated by inhibition of AP-1 activity, but importantly may also be potent inducers of apoptosis.[78] We have observed that all-*trans*-retinoic acid efficiently blocks growth-factor-mediated expression of Fos protein and AP-1 activity in breast cancer cells in vitro. Such inhibition appears to be sufficient to prevent the growth-promoting effects of estrogens, and furthermore aids the inhibitory effects of antiestrogens.[79] Such data certainly imply significant and therapeutically exploitable crosstalk between these pathways, and that combination therapy with antihormones and retinoids may be appropriate. It is noteworthy that several laboratories have developed synthetic retinoids that can selectively target AP-1 signalling without activating transcription of retinoid-regulated genes.[73,74,80–82] Indeed, since such compounds can synergize with glucocorticoids to efficiently repress phorbol-ester-induced AP-1 activity,[80] they may find an expanding role in the therapy of those endocrine-responsive and -unresponsive cancers that show increased reliance on AP-1 signalling. Finally, many naturally occurring microbial and plant extracts and their derivatives may be of future use. Of particular note are the momordins[83] and curcumin (diferuloylmethane). These agents inhibit AP-1 activity,[84–86] the latter compound inducing an unstable, hyperphosphorylated Fos protein[87] to inhibit proliferation and elicit programmed cell death.[88]

NEW THERAPEUTIC TARGETS FOR NON-CANDIDATE PATHWAYS

In addition to the above growth-related pathways in breast cancer cells, which are obvious prime targets for drug development, modern genomic and proteomic technologies are identifying many additional molecular changes in breast cancer that are potential targets for future drug development and delivery.

Of particular interest to our own group are those gene products that are normally suppressed by steroid hormones during tumour growth and that by definition are consequently upregulated by antihormonal therapies. These notably include the EGFR/ErbB2[89–92] and TGF-β.[93] We postulate that at least a portion of such gene products will be associated with enabling cancer cells to survive the effects of antihormones and thus contributing to their capacity to develop drug resistance. The strategic targeting of such survival factors thus potentially provides a highly complementary line of attack to the use of antihormones, and might be expected to significantly improve the therapeutic efficacy of such agents. Indeed, in recent experiments combining tamoxifen or fulvestrant with an EGFR-selective tyrosine kinase inhibitor, we have noted that the combination produces a much greater tumour cell kill than when the drugs are used sequentially, and can effectively control the adaption of the cells to the antihormones. Importantly, although our first priority is to identify survival factors, our initial investigations using cDNA array technology have identified gene products linked to other key cellular processes, including adhesion, immune surveillance, paracrine regulation, and angiogenesis. A number of these may also prove useful as targets for antibody-directed toxin, gene, and cell therapies.

CONCLUSIONS

Signalling through steroid hormone and growth factor pathways and their key components is far from simple, with an elaborate molecular and protein biology and a diverse regulation encompassing a network of phosphorylation cascades. It is becoming increasingly apparent that there are additional layers of complexity to such signalling, with the pathways being intimately linked rather than autonomous. Indeed, several points of productive crosstalk between steroid-hormone- and growth-factor-directed pathways have now been identified in estrogen-responsive cells, which are believed to markedly reinforce their individual cellular effects on growth and gene responses. It is thus postulated that aberrations arising in growth factor signalling pathways could dramatically influence/circumvent steroid hormone action. Certainly, altered elements of growth factor signalling pathways are a relatively common phenotypic characteristic of clinical and experimental breast cancer – a feature that correlates with the development of endocrine insensitivity in both the de novo and acquired settings. A projected paradigm, therefore, is that inhibitory agents (either synthetically or naturally derived) directed towards reducing the influence of growth factors, or their intracellular signalling pathway components, may prove to be of clinical benefit in the therapy of breast tumours exhibiting resistance to antihormonal measures. Indeed, such an approach might delay the appearance of these deleterious conditions. With the recent and continued expansion of available technologies (notably array technology and proteomics) and an increasing battery of pharmacological and molecular therapeutic agents, such targeting of aberrant growth factor signalling is now becoming a genuine possibility, and may eventually be applicable to many tumour types.

REFERENCES

1. Nicholson RI, Gee JWM, Manning DL et al. Responses to pure antioestrogens (ICI 164384 and ICI 182780) in oestrogen sensitive and resistant experimental and clinical breast cancer. *Ann NY Acad Sci* 1995; **761:** 148–63.

2. Nicholson RI, Gee JMW, Francis AB et al. Observations arising from the use of pure anti-oestrogens on oestrogen-responsive (MCF-7) and oestrogen growth-independent (K3) human breast cancer cells. *Endocr Rel Cancer* 1995; **2:** 115–21.

3. Gibson MK, Nemmers LA, Beckman WC Jr et al. The mechanism of ICI 164,384 antiestrogenicity involves rapid loss of estrogen receptor in uterine tissue. *Endocrinology* 1991; **129:** 2000–10.

4. DeFriend DJ, Howell A, Nicholson RI et al. Investigation of a new pure antiestrogen (ICI 182780) in women with primary breast cancer. *Cancer Res* 1994; **54:** 408–14.

5. McClelland RA, Manning DL, Gee JM et al. Effects of short-term antiestrogen treatment of primary breast cancer on estrogen receptor mRNA and protein expression and on estrogen-regulated genes. *Breast Cancer Res Treat* 1996; **41:** 31–41.

6. Robertson JF, Nicholson RI, Bundred NJ et al. Comparison of the short-term biological effects of 7α-[9-(4,4,5,5,5-pentafluoropentylsulfinyl)-nonyl]estra-1,3,5(10)-triene-3,17β-diol (Faslodex) versus tamoxifen in postmenopausal women with primary breast cancer. *Cancer Res* 2001; **61:** 6739–46.

7. Howell A, DeFriend D, Robertson J et al. Response to a specific antioestrogen (ICI 182780) in tamoxifen-resistant breast cancer. *Lancet* 1995; **345:** 29–30.

8. Howell A, DeFriend DJ, Robertson JF et al. Pharmacokinetics, pharmacological and antitumour effects of the specific anti-oestrogen ICI 182780 in women with advanced breast cancer. *Br J Cancer* 1996; **74:** 300–8.

9. Larsen SS, Madsen MW, Jensen BL, Lykkesfeldt AE. Resistance of human breast-cancer cells to the pure steroidal anti-estrogen ICI 182,780 is not associated with a general loss of estrogen-receptor expression or lack of estrogen responsiveness. *Int J Cancer* 1997; **72:** 1129–36.

10. Madden TA, Barrow D, McClelland RA et al. Modulation of oestrogen action by receptor gene inhibition. *Eur J Cancer* 2000; **36**(Suppl 4): S34–5.

11. Ennis BW, Lippman ME, Dickson RB. The EGF receptor system as a target for antitumor therapy. *Cancer Invest* 1991; **9:** 553–62.

12. Dean CJ, Allan S, Eccles S et al. The product of the c-erbB-2 proto-oncogene as a target for diagnosis and therapy in breast cancer. *Year Immunol* 1993; **7:** 182–92.

13. Dean C, Modjtahedi H, Eccles S et al. Immunotherapy with antibodies to the EGF receptor. *Int J Cancer* 1994; **8**(Suppl): 103–7.

14. Baselga J, Mendelsohn J. Receptor blockade with monoclonal antibodies as anti-cancer therapy. *Pharmacol Ther* 1994; **64:** 127–54.

15. Kolibaba KS, Druker BJ. Protein tyrosine kinases and cancer. *Biochim Biophys Acta* 1997; **1333:** F217–48.

16. Baselga J, Tripathy D, Mendelsohn J et al. Phase

II study of weekly intravenous recombinant humanized anti-p185HER2 monoclonal antibody in patients with HER2/neu-overexpressing metastatic breast cancer. *J Clin Oncol* 1996; **14**: 737–44.

17. Baselga J, Norton L, Albanell J et al. Recombinant humanized anti-HER2 antibody (Herceptin) enhances the antitumor activity of paclitaxel and doxorubicin against HER2/neu overexpressing human breast cancer xenografts. *Cancer Res* 1998; **58**: 2825–31.

18. Eccles SA, Court WJ, Box GA et al. Regression of established breast carcinoma xenografts with antibody-directed enzyme prodrug therapy against c-erbB2 p185. *Cancer Res* 1994; **54**: 5171–7.

19. Eccles SA, Modjtahedi H, Box G et al. Significance of the c-erbB family of receptor tyrosine kinases in metastatic cancer and their potential as targets for immunotherapy. *Invasion Metastasis* 1994; **14**: 337–48.

20. Baughman SA, Twaddell T, Glaspy JA, Slamon DJ. Phase II study of receptor-enhanced chemosensitivity using recombinant humanized anti-p185HER2/neu monoclonal antibody plus cisplatin in patients with HER2/neu-overexpressing metastatic breast cancer refractory to chemotherapy treatment. *J Clin Oncol* 1998; **16**: 2659–71.

21. Pegram MD, Lipton A, Hayes DF et al. Phase II study of receptor-enhanced chemosensitivity using recombinant humanized anti-p185HER2/neu monoclonal antibody plus cisplatin in patients with HER2/neu-overexpressing metastatic breast cancer refractory to chemotherapy treatment. *J Clin Oncol* 1998; **16**: 2659–71.

22. Ross JS, Fletcher JA. The HER-2/neu oncogene in breast cancer: prognostic factor, predictive factor, and target for therapy. *Stem Cells* 1998; **16**: 413–28.

23. Eiermann W. International Herceptin Study Group. Trastuzumab combined with chemotherapy for the treatment of HER2-positive metastatic breast cancer: pivotal trial data. *Ann Oncol* 2001; **12**: S57–62.

24. Mrsic M, Grgic M, Budisic Z et al. Trastuzumab in the treatment of advanced breast cancer: single-center experience. *Ann Oncol* 2001; **12**: S95–6.

25. Harris AL. EGF receptor as a target for therapy and interactions with angiogenesis. In: *EGF Receptor in Tumor Growth and Progression (Ernst Schering Research Foundation Workshop 19)* (Lichtner RB, Harkins RN, eds). Berlin: Springer-Verlag, 1997: 3–17.

26. Jeschke M, Wels W, Dengler W et al. Targeted inhibition of tumor-cell growth by recombinant heregulin–toxin fusion proteins. *Int J Cancer* 1995; **60**: 730–9.

27. Siegall CB, Bacus SS, Cohen BD et al. HER4 expression correlates with cytotoxicity directed by a heregulin–toxin fusion protein. *J Biol Chem* 1995; **270**: 7625–30.

28. Fiddes RJ, Janes PW, Sanderson GM et al. Heregulin (HRG)-induced mitogenic signaling and cytotoxic activity of a HRG/PE40 ligand toxin in human breast cancer cells. *Cell Growth Differ* 1995; **6**: 1567–77.

29. Osborne CK, Coronado-Heinsohn E. Targeting the epidermal growth factor receptor in breast cancer cell lines with a recombinant ligand fusion toxin. *Cancer J Sci Am* 1996; **2**: 175.

30. Casalini P, Menard S, Malandrin SM et al. Inhibition of tumorigenicity in lung adenocarcinoma cells by c-erbB-2 antisense expression. *Int J Cancer* 1997; **72**: 631–6.

31. Eisenberger MA, Sinibaldi V, Reyno L. Suramin. *Cancer Pract* 1995; **3**: 187–9.

32. Gagliardi AR, Kassack M, Kreimeyer A et al. Antiangiogenic and antiproliferative activity of suramin analogues. *Cancer Chemother Pharmacol* 1998; **41**: 117–24.

33. Kelloff GJ, Fay JR, Steele VE et al. Epidermal growth factor receptor tyrosine kinase inhibitors as potential cancer chemopreventives. *Cancer Epidemiol Biomarkers Prev* 1996; **5**: 657–66.

34. Lawrence DS, Niu J. Protein kinase inhibitors: the tyrosine-specific protein kinases. *Pharmacol Ther* 1998; **77**: 81–114.

35. Ward WHJ, Cook PN, Slater AM et al. Epidermal growth factor receptor tyrosine kinase. Investigation of catalytic mechanism, structure-based searching and discovery of a potent inhibitor. *Biochem Pharm* 1994; **48**: 659–66.

36. Wakeling AE, Barker AJ, Davies DH et al. Specific inhibition of epidermal growth factor receptor tyrosine kinase by 4-anilinoquinazolines. *Breast Cancer Res Treat* 1996; **3**: 67–73.

37. Wakeling AE, Barker AJ, Davies DH et al. New targets for therapeutic attack. *Endocr Rel Cancer* 1997; **4**: 351–5.

38. Toi M, Mukaida H, Wada T et al. Antineoplastic effect of erbstatin on human mammary and esophageal tumors in athymic nude mice. *Eur J Cancer* 1990; **26**: 722–4.

39. Umezawa K. Isolation and biological activities of signal transduction inhibitors from microorganisms and plants. *Adv Enzyme Regul* 1995; **35:** 43–53.

40. Onoda T, Iinuma H, Sasaki Y et al. Isolation of a novel tyrosine kinase inhibitor, lavendustin A, from *Streptomyces griseolavendus*. *J Nat Prod* 1989; **52:** 1252–7.

41. Clark JW, Santos-Moore A, Stevenson LE, Frackelton AR Jr. Effects of tyrosine kinase inhibitors on the proliferation of human breast cancer cell lines and proteins important in the ras signaling pathway. *Int J Cancer* 1996; **65:** 186–91.

42. Fry DW, Kraker AJ, McMichael A et al. A specific inhibitor of the epidermal growth factor receptor tyrosine kinase. *Science* 1994; **265:** 1093–5.

43. Jones HE, Dutkowski CM, Barrow D et al. New EGF-R selective tyrosine kinase inhibitor reveals variable growth responses in prostate carcinoma cell lines PC-3 and DU-145. *Int J Cancer* 1997; **71:** 1010–18.

44. Jones HE, Barrow D, Dutkowski CM et al. Effect of an EGF-R selective tyrosine kinase inhibitor and an anti-androgen on LNCaP cells: identification of divergent growth regulatory pathways. *Prostate* 2001; **49:** 38–47.

45. McClelland RA, Barrow D, Madden TA et al. Enhanced epidermal growth factor receptor signaling in MCF7 breast cancer cells after long-term culture in the presence of the pure antiestrogen ICI 182,780 (Faslodex). *Endocrinology* 2001; **42:** 2776–88.

46. Nicholson RI, Hutcheson IR, Harper ME et al. Modulation of epidermal growth factor receptor in endocrine-resistant, oestrogen receptor-positive breast cancer. *Endocrine Rel Cancer* 2001; **8:** 175–82.

47. Heimbrook DC, Oliff A. Therapeutic intervention and signaling. *Curr Opin Cell Biol* 1998; **10:** 284–8.

48. Johnson SR, Kelland LR. Farnesyl transferase inhibitors – a novel therapy for breast cancer. *Endocr Rel Cancer* 2001; **8:** 227–35.

49. Reuveni H, Gitler A, Poradosu E et al. Synthesis and biological activity of semipeptoid farnesyltransferase inhibitors. *Bioorg Med Chem* 1997; **5:** 85–92.

50. Kohl NE, Conner MW, Gibbs JB et al. Development of inhibitors of protein farnesylation as potential chemotherapeutic agents. *J Cell Biochem Suppl* 1995; **22:** 145–50.

51. Monia BP, Johnston JF, Ecker DJ et al. Selective inhibition of mutant Ha-ras mRNA expression by antisense oligonucleotides. *J Biol Chem* 1992; **267:** 19954–62.

52. Kawada M, Fukazawa H, Mizuno S, Uehara Y. Inhibition of anchorage-independent growth of ras-transformed cells on polyHEMA surface by antisense oligodeoxynucleotides directed against K-ras. *Biochem Biophys Res Commun* 1997; **231:** 735–7.

53. Scherr M, Grez M, Ganser A, Engels JW. Specific hammerhead ribozyme-mediated cleavage of mutant N-ras mRNA in vitro and ex vivo. Oligoribonucleotides as therapeutic agents. *J Biol Chem* 1997; **272:** 14304–13.

54. Umezawa K, Ohse T, Yamamoto T et al. Isolation of a new vinca alkaloid from the leaves of *Ervatamia microphylla* as an inhibitor of ras functions. *Anticancer Res* 1994; **14:** 2413–17.

55. Newmark HL. Squalene, olive oil, and cancer risk: a review and hypothesis. *Cancer Epidemiol Biomarkers Prev* 1997; **6:** 1101–3.

56. Singh SV, Mohan RR, Agarwal R et al. Novel anti-carcinogenic activity of an organosulfide from garlic: inhibition of H-RAS oncogene transformed tumor growth in vivo by diallyl disulfide is associated with inhibition of p21H-ras processing. *Biochem Biophys Res Commun* 1996; **225:** 660–5.

57. Hiramatsu T, Imoto M, Koyano T, Umezawa K. Induction of normal phenotypes in ras-transformed cells by damnacanthal from *Morinda citrifolia*. *Cancer Lett* 1993; **73:** 161–6.

58. Philip PA, Harris AL. Potential for protein kinase C inhibitors in cancer therapy. *Cancer Treat Res* 1995; **78:** 3–27.

59. Melner MH. Physiological inhibitors of protein kinase C. *Biochem Pharmacol* 1996; **51:** 869–77.

60. Kobayashi D, Watanabe N, Yamauchi N et al. Protein kinase C inhibitors augment tumor-necrosis-factor-induced apoptosis in normal human diploid cells. *Chemotherapy* 1997; **43:** 415–23.

61. McGraw K, McKay R, Miraglia L et al. Antisense oligonucleotide inhibitors of isozymes of protein kinase C: in vitro and in vivo activity, and clinical development as anti-cancer therapeutics. *Anticancer Drug Des* 1997; **12:** 315–26.

62. Geiger T, Muller M, Dean NM, Fabbro D. Antitumor activity of a PKC-α antisense oligonucleotide in combination with standard chemotherapeutic agents against various human

tumors transplanted into nude mice. *Anticancer Drug Des* 1998; **13**: 35–45.

63. Tari AM, Hung MC, Li K, Lopez-Berestein G. Growth inhibition of breast cancer cells by Grb2 downregulation is correlated with inactivation of mitogen-activated protein kinase in EGFR, but not in ErbB2, cells. *Oncogene* 1999; **18**: 1325–32.

64. Monia BP, Holmlund J, Dorr FA. Antisense approaches for the treatment of cancer. *Cancer Invest* 2000; **18**: 635–50.

65. Alessi DR, Cuenda A, Cohen P et al. PD 098059 is a specific inhibitor of the activation of mitogen-activated protein kinase kinase in vitro and in vivo. *J Biol Chem* 1995; **270**: 27489–94.

66. Amundadottir LT, Leder P. Signal transduction pathways activated and required for mammary carcinogenesis in response to specific oncogenes. *Oncogene* 1998; **16**: 737–46.

67. Hori T, Kondo T, Tsuji T et al. Inhibition of tyrosine kinase and src oncogene functions by stable erbstatin analogues. *J Antibiot (Tokyo)* 1992; **45**: 280–2.

68. Levitzki A. SRC as a target for anti-cancer drugs. *Anticancer Drug Des* 1996; **11**: 175–82.

69. Nielsen LL, Maneval DC. p53 tumor suppressor gene therapy for cancer. *Cancer Gene Ther* 1998; **5**: 52–63.

70. Ludes-Meyers JH, Liu Y, Munoz-Medellin D et al. AP-1 blockade inhibits the growth of normal and malignant breast cells. *Oncogene* 2001; **20**: 2771–80.

71. Jonat C, Rahmsdorf HJ, Park KK et al. Antitumor promotion and antiinflammation: down-modulation of AP-1 (Fos/Jun) activity by glucocorticoid hormone. *Cell* 1990; **62**: 1189–204.

72. Kerppola TK, Luk D, Curran T. Fos is a preferential target of glucocorticoid receptor inhibition of AP-1 activity in vitro. *Mol Cell Biol* 1993; **13**: 3782–91.

73. Agadir A, Shealy YF, Hill DL, Zhang X. Retinyl methyl ether down-regulates activator protein 1 transcriptional activation in breast cancer cells. *Cancer Res* 1997; **57**: 3444–50.

74. Huang C, Ma WY, Dawson MI et al. Blocking activator protein-1 activity, but not activating retinoic acid response element, is required for the antitumor promotion effect of retinoic acid. *Proc Natl Acad Sci USA* 1997; **94**: 5826–30.

75. Li BD, Liu L, Dawson M, De Benedetti A. Overexpression of eukaryotic initiation factor 4E (eIF4E) in breast carcinoma. *Cancer* 1997; **79**: 2385–90.

76. Olive M, Krylov D, Echlin DR et al. A dominant negative to activation protein-1 (AP1) that abolishes DNA binding and inhibits oncogenesis. *J Biol Chem* 1997; **272**: 18586–94.

77. Holt JT, Arteaga CB, Robertson D, Moses HL. Gene therapy for the treatment of metastatic breast cancer by in vivo transduction with breast-targeted retroviral vector expressing antisense c-fos RNA. *Hum Gene Ther* 1996; **7**: 1367–80.

78. Mangiarotti R, Danova M, Alberici R, Pellicciari C. All-*trans* retinoic acid (ATRA)-induced apoptosis is preceded by G1 arrest in human MCF-7 breast cancer cells. *Br J Cancer* 1998; **77**: 186–91.

79. McClelland RA, Nicholson RI. AP-1 signalling in antihormone resistant breast cancer. In preparation.

80. Chen JY, Penco S, Ostrowski J et al. RAR-specific agonist/antagonists which dissociate transactivation and AP1 transrepression inhibit anchorage-independent cell proliferation. *EMBO J* 1995; **14**: 1187–97.

81. Nagpal S, Athanikar J, Chandraratna RA. Separation of transactivation and AP1 antagonism functions of retinoic acid receptor alpha. *J Biol Chem* 1995; **270**: 923–7.

82. Fanjul AN, Bouterfa H, Dawson MI, Pfahl MA. Potential role for retinoic acid receptor-gamma in the inhibition of breast cancer cells by selective retinoids and interferons. *Cancer Res* 1996; **56**: 1571–7.

83. Lee DK, Kim B, Lee SG et al. Momordins inhibit both AP-1 function and cell proliferation. *Anticancer Res* 1998; **18**: 119–24.

84. Bierhaus A, Zhang Y, Quehenberger P et al. The dietary pigment curcumin reduces endothelial tissue factor gene expression by inhibiting binding of AP-1 to the DNA and activation of NF-κB. *Thromb Haemost* 1997; **77**: 772–82.

85. Xu YX, Pindolia KR, Janakiraman N et al. Curcumin inhibits IL1α and NF-α induction of AP-1 and NF-κB DNA-binding activity in bone marrow stromal cells. *Hematopathol Mol Hematol* 1997; **11**: 49–62.

86. Pendurthi UR, Williams JT, Rao LV. Inhibition of tissue factor gene activation in cultured endothelial cells by curcumin. Suppression of activation of transcription factors Egr-1, AP-1, and NF-κB. *Arterioscler Thromb Vasc Biol* 1997; **17**: 3406–13.

87. Huang TS, Kuo ML, Lin JK, Hsieh JS. A labile hyperphosphorylated c-Fos protein is induced in

mouse fibroblast cells treated with a combination of phorbol ester and anti-tumor promoter curcumin. *Cancer Lett* 1995; **96:** 1–7.

88. Kuo ML, Huang TS, Lin JK. Curcumin, an antioxidant and anti-tumor promoter, induces apoptosis in human leukemia cells. *Biochim Biophys Acta* 1996; **1317:** 95–100.

89. Dati C, Antoniotti S, Taverna D et al. Inhibition of c-erbB-2 oncogene expression by estrogens in human breast cancer cells. *Oncogene* 1990; **5:** 1001–6.

90. Chrysogelos SA, Yarden RI, Lauber AH, Murphy JM. Mechanisms of EGF receptor regulation in breast cancer cells. *Breast Cancer Res Treat* 1994; **31:** 227–36.

91. Yarden RI, Lauber AH, El-Ashry D, Chrysogelos SA. Bimodal regulation of epidermal growth factor receptor by estrogen in breast cancer cells. *Endocrinology* 1996; **137:** 2739–47.

92. deFazio A, Chiew YE, McEvoy M et al. Antisense estrogen receptor RNA expression increases epidermal growth factor receptor gene expression in breast cancer cells. *Cell Growth Differ* 1997; **8:** 903–11.

93. Knabbe C, Lippman ME, Wakefield LM et al. Evidence that transforming growth factor-β is a hormonally regulated negative growth factor in human breast cancer cells. *Cell* 1987; **48:** 417–28.

Index

Note: 'vs' indicates comparison of two or more different treatments.
Abbreviations: ER, estrogen receptor; PgR, progesterone receptor.